RESOURCES FOR THE FUTURE LIBRARY COLLECTION
POLICY AND GOVERNANCE

Volume 6

Air Pollution and Human Health

Full list of titles in the set
POLICY AND GOVERNANCE

Air Pollution and Human Health

Lester B. Lave and Eugene P. Seskin

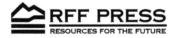

RFF PRESS
RESOURCES FOR THE FUTURE

Washington, DC • London

First published in 1977 by The Johns Hopkins University Press for Resources for the Future

This edition first published in 2011 by RFF Press, an imprint of Earthscan

Earthscan LLC, 1616 P Street, NW, Washington, DC 20036, USA
Earthscan Ltd, Dunstan House, 14a St Cross Street, London EC1N 8XA, UK
Earthscan publishes in association with the International Institute for Environment and Development

For more information on RFF Press and Earthscan publications, see www. rffpress.org and www.earthscan.co.uk or write to earthinfo@earthscan.co.uk

ISBN: 978-1-61726-058-2 (Volume 6)
ISBN: 978-1-61726-007-0 (Policy and Governance set)
ISBN: 978-1-61726-000-1 (Resources for the Future Library Collection)

A catalogue record for this book is available from the British Library

Publisher's note

The publisher has made every effort to ensure the quality of this reprint, but points out that some imperfections in the original copies may be apparent.

At Earthscan we strive to minimize our environmental impacts and carbon footprint through reducing waste, recycling and offsetting our CO_2 emissions, including those created through publication of this book. For more details of our environmental policy, see www.earthscan.co.uk.

AIR POLLUTION AND HUMAN HEALTH

Air Pollution and Human Health

LESTER B. LAVE
EUGENE P. SESKIN

With the assistance of
Michael J. Chappie

Published for Resources for the Future
By The Johns Hopkins University Press
Baltimore and London

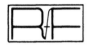

Contents

Tables

Figures

Foreword

The relationship between air pollution and human health is clearly a subject of great importance. This study of the hypothesized air pollution–health association was undertaken by the authors with the assistance of a grant from Resources for the Future. It was one of a number of independent projects that evolved in connection with RFF's quality of the environment program. The grant was made because it was felt that previous work on the nature of the relationship between air pollution and ill health had not been thorough nor persuasive in all its aspects. The grant recipients, Lester B. Lave and Eugene P. Seskin, were selected because RFF was confident of the rigor of their research methods and the neutrality of their perspective.

Now we have the results of their research project which has extended over a decade. Some readers may find that several of the conclusions presented run counter to personal experience, intuition, or, at the very least, social preference. In RFF's view, the chief danger in publishing a study of this nature is that some of its conclusions will be taken out of context and widely advertised by interested parties, without acknowledgment of the patient, almost laborious, qualifications emphasized by the authors. At the same time, RFF believes that this danger is outweighed in that publication ensures that the conclusions will be circulated where they properly belong—in the marketplace of ideas. There, they may be upheld or refuted, the sooner perhaps because of any controversy they might stimulate. For it is the hallmark of truly scientific research that investigators have—as in the present volume—made their data sources and methodology readily available in order to facilitate attempts by others at replication, and even, refutation.

Resources for the Future is interested in discovering the truth about the possible effects on human health of air pollution from both stationary and mobile sources. In supporting this study, we have discharged one of our primary obligations—to advance research and education into the relationships between people and their natural environment.

Washington, D.C.

Walter O. Spofford, Jr.
Director, Quality of the
Environment Division

Preface

Work on this book began in 1967 with a grant from Resources for the Future to Lester Lave for the purpose of estimating various aspects of the benefits that have accrued from the abatement of air pollution. Eugene Seskin joined Lave in 1968, and there were two subsequent grants from RFF in support of this joint study. This early investigation resulted in a paper, "Air Pollution and Human Health," which appeared in *Science* in 1970. Its publication received widespread attention from the public, others in the field, and the media. It also influenced the U.S. Environmental Protection Agency and other organizations in their attempts to estimate the value of air pollution abatement.

In pursuing the relationship between air pollution and human health we used a number of data sets and performed many specific analyses. Much of this work was submitted for publication as it was completed; however, this process was not entirely satisfactory. The papers appeared separately in domestic and foreign journals and edited books, ranging over such fields as economics, statistics, public health, chemistry, and mechanical engineering. As a consequence, no single audience had easy access to all the analyses. In addition, we believed that the individual analyses, while valuable, did not provide the proper perspective for examining the studies as a whole.

Thus, with the encouragement of Allen V. Kneese, who was then director of RFF's Quality of the Environment Division, we began to pull the individual studies together. Instead of merely collecting our previous articles and writing an introductory chapter to them, we felt that the addition of a lengthy chapter on theory and method was warranted. More important, we found that the individual analyses could be greatly condensed, and that they could be presented in logical order. Furthermore, the various data sets originally used for our articles were subject to re-vision and extension. Setting ourselves the task of completely reestimating all of the models, we used a standard set of data in the belief that this would provide additional clarity and uniformity to the results and con-clusions. Many of the important analyses and replications in this volume have not been published elsewhere. Given the data revisions as well as our various reexaminations, we want to point out that this book—rather than any of our previous results—reflects our current thinking as well as our most up-to-date estimates.

We hope that these studies will prove valuable to those personnel in federal, state, and local environmental protection agencies who are re-sponsible for policymaking. Both the theoretical and empirical analyses may be of interest to epidemiologists and public health professionals in the environmental health field as well as to economists working on prob-lems of applied econometrics and benefit–cost analysis. Earlier versions of this material have been used in a number of graduate and advanced undergraduate courses and we hope that this volume will be equally helpful to such students.

Washington, D.C.   Lester B. Lave
August 1977   Eugene P. Seskin

Acknowledgments

In pursuing the topic of this volume over a number of years, we have become impressed by the selflessness of the many people who commented on our work and who offered us suggestions. Our special appreciation must go to Herbert A. Simon, Allen V. Kneese, and A. Myrick Freeman III, whose valuable suggestions provided guidance throughout our research effort; to John W. Tukey whose extensive last-minute review resulted in reanalysis, which we feel greatly improved the final work; to Walter O. Spofford, Jr., whose critical examination is reflected particularly in chapters 10 and 11; and to Morton Corn whose suggestion led to this enterprise initially.

We also wish to thank a number of people for their helpful comments. They include Walter A. Albers, Jr., William J. Baumol, Blair T. Bower, Robert W. Buechley, Donald T. Campbell, Charles J. Cicchetti, Robert Dorfman, William Fairley, Benjamin G. Ferris, Jr., Kenneth M. Gaver, Martin S. Geisel, John R. Goldsmith, W. W. Holland, Johannes Ipsen, Edwin S. Mills, Frederick Mosteller, Daniel Nagin, Talbot Page, John W. Pratt, Wilson B. Riggan, Kenneth D. Rogers, Marvin A. Schneiderman, V. Kerry Smith, Theodor D. Sterling, Arthur C. Stern, and R. E. Waller.

A project such as this one cannot be carried out in the absence of excellent support staff. Linnea Freeberg furnished expert general assistance, especially in the data handling and in the literature review. Additional research assistance was provided by Katharine Doyle, Alesia Kirk, Timothy Lawrence, and Jane Meyer. Computer programming skills were provided by Michael J. Chappie, Stanley Edelstein, Mark Gelfand, Robert Gursha, and Marc Kellner. In addition, Margaret Ingram, Jo Hinkel, and Joan Tron of RFF provided valuable editorial assistance. Great patience was displayed by those who typed and retyped the manuscript: Marie

Levine, Elaine Liang, Janet Posner, Narda Rathbun, Diana Tasciotti, and Norma Ziker.

In addition to being responsible for the reestimation of the empirical work, Michael J. Chappie pointed out numerous obscurities in the writing and difficulties in the analyses—many of which he helped to rectify. His name appears on the title page in acknowledgment of these contributions.

While grateful for the criticisms and comments we have received, we retain sole responsibility for the analyses and conclusions; any errors are ours. The opinions are not necessarily those of RFF or anyone other than ourselves.

Finally, we are grateful to Resources for the Future for providing research grants for the work.

L. B. L.
E. P. S.

Background and theoretical framework

CHAPTER 1

Introduction

Air pollution is a problem of growing national and international interest. Public awareness and concern continues to rise, despite a decline in many air pollution indexes from their mid-1960 highs. Presidential messages as well as news stories have reflected the opinions of scientists and community leaders that air pollution must be abated. This concern has manifested itself at the local level by tougher antipollution ordinances (and more important, in stricter enforcement of existing ordinances) and at the federal level by the passage of the Clean Air Act of 1967 and its subsequent amendments. The enactment and enforcement of these measures have substantially increased technological research into the problem of controlling pollution emissions from automobiles and fixed sources, as well as stimulating social scientists to discuss the optimal levels of abatement and methods of achieving pollution control.[1]

A number of extreme proposals for regulating pollution emissions have been made because many policymakers misunderstand the basic physical and economic aspects of air pollution control. For example, some conservation groups advocate that all pollutants be removed from the air and that all emission of pollutants be prohibited. However, many pollutants are natural constituents of the air. Plants, animals, and natural activity would cause some pollution even without man and his technology. Animals exhale carbon dioxide, decaying vegetation produces methane, volcanic activity vents sulfur oxides, and winds ensure that there will be suspended particulates. There is no possibility of removing all pollutants from the air. Instead, the problem is one of balancing the benefits that polluters obtain from venting residuals against the damage that is incurred by society

[1] See, for example, Freeman and Haveman (1972), Kneese and Schultze (1975), and the summary in Lave and Silverman (1976).

3

as a result of the increased pollution. To find an optimum level, we must know the marginal benefits and costs associated with abatement.

Many of the effects of air pollution, though evident, are difficult to quantify or evaluate. What is the effect of air pollution on one's "life-style"? What is the value of enhanced "quality of life" as a result of air pollution abatement? Because such effects are real and likely to be important, many investigators in the past have attempted to quantify and evaluate them. We have elected to explore one aspect in detail, conjecturing that if air pollution exerts a damaging effect on health, this effect is more likely to be of policy significance than is damage to plants, animals, and materials.[2]

Our primary goal is to quantify the health benefits that would result from the abatement of air pollution. The work of many investigators (in addition to our own studies) will enter into this quantification. While we cannot estimate the total benefits with certainty, we arrive at a number of specific conclusions regarding the net benefits to society (benefits minus the associated costs) of imposing stringent emissions standards to control each compound. Estimates of total benefits (not only health benefits) and total costs will be presented in the course of the study, but our investigation will focus on the association between air pollution and health; no original research on other effects or on costs is undertaken.

FACTORS AFFECTING THE SHAPE OF THE ANALYSIS

Certain questions govern the shape of any such analysis, and must be answered at the outset: Which pollutants are pernicious? How can health status be measured? What statistical methods are most appropriate? How do measurement problems shape the analysis? And, if the effects of air pollution on health can be quantified, can they be translated into dollars?

Which pollutants are pernicious?

It is misleading to speak of air pollution as though a single substance only were involved.[3] Sulfur oxides, particulates, nitrogen oxides, carbon monoxide, and hydrocarbons are the most common of the myriad compounds emitted into the air by man. Lumping these into the single category "air pollution" ignores their different properties and obscures differences in the degree of damage that each can cause. For example, some pollutants cause atmospheric haze and impair one's visibility, others discolor fabrics, and still others cause illness. *Air pollution* is used as a summary term for

---

[2] The importance placed on health is attested to by the fact that national health expenditures in the United States for fiscal year 1972 exceeded $80 billion, or approximately 7.6 percent of the gross national product (Cooper and Worthington, 1972).

[3] A committee of the World Health Organization (WHO, 1972) developed the following definition of air pollution: ". . . the term air pollution is 'limited to the situations in which the outdoor ambient atmosphere contains materials in concentrations which are harmful to man or to his environment.' "

these compounds, but care will be taken throughout this study to examine the particular pernicious effects of each pollutant whenever possible. Our analysis focuses primarily on sulfur oxides and suspended particulates, with some attention being given to the other pollutants mentioned above. The major reasons for this are (1) the greater availability of aerometric data on sulfur oxides and suspended particulates, and (2) the relatively large body of information on the effects of these pollutants.

How can health status be measured?

The only unequivocal measurement of health status is death. All other measurements are difficult to define, let alone measure. For example, the absence rate from work due to illness will depend on such factors as the number of sick days for which the employee is paid, the individual's general job satisfaction, the exact type of work (including the level of physical and mental activity involved), an individual's perception of pain, and the value placed on leisure. Unfortunately, any measure of morbidity, whether it be its associated pain, reduction in life expectancy, or resulting disability, will be related to such factors. Even such an "objective" factor as the physical measurement of vital capacity depends on the individual's cooperation.

If death is unambiguous, mortality rates are not. Death rate statistics based on cause of death are no better than the accuracy with which the cause of death is determined; the degree of accuracy varies with the circumstances and place of death. Only a small proportion of deaths are investigated by autopsy, and very often little or no pathological information is available to the physician who must determine the cause of death. Even rates for the population at risk are difficult to determine. In most cases, deaths are recorded according to the deceased's place of residence rather than the place of occurrence. Failure to do so would lead to erroneous mortality rates, since the population at risk would be incorrect. But even if the actual place of residence were recorded, the statistics may not be completely accurate. For example, if someone moves to a new location shortly before death, the death will be associated with the new residence. If the deceased had no permanent residence, or if the residence is unknown, then the death is usually associated with the place of occurrence.

Despite the limitations associated with both morbidity and mortality data, the available figures are extremely useful when one is looking at specific types of health effects from air pollution. In particular, one would expect that mortality data would be especially relevant for ascertaining chronic, long-term health effects, while morbidity data would be especially useful in determining the acute, short-term health effects which cause illness but not death. However, because comprehensive morbidity data are not available, we had no other recourse than to concentrate exclusively on mortality data in our own empirical work.

How do measurement problems shape the analysis?

As with measures of health status, existing pollution data do not necessarily provide good measurements for our purposes. Available data are usually in the form of ambient air-quality readings for a given time period (hour, day, week, month) over a large geographical area. The local topography, location and height of buildings, weather, and location of emission sources will lead to vast (often more than tenfold) differences in the ambient air quality in various sections of a city. Consequently, the pollution measurements are, at best, remote approximations to an individual's exposure to a specific pollutant. A related issue is the actual measurement of the pollutants. For most of our period of analysis, the most extensive air pollution data were obtained for suspended particulates collected by a high-volume sampler. However, no data were available on the size distribution of the suspended particulates.[4] In some cases, the suspended particulates were analyzed for chemical composition; for example, the amount of sulfates (or other sulfur compounds) was given.[5] Only toward the latter part of the period under consideration were data on other pollutants—for example, sulfur dioxide—available on a large-scale basis. There are other difficulties with the techniques used to measure the pollution concentrations,[6] as well as problems inherent in the type and dependability of instruments used to measure the pollution levels.

Other factors hypothesized to affect mortality, such as nutritional history, are also measured poorly. For some factors, such as genetics, how and what to measure is unclear. In addition, little data are available for factors such as smoking habits.

These measurement problems will be considered in greater detail in chapter 2; however, their nature should be stressed from the outset. Virtually all measurements of health status as well as those of the factors affecting health are subject to serious measurement problems. These problems influence not only the type of analysis to be undertaken, but also the specific statistical methods to be used.

What statistical methods are appropriate?

Classically, statistical hypothesis testing is based on the assumption that a functional specification is given, that is, that the functional form of the relationship in question, as well as the relevant variables, are known. Statistical theory can then define powerful methods for testing competing

[4] The size distribution of the particulates is a crucial factor, since the ability of particulates to enter the lower respiratory tract depends on their size.

[5] The exact chemical composition of the sulfur oxides is relevant, since toxicological evidence has indicated the harmful effects of acid sulfates (Amdur, 1977). Unfortunately, no data on acid sulfates were available.

[6] For example, one method of measuring nitrogen dioxide, the Jacobs–Hochheiser method, was found to overstate considerably the true ambient level of nitrogen dioxide.

hypotheses. In examining the association between air pollution and mortality, however, the functional form of the relationship is not known, and one can only conjecture about the factors that should enter into the analysis. In addition, it is not enough to know whether air pollution is merely a cause of ill health; it is essential to know the quantitative impact of its effects.

In this context, the primary requirement for a statistical technique is that it be "robust" and "powerful."[7] Not only must it allow one to investigate questions of specification and measurement; it must also produce quantitative estimates. While a number of statistical methods are used in this study, we place primary emphasis on linear multivariable regression analysis.[8] The reader should be forewarned that the problems associated with measuring health status, ignorance of the correct specification, and measurement errors of important variables will necessitate care in the analysis and its interpretation.

Translating effects into dollars

Assuming that a quantitative relationship between air pollution and mortality can be estimated, we still must translate the implied health change (and other effects) into a common metric. This is essential if one is to address policy questions that deal with the benefits and costs of air pollution abatement. Since the natural metric for the cost side is dollars, there is good reason for using this metric to characterize benefits. However, this implies that changes in health status, as well as in the degree of damage to plants and materials, can be translated into dollars.

This translation of "physical" effects into dollars, as set forth in chapter 10, is likely to be the subject of controversy. Where a day of illness or a premature death must be translated into dollars, dispute is inevitable. While some policy decisions are possible without translation into dollars, there is no alternative to this if one wants to compare changes in health effects with the additional investment required to abate air pollution.

THE HYPOTHESIZED RELATIONSHIP

For more than forty years scientists have been accumulating evidence indicating that ill health is associated with air pollution. The scientific community has been slow to accept this evidence, however, because of

---

[7] Box and Anderson (1955) state that "to fulfill the needs of the experimenter, statistical criteria should (1) be sensitive to change in the specific factors tested, (2) be insensitive to changes, of a magnitude likely to occur in practice, in extraneous factors." These properties, usually called power and robustness, respectively, are generally agreed upon as the primary requirements of good performance in hypothesis testing.

[8] The term *multivariable* was suggested to us by John Tukey to indicate situations in which more than a single independent variable was being used, but where only a single random variable was hypothesized. We thought this term a better description of the empirical work that follows than the more common term *multivariate*.

TABLE 1.1. Typical Early Study of Air Pollution and Mortality

County or borough	Deposit index (grams per 100 m² per month)	Smoke index (milligrams per 100 m³)	Persons per acre	Bronchitis mortality[a]
Exeter (rural)	96	8	8.3	77
Salford (urban)	731	36	34.2	259

Source: Stocks (1959).
[a] Standardized mortality ratio for males. Note that Stocks is aware of the problems inherent in comparing urban and rural areas; he attempts to correct for this by controlling population density.

the methods used to gather it and the lack of studies using controls. Some early studies contrasting the mortality rates in polluted and unpolluted areas found higher death rates in the polluted regions. An example of such a comparison is illustrated in table 1.1. The problem with such an analysis is that areas with high levels of air pollution are industrialized cities, whereas the areas with low levels of air pollution are rural farming communities. Put this way, the findings are not at all surprising, since we know that people living in large cities have lower life expectancies for a host of reasons.[9]

The principal conclusion to be drawn from the literature review is that many scientists have demonstrated an "association" or link between air pollution and increased mortality rates. What can one conclude from such a link? There are four logical possibilities: (1) the association is a sampling phenomenon and occurred at random; (2) air pollution causes an increase in the mortality rate; (3) increases in the mortality rate cause air pollution; or (4) there is a "true" factor, or set of factors, that causes both air pollution and increased mortality. This true factor would give rise to a spurious correlation between air pollution and mortality.[10] For example, if automobiles were the only source of air pollution and if many deaths resulted from automobile accidents, there would be a significant correlation between air pollution and the mortality rate (across cities). To avoid this particular spurious association, the number of automobiles and such related factors as the number of miles driven and weather conditions would have to be controlled in the analysis.

We can rule out the first possibility; an enormous volume of collected evidence indicates that there is a close association between air pollution and increased mortality. We conjecture that the second possibility is correct, but we must rule out the third and fourth in order to prove it. The idea of mortality causing air pollution seems macabre: perhaps in the thirteenth century the increased mortality during Black Plague epidemics led to air pollution, but this hardly seems relevant today. Thus,

[9] See MacMahon, Puch, and Ipsen (1960, pp. 149–153).
[10] For an excellent discussion of spurious correlation, see Simon (1954).

proving that air pollution is the cause of increased mortality depends on our being able to rule out the fourth possibility—that the association is spurious.

Dramatic increases in air pollution, such as those occurring in Donora, Pennsylvania, in 1948, and in London, in 1952, have been shown to cause discomfort and even illness and death. Thus, one hypothesized relationship between air pollution and health is an acute response, in which high concentrations of air pollutants have an immediate effect on health.

A second hypothesis is that breathing polluted air, even in much lower concentrations than those which occurred in the episodes, lowers one's health status after prolonged exposure. Benzopyrene has been shown to produce cancer in laboratory animals; and other laboratory experiments have demonstrated that acute irritation can aggravate the symptoms of a chronic respiratory disease and possibly make it progressive.[11] Concentrations of the magnitude required to demonstrate these effects in the laboratory are seldom, if ever, experienced in urban air, but it is possible that long-term exposure to low levels of air pollution exacerbates existing disease or causes chronic disease. This second relationship is subtle and difficult to demonstrate.

To explore these two hypothesized relationships, we must know what factors affect health status as measured by the mortality rate of a population, as well as the causal interrelationships among those factors. Powerful tests of the hypotheses cannot be formulated without such knowledge. We must be able to evaluate methods that have been used to estimate the relationship between health status and air pollution in order to assess the confidence to be placed in each result.

FACTORS AFFECTING MORTALITY

As we noted earlier, the most readily available measure of health status is the mortality rate for a geographically defined group, such as the inhabitants of a city. A large number of factors are known to affect this index. Some of these are shown in table 1.2 and may be grouped arbitrarily into (1) physical characteristics of the population, (2) socioeconomic characteristics, (3) environmental factors, and (4) personal factors. The last is the most important set of factors, and the most difficult to control.

In order to estimate the effect of any one of these factors on the mortality rate, the others must be held constant experimentally or be controlled statistically. Only in the remote case in which a particular factor is uncorrelated with all the others could one gain unbiased estimates of its effect in an analysis involving only the mortality rate and a single factor. Thus, a difficulty with the investigation depicted in table 1.1 is that the estimated difference in mortality between the two areas may reflect

---

[11] See, for example, Saffiotti and his coauthors (1965).

TABLE 1.2. Factors Affecting Mortality

Physical	Socioeconomic	Environmental	Personal
Age distribution	Income distribution	Air pollution levels	Smoking habits
Sex distribution	Occupation mix	Radiation levels	Medical care (quality and quantity)
Race distribution	Housing density or crowding	Climatological characteristics	Exercise habits
	Differential migration	Domestic factors (home-heating equipment, heating fuels, etc.)	Nutritional history
			Genetic effects

differences in other factors affecting the death rate; one cannot reliably ascribe the entire difference to a single factor, such as air pollution.

An ideal investigation of the association between air pollution and mortality would control for all the factors shown in table 1.2. Unfortunately, many of these factors are difficult to measure conceptually (for example, genetic effects),[12] while data on other factors have not been collected (for example, smoking habits) or are poorly measured in existing statistics (for example, medical care). To prove causation, an investigation would have to control for each of the factors experimentally or statistically, explicitly or implicitly. Controlling for all factors that might influence mortality is, of course, impossible, but even though the analysis is necessarily incomplete, it can still be powerful in convincing a reviewer that the association is causal and the estimated magnitude is worthy of attention.[13]

A more helpful way to look at the information in table 1.2 is through the path-analysis diagram (figure 1.1). Mortality is hypothesized to be related to the factors in the diagram, as described by the "causal" arrows.[14] For example, both home-heating (equipment and fuels) and occupation-mix characteristics are assumed to affect both the level of air pollution and the mortality rate.[15] Genetic factors, personal habits (such as smoking

[12] Ways of measuring genetic effects include data on national origin and on cause and age of parents' deaths, and perhaps some direct observations on the individual. While the first two are a remote approximation, they are likely to exert some control for genetic factors.

[13] In the analysis that follows, we have attempted to find variables or surrogates for most of these factors. For some factors, such as genetic characteristics, we were unsuccessful; for others, such as housing density, we examined available surrogates and rejected them as inadequate.

[14] Causality itself is difficult to define for chronic disease, as is discussed in chapter 2.

[15] Home heating usually makes a direct contribution to air pollution and may also directly affect the mortality rate if it is inadequate, not properly vented, or nonexistent. Similarly, the occupation mix of an area will describe the industrial composition and thus be directly related to the types of pollutants emitted into the air. In addition, occupational accidents and exposures will directly affect the mortality rate.

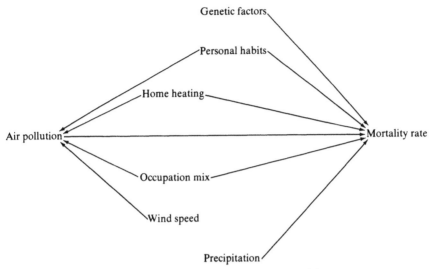

FIG. 1.1. Path analysis of the air pollution-mortality rate model.

and exercise), and precipitation are assumed to have a direct effect on the mortality rate, without having significant effects on the other factors in the model. Finally, other factors, such as wind speed, are assumed to affect the level of air pollution without noticeably affecting the mortality rate.

The path analysis makes it apparent that a simple correlation between air pollution and the mortality rate will reflect not only the hypothesized causal relationship between the two, but also the systematic influences of occupation mix and home heating, as well as the random influences of the other variables (for example, genetic effects). Although a number of replications in different settings will reduce these random influences, they will not disentangle the interdependencies among home heating, occupation mix, air pollution, and the mortality rate.

A solution to this problem is a multivariable analysis that controls statistically for the confounding factors. Strictly speaking, if items such as genetic factors, personal habits, wind speed, and precipitation were orthogonal to air pollution, there would be no need to control for them if one is interested only in estimating the effects of air pollution on mortality. (If they were orthogonal, they would exert effects independent of the effects from air pollution.) However, note that, in any given data set, one or more of these factors could be closely associated with air pollution. Thus, if one had measures of these factors, one would presumably insert them in the regression, since this would more accurately predict variations in mortality. By including these factors whenever possible, one minimizes the chance that the estimated relationship between air pollution and mortality reflects a spurious association.[16]

OUTLINE OF THE STUDY

In chapter 2 we shall explore the methods that have been used to investigate the association between air pollution and mortality, and shall provide some illustrations from the literature (a detailed literature review is presented in appendix A, pages 273–311). We argue that epidemiological rather than laboratory methods are the more powerful tools in estimating the strength of the association.

Our first set of epidemiological studies is presented in section II, which considers in detail the relationship between air pollution and mortality in the United States in 1960 (with replications for 1961 and 1969), using cross-sectional data on standard metropolitan statistical areas (SMSAs). This section is divided into five chapters. Chapter 3 relates the total mortality rate to air pollution and other variables. Chapter 4 extends this work, examining infant and other age–sex–race-adjusted total mortality rates, as well as age–sex–race-specific mortality rates, and fifteen disease-specific mortality rates. In chapter 5, additional explanatory variables are added to the original socioeconomic variables to control for occupation mix, climate, and home-heating characteristics in each area. Chapter 6 presents an analysis of suicides, venereal disease, and crime rates, with the underlying hypothesis that air pollution will not be an important explanatory variable. A partial replication of the 1960 work is performed in chapter 7, using 1969 air pollution and mortality measures and socioeconomic data from the 1970 U.S. Census. Additional tests to investigate the air pollution–mortality relationship are also presented. The chapter closes with a summary of the cross-sectional work.

Section III includes several time-series analyses of the relationship between air pollution and mortality. In chapter 8, a cross-sectional time-series analysis is presented in which twenty-six SMSAs are examined over the period 1960–69 in order to estimate the association between annual changes in air pollution and mortality rates. Chapter 9 begins with an overview of time-series mortality and morbidity studies, followed by an analysis of daily changes in pollution and climate and their association with daily changes in mortality.

Section IV investigates the implications of our findings by enumerating the benefits and costs associated with strategies of air pollution abatement. Chapter 10 presents a framework for such a benefit–cost analysis, along with estimates of the benefits and costs of air pollution abatement that is required by the 1970 amendments to the Clean Air Act. Chapter 11 summarizes our findings and presents our conclusions.

---

[16] However, from a statistical standpoint, attempting to control for all possible factors could conceivably use up all the degrees of freedom in the analysis.

CHAPTER 2

Theory and method

The central question of our study is, Does air pollution cause increased mortality? Since Hume, philosophers of science have reminded us that it is impossible to prove causation empirically.[1] A causal relationship exists only as a theoretical construct, not as a set of empirically verifiable propositions. This is true because the theoretical statement concerns the relationship between one or more causal variables and the affected dependent variable (or set of dependent variables), and it is assumed, at least implicitly, that other factors are held constant. But even in a laboratory experiment, the scientist cannot hold all other variables constant. There are forces (such as the movement of the earth) outside one's control, while other factors are assumed to be irrelevant (such as the day of the week on which the experiment is performed).

A careful experimental design must recognize the existence of four types of variables. The first are those which can be manipulated (the causal factors); the second are those which do not vary in the experimental situation (they may or may not be causal factors); the third are causal variables that are not controlled but are known to produce random effects on the dependent variable(s); and the fourth are variables systematically related to the causal factors, which might themselves contribute to the observed variation in the dependent variables or, indeed, might be the "true" causal variables. Experimentation derives its power because a large number of variables can be delegated to the second and third categories; that is, they can be held constant or randomized. When an experiment is replicated (especially by an independent investigator), the possibility that some uncontrolled variable is exerting a systematic influence on the dependent variable is greatly reduced. However, this possibility cannot be

[1] See, for example, Blalock (1964).

entirely removed. In addition, some variables may fall into the fourth category. Even a careful experimenter may not be equipped to hold all other variables constant while manipulating the variable that is hypothesized to be the causal one.

Undoubtedly, a well-designed experiment can do much to untangle the relationships among variables. The ability to replicate, to control, and to randomize gives the investigator powerful techniques, but these techniques cannot prove causation. The disturbing possibility remains that some uncontrolled variable which varies systematically with the observed one is the true causal variable.

LABORATORY VERSUS NATURAL EXPERIMENTS

In some situations, it is impractical to experiment in the laboratory. If it is hypothesized that high levels of air pollution harm people, it would not be socially acceptable to conduct laboratory experiments that expose subjects to such levels in order to measure the effects. Furthermore, long-term, low-level effects could not be discovered in a laboratory, even in the absence of ethical considerations. Finally, the hypothesized effect may be so small that it is not feasible to test for it in the laboratory (for example, a slight increase in the mortality rate of subjects with life expectancies of seventy years would require hundreds of thousands of subject-years to ascertain the relationship).

When the health effect is hypothesized to be of small magnitude, experimentation with animals is not likely to produce generalizations that can be confidently applied to humans. Differences in physiology, life span, and exposure make it difficult to extrapolate from the results of animal studies to the effects on human beings. The most useful information on the underlying physiological mechanism comes from the highly controlled laboratory animal experiments and short-term fumigation experiments on humans. However, such experimentation may still provide little direct information regarding the factors affecting disease in man. There is no alternative to evaluating natural experiments involving man; thus, we are left with an epidemiological approach to investigating the effect of air pollution on mortality. The basic task becomes one of making inferences from observational (nonexperimental) data.

A useful illustration is provided by comparing the causes of acute and chronic pulmonary diseases. In studying the prevention and cure of acute disease, the concept of causality is a powerful tool. The cause of one type of acute pneumonia is the pneumococcal bacteria; without these bacteria, the disease cannot occur, although even when the bacteria are present, other conditions must be fortuitous in order to produce the disease. While a generally rundown condition promotes pneumonia, it is not the cause.

Causality, however, may not be a useful concept in investigating the prevention and cure of chronic disease. Reduced pulmonary function might arise from a vast number of causes, ranging from acute lung disease and inadequate nutrition to the inhalation of some toxic compound. Whatever the initial cause, the failure of the body to repair the damage may be due to a set of independent factors. Furthermore, the lung damage may become progressive through a third and even larger set of contributing factors, including viral infection, occupational exposure, smoking, air pollution, or even one's genetic disposition. What, for example, is the cause of severe dyspnea in a sixty-year-old asbestos worker who smokes, lives in a large city, comes from an impoverished family, and has never received proper nutrition?[2]

Rather than attempting to find the initial cause of a chronic lung disease or the reasons for incomplete pulmonary repair, it is more useful to focus on the factors that predispose a person to the disease, aggravate the symptoms of the disease, or make the disease progressive. In the example given, all the factors named probably contributed to the dyspnea, and the absence of any factor probably would have resulted in less-severe symptoms. But the worker would not find such a conclusion helpful, nor would a public health official. They would find it more useful to know the quantitative contribution of each factor—for example, that breathing asbestos particles is ten times more detrimental than exposure to urban air pollution (at the level experienced in that particular city).

Similarly, it is more useful to determine the extent to which sulfur dioxide increases the severity and frequency of emphysema than to investigate whether high concentrations of sulfur dioxide induce the disease in white mice under controlled conditions. We are concerned primarily with estimating the effect of mitigating one of the insults, not with determining whether this insult, in isolation, can cause the disease. For this reason, an epidemiological study in which one examines human beings in their natural setting is more relevant than a laboratory experiment. But to investigate the contribution of one insult, we must control for the other factors believed to influence mortality (see table 1.2, page 10).[3] Because it is impossible to control for all such factors, a constant difficulty with such a study is the effect of uncontrolled or unobserved variables. In some cases, this effect will lend a spurious significance to the air pollution–mortality relationship; while in others, it will obscure the association.

In analyzing the results of natural experiments, one can use the four-way classification discussed on page 13. Unfortunately, both categories two (variables that do not change) and three (variables assumed to exert a random influence) are quite small. In addition, since nature does not

[2] The last two factors may have an indirect effect on dyspnea. The poverty may lead to poor nutrition, crowding, lack of indoor heating, or inadequate ventilation; and malnutrition in the formative years may have led to improper development of the body.

[3] Research is further complicated by the likelihood that pollutants interact to produce more damage than they would individually.

usually produce experiments having the scope and precision of laboratory experiments, category four (variables systematically related to the variables that may be causal) may still include a large number of variables at the end of the analysis.

The foregoing discussion has contrasted laboratory and epidemiological methods and examined the limited usefulness of causality for investigating chronic disease. Before proceeding to a more detailed consideration of these methods, a summary would be helpful. Laboratory research enables one to evaluate postulated causal variables while controlling or randomizing other factors. However, ethical considerations or the subtlety of an effect may negate this power. While laboratory methods may not be useful ways of estimating the relationship between air pollution and the incidence of disease in a population, they are essential for studying the underlying physiological mechanisms.

A study of environmental effects that are hypothesized to predispose to acute disease, impede the body's repair mechanism, or make damage progressive necessitates that we turn away from the notion of causality and focus instead on natural experiments. The question we will address is, Given the current levels of disease agents and the current demographic conditions in an area, to what extent will changes in some environmental conditions be associated with changes in the incidence of disease, as manifested by changes in mortality rates?

PREVIOUS STUDIES

The issues discussed above are particularly relevant for the analysis that follows, but they also apply to any investigation of the association between air pollution and health. Consequently, this section focuses on the methods used by past studies so that the results of such research can be properly evaluated.

An extensive literature has resulted from investigations of the relationship between air pollution and health. The literature might be classified by method (laboratory studies with animals or humans, clinical studies, population studies), by disease (bronchitis, lung cancer, etc.), by stage of the disease (morbidity versus mortality), by characteristics of the group studied (nationality, age, sex, race, etc.), by pollutant (sulfur dioxide, carbon monoxide, etc.), or by acute (day-to-day) effects versus chronic (long-term) effects. The volume of research precludes a complete literature review here. We have chosen to focus our attention on studies which offer quantitative evidence on the incidence or severity of disease and are reasonably complete in terms of controlling factors believed to affect health. We have paid little attention to laboratory experiments, since our goal is the estimation of the dose–response relationship in the general population.[4]

---

[4] The term *dose-response relationship* refers to the proportion of a given population that exhibits a specified response as a function of the dose (or concentration) of

Do the past studies prove that air pollution causes ill health? If not, how can another study hope to make a marked contribution? In appendix A (see page 273), each study considered is discussed in terms of the extent to which it controls, experimentally or statistically, for the factors listed in table 1.2 (page 10). To reiterate the obvious, no study can prove causation, since no study holds constant all of the factors hypothesized to affect the incidence of illness. Nevertheless, much is to be learned from an examination of the factors controlled in each study, the methods used, and the problems encountered.

One common method used in past research has been cross tabulations, or simple correlations, of the prevalence of a disease (or a specific mortality rate) and some index of air pollution. Recognizing the need to control for other factors affecting health, some studies cross-tabulate along several variables, while others compute partial correlations. However, even the adoption of these more sophisticated statistical procedures is unlikely to produce meaningful estimates of the air pollution–mortality relationship if the groups being compared are ill-matched. Consider, for example, a comparison of the mortality rates for coal miners and executives. Although miners are subjected to high levels of pollution, they probably exercise a great deal more than do executives. A simple comparison of the death rates (due to causes other than accidents) for the two groups would reveal little about the effect of air pollution. Similarly, the myriad factors that differ between urban and rural groups cannot be controlled completely by statistical means; one is inevitably left with a number of important uncontrolled factors that are known to vary systematically with the extent of urbanization. Thus, results such as those shown earlier in table 1.1 (page 8) must be considered as only indicative.

One improvement in method is represented by the series of studies conducted by Zeidberg and his coauthors (1961, 1963, 1964, 1967a, 1967b) in Nashville, Tennessee. For several areas within the city, they contrasted measures of health status with measures of air pollution and socioeconomic status, hypothesizing that other factors would remain constant or would vary randomly. They found mixed results in cross-tabulating respiratory disease mortality with level of air pollution and with income class. While the relationships were generally in the expected direction, they were often nonsignificant.

Failure to find a significant association might indicate that there is not a causal relationship or it might result from an inability to control important factors affecting health, from small samples, from the natural play of

---

the toxic substance. Typically, a dose-response curve will exhibit a cumulative normal or S shape, since some individuals will be relatively sensitive to the substance (and thus exhibit the response at low concentrations), while other individuals will be relatively insensitive (and thus not exhibit the response until the concentrations are quite high).

chance, or from other factors. As an illustration of the effect of small samples and of chance, under conditions where air pollution and health are causally related, consider an experimenter who randomly selects groups of ten individuals and exposes them to sulfur dioxide under controlled conditions. In a laboratory experiment, the observer would find that subjects manifest a range of responses to a carefully controlled dosage. In some groups, all subjects would display severe reactions (since all ten subjects happened to be sensitive to sulfur dioxide); in other groups, no one would display a measurable reaction (since all ten subjects happened to be insensitive to sulfur dioxide). Across a number of such experiments one would expect to observe that many would display a statistically significant number of reactions, but that some would not. A single experiment using ten subjects would not provide enough information for the investigator to draw confident conclusions about the relationship between sulfur dioxide and the subjects' symptoms.

The sample size is particularly important when a subtle irritant is involved and a number of other factors are uncontrolled. For example, in comparing the populations of areas exposed to different levels of air pollution, all factors listed in table 1.2 (page 10) are relevant. Since air pollution at current ambient levels is a subtle irritant, only a comparison between two large populations can be expected to show significantly different mortality, morbidity, or physical test results (given the variation in other factors).

Small samples were associated with the comparisons of residents of Berlin, New Hampshire, to those of Chilliwack, British Columbia (Ferris and Anderson, 1962, 1964), and those in two Pennsylvania towns (Prindle and coauthors, 1963). Since extensive evaluations were done on each resident, the sample size in each case was necessarily small, resulting in large sampling variation that precluded confident comparisons. Even in studies of this sort, where great attention is given to evaluation of the individuals and their histories, uncontrolled factors might be important. For example, neither the climates of the areas nor the ethnic origins, general habits, or occupations of the populations were controlled. We conclude that the sample size of such studies must be enlarged greatly if conclusions are to be stated with confidence—probably at prohibitive increase in cost.

A number of methods have been used to enhance the power of these investigations. One technique has been to examine an indicator of health status having a quantitative value for each member of the population, instead of examining an aggregate measure, such as mortality. For example, in the studies noted above, Ferris and Anderson gave their subjects physical examinations, including lung function tests, while in another study Schoettlin and Landau (1961) asked subjects to keep diaries on the prevalence of disease symptoms. Such procedures are expensive and, again, usually necessitate small sample sizes. In addition, irregularities in the findings might be due to a large number of factors. For example, diary studies are focused on relating day-to-day changes in symptom levels to variations in pollution concentrations. However, when air pollution levels are publicized, diary entries are likely to be biased.

These kinds of problems have led some investigators to expand the sample size so that large numbers of observations would randomize or control confounding factors. In so doing there is an underlying assumption that the important factors affecting health (or the test outcome) are controlled or vary randomly. If this is so, increasing the sample size will tend to sharpen the contrast. Replications under these conditions will tend to support the hypothesis. However, if a basic factor is not controlled, replications need not increase one's confidence in the previous results. Suppose that an investigation comparing rural and urban areas in New England finds a positive association between the level of air pollution and the incidence of venereal disease. Replications contrasting urban and rural counties in other regions of the United States, or even in other countries, will not strengthen the assertion that air pollution causes venereal disease. Here the underlying association is that urbanization and its various social and economic ramifications lead to both air pollution and venereal disease; independent replication that does not control for the effect of urbanization will not produce meaningful results. To isolate this factor, it would be more helpful to compare rural counties (or urban counties) within a region. Only by knowing the nature of the basic relationship can one design studies capable of discriminating between a spurious association and a causal one.

Other investigators have collected large samples of data on generally similar types of individuals. Examples include the work of Hammond and Horn (1958) in their analysis of death certificates for persons reportedly dying from lung cancer, that of Buell and Dunn (1967), and Buell and coauthors (1967) in their use of questionnaires sent to California veterans, and that of other researchers who have analyzed a city's population over time (to estimate the effect of day-to-day changes in pollution) or those who have analyzed the concurrent populations of several cities simultaneously.

Purifying the data by holding constant many of the factors affecting health is a classic technique in epidemiology. Reid and his coauthors (1958, 1964, 1966) have undertaken a number of studies comparing men in the same occupation (for example, postal workers who deliver mail in areas with various degrees of pollution). Such studies can be especially powerful in isolating the effects of particular pollutants (for example, automobile emissions and their effects on tunnel workers). Another related method is the examination by autopsy of accident victims in cities having different levels of air pollution, with controls introduced for such factors as age and sex. For example, Ishikawa and his coauthors (1969) compared lung tissue from individuals who had resided in Saint Louis and Winnipeg. Perhaps the ultimate attempt at controlling for confounding factors is represented by Cederlöf's study (1966) of the incidence of bronchitis in identical twins living in different environments. Yet, even a study of this sort leaves many important factors uncontrolled. While genetic factors, early nutrition, and socialization are controlled, current life-style (including exercise patterns and stress), for example, probably is not. If these factors are systematically related to urbanization, air pollution may have a spurious significance, but nothing more. While these studies help to sort out the effects of many factors, they can, at best, only help to define the nature of the association. They are not very helpful in estimating the contribution of air pollution to the incidence of bronchitis in the general population.

As the literature review in appendix A (pages 273–311) indicates, a substantial number of studies have examined the association of air pollution with mortality and with morbidity, as defined by the number of people seeking care, by work or school absence, by patient-reported acute or chronic symptoms, by ventilatory function tests, or by physicians' assessments of radiological and other physical evidence. The vast majority of this literature reports a significant association between air pollution and health. In one study or another, each of the factors hypothesized to affect health has been controlled.

The central problems with individual attempts to investigate this association have been (1) failure to control for important factors affecting health, and (2) sample sizes that are too small to lend confidence to the results. Since many of the studies exhibit both shortcomings simultaneously, it is not surprising that some have found results contrary to the weight of evidence and to our expectations. We stress the absence of controls in reviewing the literature and would merely note that in many studies the most important factors have been uncontrolled; such studies provide little evidence to confirm or deny the hypothesis of causality.

Furthermore, since investigators are more reluctant to publish negative results than positive ones, and since it is more difficult to publish results showing no association, we are probably unaware of other studies that have failed to find a strong association between air pollution and health. Although one would like to see all the evidence before reaching a conclusion, there is no alternative to evaluating the evidence at hand and allowing for the possibility of additional contrary studies.

The most complete studies evaluate a specific set of people—a particular occupation group, for example—which allows for more complete control. The comparisons made in such studies can be stated with more confidence, but they are limited in their relevance to the general population. On the other hand, the studies that have investigated effects in the general population suffer from lack of controls. Thus, one cannot have confidence that the association estimated in these studies is causal. Nonetheless, if the association were causal, these studies would allow one to estimate the magnitude of the effect.

We conclude that the studies focusing on special groups, or otherwise controlling for the most important factors, provide evidence of a causal relationship between some air pollutants (particularly sulfur oxides and suspended particulates) and health effects. The failure of any single study to control for all factors hypothesized to affect health means that no one study can be said to have proved causation. But since almost all factors are controlled in one or another of the studies, and since the relationship has been demonstrated under many circumstances, the literature suggests that the relationship is a causal one.

TESTING A CAUSAL MODEL

The following statement by Blalock (1964, page 62) provides a good indication of the nature of the analysis to follow: "It is quite correct that one can never demonstrate causality for correlational data, or in fact from any type of empirical information. Nevertheless, it is possible to make causal *inferences* concerning the adequacy of causal models, at least in the sense that we can proceed by eliminating inadequate models that make predictions that are not consistent with the data." In chapter 1 we stated our hypothesis that air pollution (sulfur oxides, suspended particulates, and, to some extent, nitrogen oxides, carbon monoxide, and hydrocarbons) causes an increase in the mortality rate. We further conjecture that the effect is a subtle one. The hypothesis will be tested by statistical investigation within a number of different settings. We will be looking for a consistent association between air pollution and mortality in each setting and seeking to "eliminate inadequate models." A few of the factors hypothesized to affect mortality will be measured directly (for example, climate), while a host of other factors will be measured via surrogates only (for example, income is represented by the proportion of poor families).[5]

We shall return frequently to the question of testing causality, although the focus of the analysis will be a detailed exploration of the effect of air pollution on mortality and attempts to estimate its magnitude. The reader should be warned at the outset that this investigation is not in the nature of a mathematical proof to a theorem. Not all of the factors hypothesized to affect mortality nor all of the measurement problems can be found, isolated, and accounted for. Testing for causality in the air pollution–mortality relationship is a slow, often tedious, process.

PROBLEMS OF ESTIMATION

Numerous problems arise in attempting to estimate the relationship between air pollution and mortality. Missing or badly measured variables can

---

[5] Other measures of income, such as median family income, were investigated but proved to be so highly correlated that only one variable was used in the analysis.

lead to biases in the estimated effects, as can social phenomenon, such as migration. We explore some of these complications in the hope that they can be dealt with directly so that, at a minimum, the direction of the bias can be determined.

If an important variable, correlated with both an explanatory variable and mortality is omitted, parameter estimates will be biased. For example, suppose that people of lower socioeconomic status smoke more than do those of a higher status. Then, since we have no measure of the rate of smoking in the population, the estimated effect of family income on mortality may reflect both poverty and the effect of greater smoking. Other variables not included in our initial analyses were sex, genetic factors, nutrition, exercise habits, medical care, housing, occupation, and weather. Some of these factors (weather, home heating, sex, race, and occupation) are considered later. However, there is little that can be done about the remaining factors except to conjecture how they might affect the parameter estimates of the included variables.

We are concerned primarily with omitted variables that would tend to bias the estimated association of mortality with air pollution. We find little reason to believe that sex distribution, genetic factors, nutrition, smoking, exercise habits, or medical care are highly correlated with air pollution in the areas we will study, although they may be correlated with other included variables.

Migration is another factor that can bias the estimated associations. Suppose, for example, that everyone in New York City who has severe asthma or another chronic respiratory disease moves to a relatively unpolluted city in the Southwest, such as Tucson. This would mean that, even if the relatively clean air in Tucson were to prolong the migrants' lives, the net effect of the migration of unhealthy people might be to raise the mortality rate in Tucson while lowering it in New York City. If there is a net migration of chronically ill persons toward unpolluted areas, the result will bias the estimated coefficients of air pollution toward zero and cause us to underestimate the association between air pollution and mortality. Carried to the extreme, so many sick people could migrate to Tucson that the resulting death rates would be higher in Tucson than in New York City, and the estimated relationship between mortality and air pollution would show that air pollution is associated with lower mortality.

Similarly, if persons with respiratory diseases move within a city to a less-polluted area or install devices in their present homes to filter out pollution, the mortality rate is likely to fall. Behavior of this sort will affect the estimated association with air pollution. Insofar as such actions take place with greater frequency in more-polluted cities, the mortality rate in these cities will be lower than expected, and one will tend to underestimate the effect of air pollution. In addition, since people will respond differently within cities, the relationship between air pollution and mortality may be obscured and the precision with which we can estimate it impaired.[6]

Another problem arises from the fact that we have no measure of cumulative exposure of the population or of individuals.[7] Suppose that the "true" relationship between air pollution and mortality can be illustrated by Equation 2.1:

$$MR = \alpha_0 + \alpha_1 P + \alpha_2 S + \mu \qquad\qquad 2.1$$

where MR is the mortality rate, P is the cumulative exposure of air pollution that the population has experienced, S is a socioeconomic index, and μ is an error term, while α_0, α_1, and α_2 are the coefficients to be estimated. If the only available measure of air pollution is the current level of pollution (denoted P^*), then estimating the equation with P^* instead of P will lead to a number of difficulties. Provided that air pollution has been constant over time, P^* will be proportional to P, and the significance test of the estimated coefficient a_1 will be appropriate. However, if air quality has been worsening in some cities and improving in others, P and P^* will not be as closely related, and neither the estimated coefficient nor its statistical significance will reflect the true effect of air pollution on mortality.[8] A number of possible cases could be explored but, in the absence of relevant data, little would be accomplished. Furthermore, if air pollution has been generally worsening, estimation with P^* instead of P (even if they are still proportional) will mean that we are again underestimating the true effect of air pollution. If current mortality is assumed to be related not only to current pollution, but also to the lower levels of pollution prevailing in the past, the coefficient of pollution will be biased downward. The resulting underestimate could have significant policy implications. Despite all of these difficulties, we are left with no alternative but to assume that the current measures of air pollution are characteristic of those past levels, which are, in fact, related to current deaths.

Another serious issue involves the possible error associated with air pollution measurements. In general, a single sampling station in a region generates readings that are reported as biweekly samples. Since pollution concentration varies greatly with terrain, it is an heroic assumption, when making comparisons across areas, to regard these figures as representative of an entire SMSA. In addition, measuring instruments change over time

[6] It is, of course, possible that some of these adjustments might lead to an overestimate of the effects of air pollution, but in most cases it would seem that the bias would be toward underestimation.

[7] Air pollution data on more than a handful of cities date from the late 1950s and the beginning of the National Air Sampling Network.

[8] Areas with net in-migration are extreme instances in which P and P^* are unrelated, since the migrants will have been affected by the air quality of their former residence.

and differ across cities, and some of them have little reliability. At best, the air pollution variables based on such sampling are a remote approximation to the true current and cumulative exposure to air pollution experienced by individuals. Errors in variables will cause the estimated coefficient to be biased and inconsistent; and there is a relatively strong, but not certain, presumption that the coefficient will be underestimated.

As a simple example, consider a version of the model in Equation 2.1 that includes only one explanatory variable: $MR = \alpha_0 + \alpha_1 P + \mu$. Now suppose that $P*$ is measured with error; that is, observed pollution $P*$ is equal to "true" pollution P' plus a random factor or error of observation ϵ; $P* = P' + \epsilon$. The least-squares estimate of a_1 is given by[9]

$$a_1 = \frac{\Sigma MR \cdot P}{\Sigma P^2} = \frac{\Sigma MR \cdot P' + \Sigma MR \cdot \epsilon}{\Sigma P'^2 + 2\Sigma P' \cdot \epsilon + \Sigma \epsilon^2}$$

On the assumption that the error ϵ is distributed independently of the true values (that is, that the error in measuring pollution is independent of both the true level of pollution and the mortality rate, $\Sigma P' \cdot \epsilon = \Sigma MR \cdot \epsilon = 0$. Then, the least-squares estimate simplifies to

$$a_1 = \left| \frac{\Sigma MR \cdot P'}{\Sigma P'^2 + \Sigma \epsilon^2} \right| < \left| \frac{\Sigma MR \cdot P'}{\Sigma P'^2} \right|,$$

the right-hand term corresponding to the least-squares estimate when the true value of pollution is observed.[10] Thus, a_1 (the estimated coefficient), when $P*$ is measured with error, is smaller than the corresponding coefficient when $P*$ is measured accurately.

Another source of bias is the relationship between air pollution exposure within an SMSA and socioeconomic factors, such as income and race. Freeman (1972) has shown that nonwhite residential areas have higher pollution levels than do white residential areas. In the absence of measurements of individual exposure, the socioeconomic variables of income and race may be confounded with any effect of air pollution variables.

To illustrate, suppose that we are estimating Equation 2.1 with $P*$ (current pollution) substituted for P (cumulative pollution) under the assumption that the model is applicable to all socioeconomic groups. Let P^o ($<P*$) be the actual level of air pollution to which high-income whites are exposed and P_o ($>P*$) be the actual level of air pollution to which low-income blacks are exposed. Then, using the available measure of air pollution $P*$ will mean that the estimates corresponding to the socioeconomic variables of income and race will be biased, since they will incorporate the effects of differences in the exposures of the two groups. More important, the true effects of air pollution will be confused with the esti-

---

[9] In this formulation, the variables are expressed as deviations from means.
[10] The general case is treated by Johnston (1972, pp. 281–283).

mated effects of income and race (the two socioeconomic characteristics distinguishing the groups).

A closer look at a model of the death process will provide insight into another aspect of the problem with which we are dealing. The number of deaths occurring in an area during a specific period is often assumed to follow a Poisson distribution. This assumption could be used to specify the functional form of our regressions, since the distribution can be expressed analytically. However, determining the functional form on the basis of an assumed Poisson distribution seems a pedantic refinement, given our general ignorance of other important matters regarding the association between air pollution and mortality.

The assumption is useful for examining the degree of variation inherent in our data. The mean population of the 117 SMSAs which constituted our initial data base was approximately 800,000,[11] and the mean total mortality rate was about 900 per 100,000, with a standard deviation of about 150 per 100,000. An area of this size would experience a standard deviation in the mortality rate of only 10.6 per 100,000 if the underlying process followed a true Poisson distribution.[12] Thus, the observed standard deviation across the 117 SMSAs was approximately fourteen times as large as the variation that would be expected if the underlying process were a Poisson distribution and each area had a population of 800,000. (Note that an area with 10 million persons would be associated with a standard deviation of 3 per 100,000, while an area with 50,000 would be associated with a standard deviation of about 42 per 100,000.)

This type of calculation serves to place an upper bound on the sum of squares that might be accounted for by our regressions. Since the computation shows that about 7 percent of the observed variation would be inherently random, it follows that one would not expect to "explain" more than about 93 percent of the variation by the regressions.

We have discussed the estimation difficulties caused by our lack of a priori knowledge of the "true" specification of the relation, omitted variables, errors of observation, and systematic biases. These problems all tend to obscure the air pollution–mortality relationship and to bias the estimated relationship toward statistical nonsignificance. If, in spite of these problems, air pollution appears to have a significant association with mortality, the interpretation would seem to be that the underlying relation deserves further attention. We shall present the first of our estimates in chapter 3. Needless to say, the estimated parameters are to be viewed with caution.

[11] The selection of SMSAs was based on the availability of pollution data. A listing of SMSAs in the analysis appears in appendix C.

[12] This follows since there would be 7,200 expected deaths per year with a standard deviation of approximately 85, which is equal to a standard deviation of 10.6 per 100,000.

Cross-sectional analysis of U.S. SMSAs, 1960, 1961, and 1969

CHAPTER 3

Total U.S. mortality, 1960 and 1961

Sections II and III will explore the empirical association between air pollution and health status (as measured by mortality). Much of the analysis will focus on whether the empirical evidence is consistent with a causal relationship. At the same time, a major output of the analysis will be a quantitative estimate of the dose–response relationship between air pollution (as measured primarily by sulfates and suspended particulates) and mortality.

The second hypothesized relationship between air pollution and mortality, discussed in chapter 1, was that long-term exposure to low levels of pollution adversely affects health. Two different types of analyses might be used to explore this hypothesis. The first would involve an investigation of a measure of health status across areas having different qualities of ambient air. The second would involve an analysis of a measure of health status within a single location experiencing changing air quality over a period of time. Of the two, it seems likely that one would observe larger differences in air quality across different places than within a single place over time. Thus, cross-sectional analysis of areas with differing pollution levels at a given time offers a greater possibility of isolating pollution effects should they exist.

Specifically, this chapter is based on analysis of annual cross-sectional data for 117 SMSAs in the United States.[1] We have sought to avoid the more obvious fallacies associated with comparing urban and rural places by using these large metropolitan areas as our units of observation. The statistical method used to analyze these data is linear multivariable re-

---

[1] Actually, standard economic areas (SEAs) were used as the unit of observation for the New England region because of the methods employed in data collection (see appendix C).

gression analysis. We begin by reporting analyses of total mortality, using socioeconomic variables to control for population density, racial composition, age distribution, income, and population. Air pollution will be represented by the measured levels of sulfates and suspended particulates.[2]

METHOD

Since we had little a priori knowledge as to which measures of air pollution or which socioeconomic variables would be important, many were used in the analysis. In Equation 3.1 the total 1960 mortality rate was regressed on socioeconomic and air pollution variables across 117 SMSAs.[3]

$$MR = 343.381 + 0.473 \text{ } Min \text{ } S + 0.173 \text{ } Mean \text{ } S + 0.028 \text{ } Max \text{ } S$$
$$(1.67)(0.53)(0.25)$$

$$+ \text{ } 0.199 \text{ } Min \text{ } P + 0.303 \text{ } Mean \text{ } P - 0.018 \text{ } Max \text{ } P + 0.083 \text{ } P/M^2$$
$$(0.32)(0.71)(-0.19)(1.54)$$

$$+ \text{ } 6.880 \geq 65 + 0.396 \text{ } NW + 0.038 \text{ } Poor - 0.276 \text{ } Log \text{ } Pop$$
$$(16.63)(3.82)(0.26)(-1.38)$$

$$+ \text{ } e (R^2 = 0.831) 3.1$$

where MR is the total mortality rate in the area, $Min \text{ } S, \text{ } Mean \text{ } S,$ and $Max \text{ } S$ are the smallest, the arithmetic mean, and the largest, respectively, of the twenty-six biweekly sulfate readings; $Min \text{ } P, \text{ } Mean \text{ } P,$ and $Max \text{ } P$ are the smallest, the arithmetic mean, and the largest, respectively, of the twenty-six biweekly suspended particulate readings; P/M^2 is the population density in the SMSA; ≥ 65 is the percentage of the SMSA population aged sixty-five and older; NW is the percentage of the SMSA population who are nonwhite; $Poor$ is the percentage of the SMSA families with incomes below the poverty level; $Log \text{ } Pop$ is the logarithm of the SMSA population;[4] and e is an error term. The scaling of the variables is reported in table D.1 (pages 321–324), along with their means and standard deviations. The figures shown in parentheses below the regression coefficients are the t statistics. Table 3.1 also reports the sums of elasticities about the mean. Each elasticity is equal to $100 \times b \text{ } (\overline{X}/\overline{Y})$, where b is the estimated coefficient and $\overline{X}$ and $\overline{Y}$ are the means of the independent and dependent variables, respectively.

The results are encouraging in that more than 83 percent of the variation in the total mortality rate across these 117 SMSAs was accounted

---

[2] As discussed earlier, the most complete air pollution data available were for suspended particulates. Sulfate data were available for most of the same SMSAs. When no 1960 data existed, data from the closest year (usually 1959 or 1961) were used as surrogates.

[3] Equation 3.1 corresponds to regression 3.1-1 in table 3.1.

[4] Population was transformed into logarithms, since it seemed unlikely that it would have a linear relationship to the mortality rate. New York City is twice as large as Chicago and a hundred times as large as the smallest SMSA; while "urbanness" rises from the smallest to the largest SMSA, one would hardly expect it to rise 100-fold. The logarithmic transformation emphasizes the differences in population among the smaller SMSAs and tends to play down the New York City–Chicago difference.

TABLE 3.1. Total Mortality Rates, 1960

	3.1-1	3.1-2
R^2	.831	.828
Constant	343.381	301.205
Air pollution variables		
Min S	.473	.631
	(1.67)	(2.71)
Mean S	.173	
	(.53)	
Max S	.028	
	(.25)	
Sum S elasticities	5.04	3.27
Min P	.199	
	(.32)	
Mean P	.303	.452
	(.71)	(2.67)
Max P	−.018	
	(−.19)	
Sum P elasticities	4.37	5.85
Socioeconomic variables		
P/M^2	.083	.089
	(1.54)	(1.71)
≥ 65	6.880	7.028
	(16.63)	(18.09)
NW	.396	.422
	(3.82)	(4.32)
Poor	.038	−.002
	(.26)	(−.02)
Sum SE elasticities	70.07	71.03
Log Pop[a]	−.276	−.212
	(−1.38)	(−1.12)

Note: Both regressions are based on data for 117 SMSAs. The numbers in parentheses below the regression coefficients are *t* statistics.

[a] The population variable (Log Pop) is not included in the summed elasticities of the socioeconomic variables, since the transformation to logarithms means that the regression coefficient can be interpreted directly as an elasticity.

for by the eleven independent variables ($R^2 = 0.831$). The estimated coefficients for the air pollution variables were disappointing in that none had a statistically significant coefficient,[5] and one coefficient was negative;

[5] A variable will be termed statistically *significant* if the probability that its coefficient differs from zero is greater than 0.95. When we use the term *approached statistical significance,* we are making a judgment that the estimated *t* statistic would have called for rejection of the null hypothesis of no association (that is, a coefficient equal to zero) at a lower level of significance.

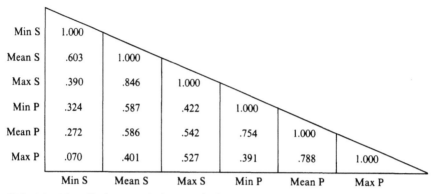

	Min S	Mean S	Max S	Min P	Mean P	Max P
Min S	1.000					
Mean S	.603	1.000				
Max S	.390	.846	1.000			
Min P	.324	.587	.422	1.000		
Mean P	.272	.586	.542	.754	1.000	
Max P	.070	.401	.527	.391	.788	1.000

FIG. 3.1. Air pollution correlation matrix for 1960.

however, the six variables made a statistically significant contribution as a group.[6] These results are partially explained by the high correlation between the six measures of air pollution, as is shown in figure 3.1. Such multicollinearity has the effect of increasing the standard errors of the estimated coefficients and of impairing the accuracy with which individual coefficients can be estimated. A more complete discussion of this regression appears below.

One conventional approach to regression estimation involves dropping superfluous variables in order to derive an equation which contains coefficients with predicted signs, plausible magnitudes, and statistical significance. Since our interest was centered on the air pollution variables, we initially retained only those whose coefficients were positive and exceeded their standard errors, with the further constraint that at least one sulfate measure and one particulate measure were retained. In reestimating the relationship, we often found that the retained air pollution variables were now significant (which is not surprising, since the pollution variables were highly correlated). Sometimes the retained air pollution variable contributed little to the statistical significance of the regression. Such variables were eliminated, subject to the restriction that at least one air pollution variable be retained in the final equation. This technique was used throughout our analyses of other mortality rates. (The five basic socio-

[6] As part of the analysis we examined the total effect of the pollution variables by comparing a regression including the socioeconomic variables only with a regression including the six pollution variables as well. Adding additional explanatory variables to a regression cannot lower the explanatory power (R^2) and generally increases it. To test whether the increase in R^2 is statistically significant, the decrease in the residual sum of squares (divided by the number of additional variables) is divided by the residual sum of squares (divided by the degrees of freedom). This ratio of mean reduction in residual squares to mean residual squares is distributed according to F. For the 1960 total mortality rate, $F = 3.71$, with 6 and 105 degrees of freedom. Since $F_{0.05} = 2.18$, with 6 and 120 degrees of freedom, the result indicated that the pollution variables added significantly to the explanatory power of the regression.

economic variables were retained throughout.) Because these relations are estimated ad hoc, they must be viewed with care.

Equation 3.1, containing all six pollution variables, is reported in table 3.1 as regression 3.1-1. (Note that all regressions are numbered according to the table in which they appear.) Regression 3.1-2 represents a similar specification but includes only the two most significant air pollution variables (Min S and Mean P). As expected, there was little loss in explanatory power when the other four measures of air pollution were deleted [R^2 decreased from 0.831 to 0.828; the F statistic ($F = 0.40$) computed to examine this loss confirmed the nonsignificance of it]. Each of the coefficients of the two remaining air pollution variables was statistically significant and approximately equal in magnitude to the sum of the three variables it represented.

PRINCIPAL COMPONENT ANALYSIS

A less-arbitrary procedure for reducing the size of the equation was also examined. As shown in figure 3.1, the six air pollution measures tended to be highly correlated. One method for circumventing the collinearity problem is to perform a principal component analysis on the pollution variables and to replace the pollution measures with the resulting components in the regressions.[7] We have explored this method with the 1960 data. First, we found the principal components of all six pollution measures; then we found the principal components of the suspended particulate and sulfate measures separately (table 3.2). The first principal component explained 59.5 percent of the variation in the six variables, 74.8 percent of the variation in the sulfate measures, and 76.8 percent of the variation in the suspended particulate measures. The corresponding figures for the first two components together were 78.3 percent, 96.1 percent, and 97.1 percent, respectively.

Four regressions are reported in table 3.2 for the total 1960 mortality rate. Regression 3.2-1 used the original six air pollution variables and is shown for comparison; regression 3.2-2 used the two most significant air pollution variables; regression 3.2-3 used the first two principal components extracted from all six pollution measures; and regression 3.2-4 used the first two principal components from the separate analyses of the sulfate and suspended particulate measures. In addition to these components, the five socioeconomic variables were included.

Comparing regression 3.2-2 with regressions 3.2-3 and 3.2-4, one notes little or no difference between using the principal components and using the ad hoc method of selecting pollution variables. The statistical significance of the principal components of the air pollution variables was vir-

---

[7] For a discussion of principal component analysis (sometimes called principal factor analysis), see Harman (1967, pp. 154–191). By construction, principal components are uncorrelated with each other.

TABLE 3.2. Principal Components Analysis of Total Mortality Rates, 1960

	3.2-1	3.2-2	3.2-3	3.2-4
R^2	.831	.828	.829	.830
Constant	343.381	301.205	442.990	422.785
Air pollution variables				
Min S	.473	.631		
	(1.67)	(2.71)		
Mean S	.173			
	(.53)			
Max S	.028			
	(.25)			
Sum S elasticities	5.04	3.27		
Min P	.199			
	(.32)			
Mean P	.303	.452		
	(.71)	(2.67)		
Max P	−.018			
	(−.19)			
Sum P elasticities	4.37	5.85		
Principal components (sulfates and suspended particulates)				
SP$_1$			30.763	
			(4.58)	
SP$_2$			10.617	
			(1.47)	

Note: All regressions are based on data for 117 SMSAs. The numbers in parentheses below the regression coefficients are *t* statistics. Elasticities are not given for the principal components since by construction their means and elasticities are equal to zero.

Principal components:

    Three sulfate and three suspended particulate measures

        Cumulative proportion of variance explained by component:

            SP$_1$ = 0.595   SP$_2$ = 0.783

        Eigenvalues:

            1 = 3.5726   2 = 1.1275

        Eigenvectors:

	1	2
Min S	0.5377	0.7106
Mean S	0.8786	0.3459
Max S	0.8227	0.1519
Min P	0.7648	−0.1040
Mean P	0.8695	−0.3813
Max P	0.7028	−0.5689

    Three sulfate measures

        Cumulative proportion of variance explained by component:

            S$_1$ = 0.748   S$_2$ = 0.961

TABLE 3.2. (*Continued*)

	3.2-1	3.2-2	3.2-3	3.2-4
Principal components (sulfates)				
S_1				22.514 (2.56)
S_2				−7.807 (−1.10)
Principal components (suspended particulates)				
P_1				13.050 (1.59)
P_2				−3.148 (−.46)
Socioeconomic variables				
P/M^2	.083 (1.54)	.089 (1.71)	.089 (1.71)	.084 (1.59)
≥ 65	6.880 (16.63)	7.028 (18.09)	6.836 (17.14)	6.869 (16.97)
NW	.396 (3.82)	.422 (4.32)	.385 (3.97)	.388 (3.93)
Poor	.038 (.26)	−.002 (−.02)	.054 (.37)	.044 (.30)
Sum SE elasticities	70.07	71.03	69.97	69.86
Log Pop	−.276 (−1.38)	−.212 (−1.12)	−.297 (−1.60)	−.263 (−1.34)

Note (*continued*)

Eigenvalues:

$\quad\quad 1 = 2.2449 \quad\quad\quad 2 = 0.6387$

Eigenvectors:

	1	*2*
Min S	0.7403	−0.6671
Mean S	0.9581	0.1275
Max S	0.8825	0.4212

Three suspended particulate measures

Cumulative proportion of variance explained by component:

$\quad\quad P_1 = 0.768 \quad\quad\quad P_2 = 0.971$

Eigenvalues:

$\quad\quad 1 = 2.3036 \quad\quad\quad 2 = 0.6091$

Eigenvectors:

	1	*2*
Min P	0.8134	−0.5678
Mean P	0.9738	0.0166
Max P	0.8328	0.5352

35

tually identical to the significance of the air pollution variables when they were used. The coefficients of the socioeconomic variables and their statistical significance were essentially unchanged. Thus, we concluded that little would be gained by using the principal components in place of the air pollution variables. On the contrary, interpretation of the principal components is somewhat more difficult than interpretation of the untransformed pollution measures.

IMPLICATIONS OF THE REGRESSIONS

Because there is no diagnostic problem and little or no reporting problem involved, the mortality data for total deaths are more accurate and complete than data for any of the subcategories. Thus, an analysis of total mortality is a good place to begin our study, and it serves as a reference point for analyses of other data sets. It should be noted, however, that the accuracy and completeness of these data come at some cost because they are so aggregated.[8] Age-specific analysis is needed if the effect of air pollution on life expectancy is to be calculated;[9] it is also desirable to determine which particular diseases are associated with air pollution. Disease-specific mortality rates are analyzed in chapter 4.

The estimates from a multivariable regression are not to be taken as proof of causation, but as evidence of associations that may or may not indicate a causal relation. Thus, we will speak of the *association* between a single variable, such as suspended particulates, and the mortality rate, holding other factors constant. These are not statements of causation, but are merely indications of the magnitude of the observed association.

In regression 3.1-1 (see Equation 3.1) the total mortality was regressed on all of the air pollution and socioeconomic variables. The multicollinearity among the air pollution variables and the resulting nonsignificance of the estimated coefficients make their interpretation somewhat difficult. In regression 3.1-2, only the most significant sulfate and suspended particulate measures were retained.

Over 83 percent of the variation was accounted for by the eleven independent variables in regression 3.1-1. As expected, the most significant variable was the percentage of the population aged sixty-five and older

[8] The mortality rates are not adjusted for age, race, or sex. Age and race are partially accounted for by including explanatory variables for the proportion of the population aged sixty-five and older and the proportion who are nonwhite. However, these two variables may not be satisfactory controls for the failure to use standardized mortality rates. In chapter 4, we shall analyze age–sex–race-adjusted and age–sex–race-specific death rates. As a final control, principal components for the age–sex–race mix of the area are added as explanatory variables.

[9] In addition, since areas in the Northeast tend to have both the highest levels of air pollution (sulfates and suspended particulates) and the greatest proportion of older people, age-specific mortality rates can also be used to examine the possibility of a spurious association. We note, however, that the simple correlation between the minimum biweekly sulfate reading and the proportion of people sixty-five and older was only 0.31 for the 1960 data.

(≥ 65). The implication of the estimated coefficient is that an increase of one percentage point in the proportion of the population aged sixty-five and older (raising the mean of the scaled variable from 83.9 to 93.9) was associated with a rise in the total death rate of 68.8 per 100,000 (from a mean of 912.3 to 981.1).

The percentage of nonwhites in the population (NW) was also a significant variable. An increase of one percentage point in the concentration of nonwhites (raising the mean of the scaled variable from 124.8 to 134.8) was associated with an increase in the total death rate of 4.0 per 100,000. Population density (P/M^2) approached statistical significance; an increase of 100 persons per square mile (from a mean of 70.0 to 80.0) was associated with an increase in the total death rate of 0.8 per 100,000.

The percentage of poor families in the population (Poor) was not statistically significant. The implication of its coefficient was that an increase of one percentage point in the proportion of poor people (raising the mean of the scaled variable from 181.1 to 191.1) was associated with an increase in the total mortality rate of 0.4 per 100,000. The population variable (Log Pop) was also statistically nonsignificant; a 10 percent increase in the log of the population was associated with a decrease of 0.03 per 100,000 in the total mortality rate.

The most significant pollution variable was the minimum biweekly sulfate reading (Min S). An increase of 1 μg per cubic meter in the Min S reading (raising the mean of the scaled variable from 47.2 to 57.2) was related to an increase of 4.7 per 100,000 in the total death rate; increases in the arithmetic mean (Mean S) and the maximum (Max S) of the biweekly sulfate readings were also related to increases in the mortality rate. The mean arithmetic level (Mean P) was the most significant of the suspended particulate variables. An increase of 10 μg per cubic meter in the mean level of suspended particulate pollution (from a mean of 118.1 to 128.1) was related to an increase of 3.0 per 100,000 in the total mortality rate. An increase in the smallest biweekly suspended particulate reading was related to an increase in the mortality rate, while an increase in the largest biweekly suspended particulate reading was associated with a decrease in the mortality rate.

While one should be cautious not to overinterpret the results, the fact that the mean, minimum, or maximum measure of air pollution was most significant does have possible implications. The mean level is an approximation to the average exposure. Significance of this measure could be interpreted as saying that the "average" exposures were closely associated with the mortality rates. Significance of the minimum measure might imply that areas with the "highest" minimums, that is, those areas that never experienced relatively low levels of air pollution, had the highest mortality rates. Significance of the maximum measure would imply that areas with the worst air pollution levels (at some time during the year) had the highest mortality rates.

TABLE 3.3.   Estimated Percentage Change in Total Mortality Rates, 1960

10 percent change in	Percentage change	Deaths per 100,000
All S together	0.50	4.60
All P together	0.44	3.99
P/M²	0.06	0.58
≥65	6.33	57.70
NW	0.54	4.94
Poor	0.08	0.69
Log Pop	−0.28	−2.52

Note: Estimates are based on regression 3.1-1.

Since the estimated coefficients depend directly on the measurement units, it is helpful to restate the implications of the estimated regression as elasticities, or in unit-free terms. The sum of elasticities for sulfates, suspended particulates, and socioeconomic variables (excluding Log Pop) are reported in table 3.1, along with the regressions. Table 3.3 outlines the change in total mortality associated with a 10 percent change in the mean value of each of the independent variables from regression 3.1-1. For example, a 10 percent decrease in the percentage of those aged sixty-five and older in the population (0.8 percentage points) was associated with a reduction of 6.33 percent in the total death rate (57.7 per 100,000). The interpretations for the other variables are similar. The evidence in table 3.3 suggests that the association between air pollution and mortality is significant and of substantial magnitude.

JACKKNIFE ANALYSIS

One question which arises in this type of analysis is, To what extent do the results depend on "extreme" observations? In order to examine the sensitivity of the results to observations from one or two SMSAs, we performed the so-called jackknife tests.[10]

First, the 117 observations were arranged according to the value of the mean suspended particulate variable, and thirteen subsets of 108 observations were formed by dropping the first nine observations, then the second nine, and so on. Then, the same specification as that in regression 3.1-2 was estimated for each of the thirteen data sets. Table 3.4 reports the regression coefficients for the entire sample (from regression 3.1-2), the jackknife estimates, and 95 percent confidence intervals for the estimates.[11]

---

[10] See Mosteller and Tukey (1969) who report that the term "jackknife is intended to suggest the broad usefulness of a technique as a substitute for specialized tools that may not be available, just as the Boy Scout's trusty tool serves so variedly."

[11] The jackknife estimate (j) for a regression coefficient is calculated

$$j = \sum_{i=1}^{n} \frac{nb_n - (n-1)b_i}{n}$$

TABLE 3.4.   Jackknife Analysis of Total Mortality Rates, 1960

	Whole sample[a]	Jackknife	
		Estimate[b]	95 percent confidence interval
Constant	301.205	267.383	(−125.440, 660.206)
Air pollution variables			
Min S	.631	.616	(−.124, 1.356)
Mean P	.452	.451	(.342, .560)
Socioeconomic variables			
P/M²	.089	.004	(−.221, .227)
≥65	7.028	6.933	(5.261, 8.605)
NW	.422	.417	(.179, .655)
Poor	−.002	−.017	(−.480, .447)
Log Pop	−.212	−.124	(−.531, .283)

[a] Estimates correspond to those for regression 3.1-2.
[b] Estimates based on thirteen groups of 108 observations sorted on Mean P.

Jackknife estimates were also calculated, using two similar procedures (not reported in table 3.4): (1) by arranging the observations according to the value of the Poor variable, and (2) by arranging the observations according to the value of the total mortality rate variable. In addition, another method of omitting observations was applied to the data sets. It entailed the creation of subsets of 108 observations, formed by eliminating every thirteenth observation starting with the first, eliminating every thirteenth observation starting with the second, and so on; this method was used to calculate 95 percent confidence intervals for the estimates, as is shown in table 3.4.

The first procedures were designed to examine whether systematic effects existed because SMSAs had high or low measured pollution, large or small populations of poor persons, or high or low total mortality rates. The second procedure (elimination of every thirteenth observation) allowed for a larger element of chance.

The results of all the jackknife tests were quite similar. In general, the 95 percent confidence interval was smaller than a 95 percent interval calculated by the estimated standard error in least-squares regression. The estimates for the subsets of 108 observations were quite similar to the estimates for the entire sample, indicating that the results are not sensitive to a few extreme observations. These results, and the fact that they are relatively stable when the observations are sorted on different variables or

where n is the number of subsamples (regressions estimated), b_i is the coefficient from the ith subsample and b_n is the coefficient estimated from the whole sample. The confidence interval is $j \pm \sqrt{\text{variance}}$ $(t_{0.975})$, where the variance is

$$\text{Var} = \sum_{i=1}^{n} \frac{(j - nb_n + (n-1)b_i)^2}{n-1}$$

when another elimination scheme is used, give us confidence that the least-squares estimates do indeed summarize the data well.

REESTIMATION WITH 1961 DATA

To corroborate our original findings, we reestimated the regressions with 1961 data. (Reestimation using 1969 data is discussed in chapter 7.) The 1961 replication had two major data problems: the lack of accurate population figures and the lack of air pollution data.

The 1960 population figure was taken from the U.S. Census and is presumed to be reasonably accurate. No census was taken in 1961; hence, we used interpolated values based on the 1960 and 1970 censuses. Since the mortality rate is determined by dividing the number of deaths by the population at risk, we had an accurate measure of the numerator for 1961 but not of the denominator. Insofar as the population changed in a way other than that characterized by the interpolated estimates, the 1961 rates are subject to error. For example, suppose that the population in a specific SMSA increased from 1960 to 1961 but decreased from 1960 to 1970. Then our procedure will overestimate the 1961 mortality rate. Since such changes are not likely to be important, we believe that the 1961 estimates are good approximations of the true mortality rates. Furthermore, so long as the air pollution levels are not systematically related to the errors in the population estimates, the effects on the estimated association with pollution should not be serious. The effects on the coefficients for the socioeconomic variables could be more important.[12] Between 1960 and 1961 southwestern cities were growing more rapidly than those in the Northeast. At the same time, areas in the Southwest had relatively few persons aged sixty-five and older and relatively low levels of air pollution. Thus, the 1961 estimated coefficients for the socioeconomic variable representing the proportion of those aged sixty-five and older, as well as for the air pollution variables, may reflect a slight downward bias.

The other problem with the 1961 replication was the lack of pollution data. Only one-third of the SMSAs had 1961 sulfate data, while two-thirds had 1961 suspended particulate data. For the remaining SMSAs, we used the 1960 data.

In view of these difficulties with the 1961 data, our primary interest was in whether there would be general similarity between the 1960 and 1961 results, particularly with regard to the estimated coefficients for air pollution variables. If the 1960 results were artifacts of that particular sample, one would expect to observe generally lower coefficients of determination (R^2) for the 1961 results and lower significance levels for the estimated

---

[12] Socioeconomic data for 1961 were based on linear interpolations of 1960 and 1970 values. However, for six SMSAs, the 1960 values were used because 1970 figures could not be obtained for an identical geographical area.

coefficients. For example, assume that the true model explaining mortality is

$$MR = \beta_0 + \beta_1 X + \beta_2 Y + \zeta \qquad 3.2$$

rather than the model shown in Equation 2.1 (see page 23). If, in 1960, X were highly correlated with P, and Y were highly correlated with S, we would not expect that the ad hoc procedures used to obtain the 1960 results could determine whether P were acting as a surrogate for X and whether S were acting as a surrogate for Y. In general, there is no conclusive test as to whether P and S are the so-called true (causal) explanatory variables or only proxies for the true variables. However, replication in a different setting, or for another time period, should provide some insight. If the relationships between (P, S) and (X, Y) occurred by chance, we would not expect them to occur in a replication. Thus, estimating Equation 2.1 with a different data sample should result in coefficients differing substantially from those estimated with the original sample, both in magnitude and significance.[13]

If the associations between (P, S) and (X, Y) were systematic, we could determine whether our original equation (Equation 2.1) represents the "true causal" relationship by investigating areas in which P and S were not closely associated with X and Y. Unfortunately, it is extremely difficult to construct such pure contrasts. For example, one must be careful not to select areas that are also characterized by either high or low standardized mortality rates, since they would produce misleading results.

Because our analysis of the effects of air pollution on mortality is also subject to both measurement difficulties and possible misspecification problems, one would expect the parameter estimates to exhibit some change in the replications we undertake, but the change will not be great if the causal variables are present.

Regression 3.5-2 represents the same specification as regression 3.1-2 (reproduced in table 3.5 as regression 3.5-1), with the 1961 data substituted. Since R^2 increased and the estimated coefficients exhibited little change (the decreased significance of the sulfates, in contrast to the increased significance of suspended particulates, could be attributed to the lack of comprehensive 1961 pollution data), the 1961 replication may be taken as evidence that the 1960 result was not merely an artifact of the particular sample.[14]

---

[13] Even if the associations were systematic, that is, $P = \alpha X + \mu$ and $S = \beta Y + v$, we would still expect the random components (μ and v) to vary from one sample to another; hence, the parameter estimates would differ in various replications.

[14] The F value for testing the effect of adding all six pollution variables to a 1961 regression with only the socioeconomic variables was 5.06, with 6 and 106 degrees of freedom. We also computed an F ratio to test the hypothesis that the structure differed between 1960 and 1961. $F = 0.85$, with 8 and 226 degrees of freedom. Since $F_{0.05}$ (8 and 200) $= 1.98$, we concluded that the coefficients were equivalent.

TABLE 3.5.   Alternative Specifications of Total Mortality Rates, 1960 and 1961

	1960	1961	Log-log	Quadratic	Dummy variable[a]	Linear spline[b]	Mean P split High[c]	Mean P split Low[d]	Census regions[e]	Migration	Migration split High[f]	Migration split Low[g]
	3.5-1	3.5-2	3.5-3	3.5-4	3.5-5	3.5-6	3.5-7	3.5-8	3.5-9	3.5-10	3.5-11	3.5-12
R^2	.828	.823	.787	.842	.841	.843	.906	.826	.862	.854	.804	.882
Constant	301.205	379.633	152.891	400.190	403.638	398.849	250.759	647.343	352.151	380.437	435.160	474.549
Air pollution variables												
Min S	.631 (2.71)	.456 (1.87)	.032 (3.06)	1.084 (1.40)		−.636 (−.38)	.167 (.74)	.917 (1.82)	.376 (1.50)	.428 (1.95)	.305 (.83)	.330 (1.42)
$(Min\ S)^2$				−.130 (−3.09)								
Mean P	.452 (2.67)	.516 (2.90)	.039 (1.65)	−.214 (−.25)		.113 (.06)	.277 (1.23)	−.731 (−1.24)	.559 (3.10)	.432 (2.76)	.293 (1.46)	−.021 (−.10)
$(Mean\ P)^2$				.130 (.46)								
Mean S × Min P				.095 (1.69)								
Sum of AP elasticities	9.12	8.98	7.08	6.70	4.52	5.84	5.51	−3.02	9.18	7.82	5.40	1.65
Socioeconomic variables												
P/M^2	.089 (1.71)	.125 (2.35)	.024 (1.91)	.134 (2.53)	.110 (2.23)	.110 (2.09)	.093 (2.13)	.402 (.86)	.054 (1.09)	.068 (1.40)	.361 (.11)	−.026 (−.55)
≥65	7.028 (18.09)	7.057 (17.59)	.558 (14.58)	6.799 (17.64)	6.822 (17.28)	6.895 (17.74)	8.535 (16.85)	6.592 (12.40)	6.288 (15.26)	6.560 (17.51)	5.610 (12.31)	6.722 (11.10)
NW	.422 (4.32)	.342 (3.40)	.007 (.71)	.372 (3.87)	.350 (3.53)	.382 (3.89)	.447 (4.21)	.727 (3.74)	.496 (4.85)	.404 (4.48)	.557 (4.35)	.777 (5.51)
Poor	−.002 (−.02)	−.048 (−.31)	.088 (3.26)	.015 (.11)	.010 (.07)	−.000 (−.00)	.203 (1.30)	−.614 (−2.15)	.156 (.90)	−.057 (−.43)	−.356 (−1.89)	−.386 (−1.67)
Sum of SE elasticities	71.03	71.39	45.17	68.93	68.55	69.46	86.32	62.20	68.10	65.23	52.47	63.91
Log Pop	−.212 (−1.12)	−.360 (−1.90)	−.007 (−.62)	−.314 (−1.66)	−2.79 (−1.50)	−.306 (−1.53)	−.303 (−1.50)	−.505 (−1.48)	−.257 (−1.36)	−.179 (−1.02)	−.118 (−.39)	−.037 (−.18)
Migration										−.109 (−4.41)	−.044 (−1.54)	−.726 (−4.86)

42

Note: Unless otherwise specified, the regressions are based on data for 117 SMSAs. The numbers in parentheses below the regression coefficients are t statistics.

a The air pollution dummy variables were defined as follows:
DS₁ = 1 if Min S ≤ 25 (μg per cubic meter × 10), 0 otherwise
DS₂ = 1 if 25 (μg per cubic meter × 10) < Min S ≤ 47 (μg per cubic meter × 10), 0 otherwise
DS₃ = 1 if 47 (μg per cubic meter × 10) < Min S ≤ 70 (μg per cubic meter × 10), 0 otherwise
DS₄ = 1 if 70 (μg per cubic meter × 10) < Min S, 0 otherwise
DP₁ = 1 if Mean P ≤ 75 μg per cubic meter, 0 otherwise
DP₂ = 1 if 75 μg per cubic meter < Mean P ≤ 111 μg per cubic meter, 0 otherwise
DP₃ = 1 if 111 μg per cubic meter < Mean P ≤ 165 μg per cubic meter, 0 otherwise
DP₄ = 1 if 165 μg per cubic meter < Mean P, 0 otherwise.

For estimation purposes DS₁ and DP₁ were excluded. The regression coefficients and t statistics for the remaining dummy variables were:

DS_2	26.866	DP_2	−18.252
	(1.63)		(−.86)
DS_3	61.052	DP_3	19.444
	(3.28)		(.87)
DS_4	60.468	DP_4	42.405
	(2.82)		(1.57)

b The air pollution linear spline variables were defined as follows:
Min S₁ = Min S − 25 (μg per cubic meter × 10) if Min S ≥ 25 (μg per cubic meter × 10), 0 otherwise
Min S₂ = Min S − 47 (μg per cubic meter × 10) if Min S ≥ 47 (μg per cubic meter × 10), 0 otherwise
Min S₃ = Min S − 70 (μg per cubic meter × 10) if Min S ≥ 70 (μg per cubic meter × 10), 0 otherwise

Mean P₁ = Mean P − 75 μg per cubic meter if Mean P ≥ 75 μg per cubic meter, 0 otherwise
Mean P₂ = Mean P − 111 μg per cubic meter if Mean P ≥ 111 μg per cubic meter, 0 otherwise
Mean P₃ = Mean P − 165 μg per cubic meter if Mean P ≥ 165 μg per cubic meter, 0 otherwise.

The regression coefficients and t statistics were:

Min S₁ =	3.804	Mean P₁ =	.202
	(1.63)		(.09)
Min S₂ =	−3.597	Mean P₂ =	.428
	(−1.95)		(.45)
Min S₃ =	.448	Mean P₃ =	−.443
	(.33)		(−.46)

c Based on fifty-eight SMSAs with Mean P ≥ 113 μg per cubic meter.
d Based on fifty-nine SMSAs with Mean P ≤ 112 μg per cubic meter.
e The estimated effects of the census region variables were defined so that they summed to zero. The estimates were as follows:

New England	74.182
Mid-Atlantic	77.717
Eastern North Central	3.240
Western North Central	−10.290
South Atlantic	−26.054
Eastern South Central	−49.811
Western South Central	−40.827
Mountain	−31.639
Pacific	3.481

f Based on fifty-eight SMSAs with 1950 to 1960 population increase ≥ 25 percent.
g Based on fifty-nine SMSAs with 1950 to 1960 population increase < 25 percent.

ALTERNATIVE SPECIFICATIONS

Most research relating air pollution to mortality has assumed a linear relationship. At best, this assumption should be interpreted as an approximation over a limited range to a much more complicated function. We also examined alternative specifications. The first was a comparison of the linear model with a log-log specification. In regression 3.5-3, all variables of the basic linear model (reproduced as regression 3.5-1) were transformed into logarithms. The coefficients of the pollution variables Min S and Mean P were 0.032 and 0.039, respectively, in the log-log formulation. These estimated coefficients are analogous to elasticities calculated from a linear model.

In regression 3.5-4, a quadratic model was fit (augmenting regression 3.5-1 by squared values of the pollution variables as well as the product of Mean P and Min S). The three quadratic terms do add significantly to the explanatory power of the regression ($F = 3.21$, with 3 and 106 degrees of freedom). Presumably because of the collinearity among the pollution variables, only (Min S)^2 was statistically significant. Ignoring significance for the moment, the magnitude of the coefficients suggests that the effect of sulfates rises less than linearly, while that of suspended particulates rises more than linearly. The quadratic formulation is somewhat difficult to interpret and is highly sensitive to the coefficient estimates (which are imprecisely estimated due to multicollinearity). For now, we shall continue to rely on the simple linear specification, while noting that the effect of air pollution may not be linear. (In chapter 7, we reconsider alternative specifications in analyzing the 1969 data.[15])

A more general way of examining the functional form of the relationship is to approximate it over segments of the range of air pollution levels. For example, we split the measured values of minimum sulfates and mean suspended particulates into four roughly equal groups and approximated the functional form within each group. Two methods were used. The first, a dummy variable procedure, estimated the mean total mortality rate within each of the groups for sulfates and suspended particulates (controlling statistically for the socioeconomic variables).[16] The second used a linear spline to approximate the relationship across the four groups. A

---

[15] Models were also tried in which the air pollution variables were represented by third-degree polynomials (not reported). However, these alterations in the functional form of the relationship between pollution and mortality failed to result in significant increases in the explanatory power of the regressions.

[16] Computational difficulty arises from the use of dummy variables. Since each of the pollution variables must be in one of the quartiles, the sum of the four dummy variables is equal to one for each entry. Thus, including all the dummy variables would preclude inverting the matrix of cross products and make it computationally impossible to derive estimates of the regression coefficients. A simple solution to this difficulty is to exclude one of the variables. The estimated regression coefficient of an included variable is then interpreted as the difference between the coefficient of the variable and the coefficient of the excluded one. Suppose we have a set of dummy variables S_1, S_2, S_3. Each takes on a value of zero or 1 for a given observation and $S_1 + S_2 + S_3 = 1$ for each observation. We wish to estimate the regression $Y = \beta_0 +$

linear spline estimates a linear relationship between air pollution and mortality within each of the quartiles and constrains the linear segment to meet at the boundary between quartiles.

The results of applying the first method, using step functions to approximate the air pollution–mortality relationship, are reported in regression 3.5-5 and shown in figures 3.2 and 3.3. For the sulfate measure, the height of the first step is set equal to zero, that of the second step is estimated to be 26.9, that of the third step 61.1, and that of the fourth step 60.5. Thus, as Min S rises above 25 (μg per cubic meter $\times$ 10) into the range 26–47, the mortality rate is estimated to increase by 26.9 per 100,000; as Min S rises above 47 (μg per cubic meter $\times$ 10) into the range 48–70, the mortality rate is estimated to increase by 34.2 per 100,000; and as Min S rises above 71 (μg per cubic meter $\times$ 10), the mortality rate is estimated to decrease by 0.6 per 100,000.

A step function is also estimated for suspended particulates. The height of the first step is set equal to zero, that of the second step is estimated to be -18.3, that of the third step is estimated to be 19.4, and that of the fourth step is estimated to be 42.4. Thus, as Mean P rises above 75 μg per cubic meter (into the range 76–111), the mortality rate is estimated to decrease by 18.3 per 100,000; as Mean P rises above 111 μg per cubic meter (into the range 112–165), the mortality rate is estimated to increase by 37.7 per 100,000; as Mean P rises above 165 μg per cubic meter, the mortality rate is estimated to increase by 23.0 per 100,000.

These results agree with those of the quadratic specifications; the effect of sulfates rises less than linearly while that of suspended particulates rises more than linearly. To determine whether the dummy variable specification had greater explanatory power than the basic linear specification, an

---

$\beta_1 S_1 + \beta_2 S_2 + \beta_3 S_3$. But the matrix of cross products will be singular, and estimation by simple, least-squares techniques will be impossible. However, substitution is possible: $S_3 = 1 - S_1 - S_2$, so that $Y = \beta_0 + \beta_1 S_1 + \beta_2 S_2 + \beta_3(1 - S_1 - S_2)$, which simplifies to $Y = (\beta_0 - \beta_3) + (\beta_1 - \beta_3)S_1 + (\beta_2 - \beta_3)S_2$. Thus, one would estimate $Y = \alpha_0 + \alpha_1 S_1 + \alpha_2 S_2$. It is then easy to interpret the coefficients relative to any excluded variable. The estimated coefficients take the form: $\alpha_i = \beta_i - \beta_3$, when S_3 is the excluded variable. If we would rather exclude S_2, the relation need not be reestimated; the new parameter estimates can be derived for estimating $Y = \gamma_0 + \gamma_1 S_1 + \gamma_3 S_3$, where $\gamma_i = \beta_i - \beta_2 = \alpha_i - \alpha_2$, since $\alpha_i - \alpha_2 = (\beta_i - \beta_3) - (\beta_2 - \beta_3) = \beta_i - \beta_2$. Significance tests are a more difficult problem. The value of the t statistic corresponding to an estimated coefficient is used to test the difference between the effect of variable S_i and the excluded variable; a significant value of t indicates that the two variables have different effects. In the above notation, testing the significance of α_1 is equivalent to testing whether β_1 is significantly different from β_3. If one were to choose to exclude an S_i whose β_i is different from the other βs, all of the α_is would be significant. In transforming the estimated coefficients to exclude a different variable, the standard error of the coefficient will change, and it is not simple to derive the new standard error of the coefficient. For our purposes, it is not as important to derive significance tests for individual coefficients as it is to determine whether the set of variables makes a significant contribution to the explanatory power of the regression; this is done via an F test, which is unaffected by the particular variable we decide to exclude.

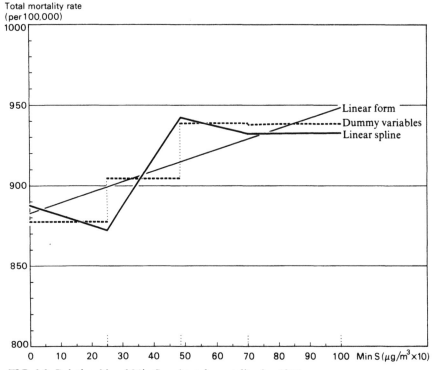

FIG. 3.2. Relationship of Min S and total mortality for 1960.

F test was used.[17] $F = 2.49$, with 4 and 105 degrees of freedom, which was very close to the critical value ($F_{0.05} = 2.45$, with 4 and 120 degrees of freedom). Thus, the explanatory power of the dummy variable formulation was very close statistically to the simple linear specification. Nevertheless, the contribution of the two air pollution variables to the regression with only socioeconomic variables was greater ($F = 10.58$) than the contribution of the six dummy variables to the regression with only socioeconomic variables ($F = 5.38$), accounting for degrees of freedom.

Regression 3.5-6 reports estimates of a linear spline for the two air pollution variables. The same groups used in the previous specification were used to define three new air pollution variables for Min S and the same for Mean P. The first variable for Min S was Min S − 25 μg per cubic meter ($\times$ 10), if Min S were greater than, or equal to 25, but otherwise it was zero. The second variable was Min S − 47, if Min S were greater than, or equal to 47, but otherwise it was zero. The third variable was Min S − 70, if Min S were greater than, or equal to 70, but otherwise it was zero. The

---

[17] Strictly speaking, this is not a correct test, since the linear model is not a subset of the dummy variable model.

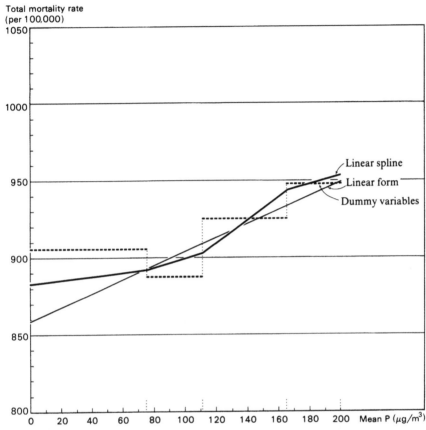

FIG. 3.3. Relationship of Mean P and total mortality for 1960.

critical values for the Mean P variables were 75, 111, and 165 μg per cubic meter; and the variables were constructed similarly.

Figures 3.2 and 3.3 illustrate these results for the two air pollution measures. For Min S, the effect on total mortality is greatest in the second quartile and nonsignificant otherwise (figure 3.2). For Mean P, the linear spline is similar to the simple linear form (figure 3.3).

To test whether the explanatory power of this formulation was significantly greater than that of the simple linear model, we again employed an F test. $F = 1.71$, with 6 and 103 degrees of freedom, indicating that this formulation was not significantly "better" at explaining the variation in total mortality.

As a final test of the linearity of the relationship, we divided the sample in half on the basis of suspended particulate levels. Regression analysis provides a linear approximation to the true relationship over the range of observations. If the relationship being analyzed is not well approximated by a linear relationship, then regression estimates for each half of the sample should be quite different. The resulting estimates, shown in regressions 3.5-7 and 3.5-8, do appear to be somewhat different. To check this further, we calculated an F test which compared the explanatory powers of these two regressions with that of the analogous regression based on the whole sample (regression 3.5-1). The F statistic of 4.26, with 8 and 101 degrees of freedom, was sufficient to indicate that the two sets were different.

We also divided the sample in half on the basis of the Min S readings and repeated this test (not reported). $F = 2.15$, with 8 and 101 degrees of freedom. Since $F_{0.05} = 2.02$, with 8 and 120 degrees of freedom, we cannot again reject the hypothesis that the two sets were different, although the F statistic was quite close to the critical value.

With a sufficient number of observations and enough perseverance, one can usually find several functional forms that appear superior to a simple linear model (even if the linear specification is "correct"). We concluded that on the basis of the tests above, linearity was not rejected.

OTHER SPECIFICATIONS

In an attempt to look for systematic effects on the pollution coefficients by areas of the country, we employed a set of dummy variables for the nine census regions of the United States. Each of the nine dummy variables was assigned a value of zero or one, depending on whether the SMSA was in that census region. For example, for Los Angeles, eight of the dummy variables were set equal to zero, while the dummy variable representing the Pacific region was set equal to one.[18]

The addition of the dummy variables in regression 3.5-9 significantly increased the explanatory power over that of regression 3.5-1 ($F = 3.09$, with 8 and 101 degrees of freedom); however, the pollution coefficients were not substantially affected. The coefficients of Min S and Mean P were 0.376 and 0.559, respectively. Since the dummy variables are surrogates for all the factors that differ among regions, it is difficult to interpret them. In view of the stability of the pollution coefficients, and the difficulties with interpretation, we again felt that the simple linear specification dominated.

As discussed previously, migration complicates our task of estimating the effect of air pollution on mortality for a number of reasons. Since Americans are highly mobile, we tried to analyze the effect of migration by including a variable that measured the change in an SMSA's population from 1950 to 1960. Regression 3.5-10 shows the effect of the migration variable. It was quite significant, increasing the explanatory power of the basic regression from 0.828 to 0.854. The coefficient indicated that the

---

[18] These dummy variables are reported so that the sum of regional effects is zero; thus, each coefficient is relative to all others.

fastest-growing SMSAs had relatively lower death rates, presumably due to their better climates and younger age distributions.[19] The coefficients of the pollution and socioeconomic variables exhibited little change.

As a more sensitive test of the effect of migration, we divided the sample in half, with one-half representing the fastest-growing SMSAs and the other half representing the slowest-growing areas. The basic model was estimated for each half (see regressions 3.5-11 and 3.5-12) and then compared with the original regression. The resulting F statistic of 5.29, with 9 and 99 degrees of freedom, was statistically significant, indicating that dividing the sample contributed to the explanatory power of the model. When the means and standard deviations of the variables in the two sub-samples were closely examined, a marked difference was found in the socioeconomic factors (see table D.2, pages 325–326); the SMSAs with low migration rates had relatively older populations and fewer nonwhites. There was little difference in the Mean P coefficients but some discrepancy in the Min S coefficients.

Consequently, we hypothesized that the greater explanatory power of the model estimated separately on the two subsamples was due more to differences in the effect of socioeconomic characteristics than to differences in the effect of air pollution levels. We tested this hypothesis by estimating two further models, using the pooled data (not reported). In the first, we split the socioeconomic variables into two sets to allow their effects to differ between areas of high migration and areas of low migration; one set took on the actual values of the socioeconomic variables if the SMSA had little population change, or each variable was given a value of zero if population changed a great deal, while the other set took on the actual values if the SMSA population changed a great deal, otherwise zero values were assigned to the variables. In the second, two sets of air pollution variables were employed on a similar basis. We then calculated two F ratios, using each of these models and the regression estimated from the whole sample. The F statistic of 4.24, with 5 and 103 degrees of freedom, computed from using the model with separate socioeconomic variables, was significant, indicating that the effect of these socioeconomic factors on the mortality rate differed between areas with different migration rates. The F

---

[19] Migration is most common among young people; hence, areas that lose population tend to have an older age distribution, whereas those which gain population tend to have a younger age distribution. Over the period 1965–70, the percentage of persons moving from one county to another was as follows:

Age	Percentage	Age	Percentage	Age	Percentage
All ages	17.1	30–34	23.8	55–59	8.0
5–9	19.1	35–39	18.1	60–64	8.2
10–14	14.6	40–44	13.4	65–69	9.0
15–19	17.2	45–49	10.8	70–74	7.9
20–24	34.2	50–54	9.0	75 and older	7.9
25–29	31.8				

See U.S. Bureau of the Census (1973).

statistic of 1.14, with 2 and 106 degrees of freedom, computed from using the model with separate air pollution variables, was not significant, indicating that the effect of air pollution was the same in areas of high migration as it was in low ones. Thus, our hypothesis was confirmed that the greater explanatory power was due to differences in the effects of the socioeconomic factors between areas with different migration rates.

INTERACTIONS BETWEEN THE SOCIOECONOMIC AND AIR POLLUTION VARIABLES

Interdependence among the independent variables impedes our ability to obtain good estimates of the association.[20] Least-squares regression estimates continue to be unbiased in the presence of multicollinearity; however, the dispersion of the estimates (the standard error) increases. One can adopt an estimation procedure known to produce estimates biased against showing significance for the air pollution variables. This procedure involves reestimating the relationship by omitting the air pollution variables. The residual of this equation is then regressed on the air pollution variables.

Thus, in stage one, the mortality rate (MR) was regressed on the socioeconomic variables (SE):[21]

$$MR = \alpha + \beta SE + \epsilon \qquad\qquad 3.3$$

and in stage two, the estimated residual, $e,$ or unexplained portion of the variation in mortality rates, was regressed on the air pollution variables (AP):

$$e = \gamma + \delta AP + \mu \qquad\qquad 3.4$$

If SE and AP are orthogonal, the estimated coefficients b and d will be identical to the figures in Equation 3.1. Insofar as the air pollution variables are correlated with the socioeconomic variables, this two-stage procedure will increase the magnitude and significance of the estimated coefficients for the socioeconomic variables, while biasing the estimated coefficients for the air pollution variables toward zero and reducing their significance.

This two-stage procedure has been carried out for the total mortality rate, with estimates shown in Equations 3.5 and 3.6.

---

[20] Laboratory investigations have found an important interaction between suspended particulates and sulfur dioxide, where the latter is absorbed into the particle and passes through the respiratory system (see Amdur, 1977). The importance of this interaction cannot be tested with our data, since the sulfate measure is determined by a chemical analysis of the particulates; that is, the sulfate variable is measured in terms of the presence of sulfur in the particulates.

[21] In the discussion which follows, SE and AP represent sets of socioeconomic and air pollution variables, respectively; hence, β and δ represent sets of corresponding coefficients and b and d represent sets of corresponding estimates.

$$MR = 361.908 + 0.160\,P/M^2 + 7.079 \geq 65 + 0.366\,NW + 0.004\,Poor$$
$$ (3.01) \qquad (18.36) \qquad (3.62) \qquad (0.03)$$

$$- 0.178\,Log\,Pop + e$$
$$(-0.92) \hspace{10cm} 3.5$$

$$e = -71.605 + 0.499\,Min\,S + 0.407\,Mean\,P + u \hspace{3cm} 3.6$$
$$ (2.49) \qquad\quad (2.66)$$

A reduction in R^2 for the second-stage equation is to be expected (in Equation 3.5, $R^2 = 0.795$; in Equation 3.6, $R^2 = 0.137$). The implication of Equation 3.6 is that, after accounting for the socioeconomic variables significantly associated with the mortality rate, the two air pollution variables account for almost 14 percent of the remaining variation in the mortality rates. The estimated coefficients of the air pollution variables retain their significance, and the parameter estimates differ little from the results reported in Equation 3.1.[22]

CONCLUSION

We have investigated various problems in estimating the relationship between air pollution (as measured by sulfates and suspended particulates) and health (as measured by mortality), including uncertainty as to the correct specification, lack of data on crucial variables, errors in the measurement of variables, and the possibility of systematic biases. These problems tend to obscure the effect of air pollution on mortality by biasing the association toward numerical and statistical nonsignificance.

The 1960 total mortality rate across SMSAs was analyzed, and the effect of sulfate and suspended particulate pollution was estimated. A jack-knife analysis indicated that the pollution estimates were not sensitive to extreme observations. Various specifications were examined; and while several had greater explanatory power, we concluded that none appeared clearly to dominate a simple linear relationship. Quadratic, dummy variable, linear spline, and split-sample specifications indicated that a linear relationship between the pollution variables and the mortality rates could be improved upon, but missing variables and other difficulties persuaded us to focus on the simple linear formulation. There was no evidence from these specifications of some threshold level of air pollution below which there were no mortality effects, at least within the range of our data. In an effort to account for the effects of geographical location, regional dummy variables were added, but the pollution variables were not greatly

---

[22] This also provides evidence that the effects of air pollution on mortality are not artifacts of a spurious association arising from collinearity between air pollution measures and the variable representing the percentage of the population aged sixty-five and older.

affected. In addition, the effects of migration were explored in two ways: (1) by adding a variable measuring the change in the SMSA population from 1950 to 1960, and (2) by splitting the sample in half. There was little effect on the estimated effects of air pollution. Finally, a two-stage procedure, known to bias the estimates of the pollution coefficients toward zero, was implemented. Air pollution remained an important factor in explaining variation in the total death rate across the United States.

These 1960 cross-sectional results, together with the principal component analysis and the 1961 replication, demonstrate a significant, robust association between both sulfates and suspended particulates, and the total mortality rate. Further exploration is warranted.

CHAPTER 4

Disaggregated mortality rates, 1960 and 1961

In chapter 3 we discussed the analysis of total 1960 mortality rates for 117 SMSAs in the United States. There remains the possibility that some of the results might have been distorted because total deaths was used as the dependent variable. By examining age- and disease-specific death rates one can attempt to estimate the effects of air pollution on life expectancy and perhaps shed some light on how air pollution affects health. Using the same methods and general data base as that utilized in chapter 3, we will now examine infant, age–sex–race-adjusted, age–sex–race-specific, and disease-specific mortality rates.

UNADJUSTED INFANT RATE

Complete 1960 and 1961 mortality data (per 10,000 live births) were available for infants under one year of age.[1] Regressions 4.1-1 and 4.1-2 (table 4.1) report the 1960 results across 117 SMSAs for the infant mortality rate. Regression 4.1-1 contains all six air pollution measures as well as all five socioeconomic variables used in the previous analysis. The statistically significant socioeconomic variables were the percentage of nonwhites and the percentage of poor families in the population. [A 10 percent decrease in each of the four socioeconomic variables (not including Log Pop) was associated with a 1.67 percent decrease in the death rate.] At the same time, a 10 percent decrease in all three sulfate measures was associated with a 0.04 percent increase in the mortality rate for infants under one year of age. A 10 percent decrease in all three suspended particulate measures was associated with a 0.74 percent decrease in the infant mortality rate. In regression 4.1-2, four air pollution measures were omit-

---

[1] An earlier analysis (Lave and Seskin, 1973) examined the fetal death rates during the years 1960 and 1961 and those for infants under twenty-eight days of age.

TABLE 4.1. Infant Mortality Rates, 1960 and 1961

	Unadjusted			Race-adjusted			White		Nonwhite	
	1960		1961	1960		1961	1960		1960	
	4.1-1	4.1-2	4.1-3	4.1-4	4.1-5	4.1-6	4.1-7	4.1-8	4.1-9	4.1-10
R^2	.563	.544	.549	.193	.180	.255	.097	.080	.199	.197
Constant	205.428	202.281	198.133	197.292	196.098	195.176	198.579	197.959	188.868	185.587
Air pollution variables										
Min S	.053 (.49)	.082 (.91)	−.012 (−.14)	.162 (1.29)	.176 (1.72)	.088 (1.07)	.065 (.55)	.082 (.85)	.622 (1.28)	.624 (1.57)
Mean S	.130 (1.05)			.073 (.51)			.091 (.67)		−.021 (−.04)	
Max S	−.072 (−1.69)			−.046 (−.95)			−.053 (−1.14)		−.016 (−.08)	
Sum S elasticities	−0.39	1.52	−0.23	1.70	3.31	1.69	0.04	1.74	6.21	7.70
Min P	.214 (.90)			−.001 (−.00)			−.049 (−.19)		.239 (.22)	
Mean P	.045 (.28)	.130 (1.98)	.158 (2.54)	.262 (1.40)	.207 (2.76)	.160 (2.66)	.154 (.87)	.095 (1.34)	.789 (1.08)	.748 (2.58)
Max P	.014 (.36)			−.013 (−.29)			−.009 (−.22)		−.032 (−.19)	
Sum P elasticities	7.35	6.07	7.17	10.94	9.71	7.37	6.06	5.01	25.00	23.11
Socioeconomic variables										
P/M²	.004 (.20)	.009 (.46)	.004 (.20)	−.007 (−.31)	−.004 (−.19)	−.003 (−.15)	−.000 (−.02)	.003 (.14)	−.041 (−.44)	−.039 (−.44)
≥65	−.090 (−.57)	−.064 (−.42)	−.023 (−.16)	−.012 (−.06)	−.005 (−.03)	−.128 (−.95)	−.137 (−.79)	−.133 (−.82)	.609 (.86)	.624 (.94)
NW	.175 (4.41)	.193 (5.10)	.151 (4.27)	.028 (.61)	.034 (.80)	−.036 (−1.05)	−.065 (−1.51)	−.059 (−1.46)	.478 (2.68)	.487 (2.92)
Poor	.154 (2.70)	.144 (2.59)	.191 (3.49)	.113 (1.71)	.111 (1.77)	.209 (3.95)	.127 (2.05)	.128 (2.14)	.043 (.17)	.034 (.14)
Sum SE elasticities	16.70	17.87	20.03	8.90	9.43	8.30	1.52	2.13	30.22	30.48
Log Pop	−.020 (−.27)	−.023 (−.31)	−.027 (−.41)	−.000 (−.00)	−.002 (−.02)	.016 (.25)	.015 (.18)	.011 (.14)	−.073 (−.21)	−.066 (−.20)

Note: All regressions are based on data for 117 SMSAs. The numbers in parentheses below the regression coefficients are t statistics.

54

ted; Mean P became statistically significant. Decreases of 10 percent in the sulfate, suspended particulate, and the four socioeconomic variables were now associated with 0.15, 0.61, and 1.79 percent decreases, respectively, in the death rate for infants under one year. F tests indicated that the addition of the six air pollution variables in regression 4.1-1 did not contribute significantly ($F = 1.90$), while the addition of the two pollution variables in regression 4.1-2 contributed significantly to the explanatory power in the equations ($F = 3.28$). A 1961 replication of regression 4.1-2 is shown in regression 4.1-3; the results are in general agreement.

To place the estimated effect of air pollution in perspective, we compared the effect on infant mortality of decreasing air pollution with the effect of decreasing the proportion of poor families in the population. The reduction in the infant mortality rate, associated with a 10 percent decrease in both Min S and Mean P, was 0.76 percent (regression 4.1-2) compared with a 1.02 percent reduction associated with a corresponding decrease in Poor. Thus, we conclude that the estimated impact of a decrease in air pollution was large, both in absolute value and in comparison with the estimated effects of other factors that could be affected by government policy.

AGE–SEX–RACE-ADJUSTED RATES

As previously noted, age, sex, and racial distributions of the population are likely to be significant factors influencing the mortality rate of an area. In our initial work, we attempted to account for age and race by including two regressors, the percentage of the population aged sixty-five and older and the percentage of nonwhites. It may not be sufficient to use only these two explanatory variables to control for age and racial differences in the populations of SMSAs. One alternative would be to include detailed demographic information as explanatory variables (that is, detailed measures of the age, sex, and racial composition of the population). However, with nine age groups, two sex classifications, and two racial groups, thirty-six variables would be required. Not only would numerical accuracy in estimation be affected, but also many degrees of freedom would be lost. In addition, the correlation between the thirty-six groups would guarantee multicollinearity problems. (We use a modification of this approach later in this chapter.) A more direct way to control for variations in demographic composition is to recalculate the mortality rate in each SMSA as if the population had demographic characteristics identical to those of the entire United States.[2] Here we analyze these standardized mortality rates. First, we

[2] The procedure, called the direct method of adjustment, uses the following age groups: newborn to four, five to fourteen, fifteen to twenty-four, twenty-five to thirty-four, thirty-five to forty-four, forty-five to fifty-four, fifty-five to sixty-four, sixty-five to seventy-four, and seventy-five and older. For details, see Duffy and Carroll (1967,

examined race-adjusted infant mortality rates, then we disaggregated the total mortality rate by age, sex, and race (adjusted by age) in an effort to isolate further the effects of these characteristics.

Race-adjusted infant mortality

The race-adjusted infant mortality rate is analyzed in regressions 4.1-4, 4.1-5, and 4.1-6. Direct adjustment of the mortality rate for race provides a more satisfactory basis for controlling the race distribution across SMSAs than does using the percentage-of-nonwhite variable,[3] although it does involve a loss in explanatory power, as shown in regression 4.1-4. Regression 4.1-2 was replicated by regression 4.1-5; Mean P retained its significance, and Min S approached statistical significance. In addition, F statistics for regressions 4.1-4 ($F = 2.76$) and 4.1-5 ($F = 7.56$) indicated that the air pollution variables contributed significantly to the explanatory powers of the equations.

The effects of air pollution were also enhanced in these regressions, while those of the socioeconomic factors were reduced. The estimated decreases in the infant mortality rate associated with 10 percent decreases in the sulfate and suspended particulate measures and the socioeconomic factors were 0.17, 1.09, and 0.89 percent, respectively, in regression 4.1-4; and 0.33, 0.97, and 0.94 percent, respectively, in regression 4.1-5. Thus, in these regressions the air pollution variables were together more closely associated with the infant death rate (adjusted for race) than were the socioeconomic factors.

Finally, regression 4.1-6 reports a 1961 replication of regression 4.1-5. Again, the results were similar, although the effects of air pollution (particularly sulfates) were reduced slightly (Mean P retained its significance). To test whether the coefficients in the two years were identical, we aggregated the 1960 and 1961 data sets and estimated the same specification. An F statistic was then computed to determine whether the explanatory power of the two regressions was greater than that of the single regression for the aggregated data set. The F statistic of 0.49, with 8 and 218 degrees of freedom, was statistically nonsignificant.

With data on mortality by race, it was also possible to analyze white and nonwhite infant death rates separately. Regressions 4.1-7 and 4.1-8 represent the same specifications as regressions 4.1-1 and 4.1-2, using

---

pp. vi–vii). The age groups analyzed were all ages, under one year, newborn to fourteen, fifteen to forty-four, forty-five to sixty-four, and sixty-five and over. (See also appendix B.)

[3] Nevertheless, we retained the same explanatory variables in analyzing the adjusted mortality rates. For example, the percentage-of-nonwhite variable was retained, since we felt that it might be exerting an independent effect on the mortality rate in addition to its role in controlling for the population at risk; that is, a concentration of nonwhites could indicate a geographically concentrated group with poor housing or high crime rates.

the white infant mortality rate as the dependent variable, while regressions 4.1-9 and 4.1-10 represent the same specification, using the nonwhite infant mortality rate. Comparing these race-specific regressions, it appears that mortality rates for nonwhite infants are better explained than' are those for white infants (R^2 was significantly greater for nonwhites in both cases). The percentage of poor families in the SMSA was the only statistically significant variable in regressions 4.1-7 and 4.1-8, while the percentage of nonwhites in the SMSA was statistically significant in regressions 4.1-9 and 4.1-10, and mean suspended particulates was significant in regression 4.1-10. The addition of the two air pollution variables did increase the explanatory power for the regression involving nonwhite infants ($F = 6.49$) but not for white infants ($F = 1.80$). These results corroborate and extend the earlier analysis.

Age–sex–race-adjusted total mortality

Detailed age–sex–race-specific mortality rates can be calculated for census years. We have calculated these rates for 1960 and use them in the analysis that follows. Duffy and Carroll (1967) also tabulate such detailed rates, although they averaged the rates over the three years, 1959–61, in order to avoid individual age–sex–race groups with extremely small numbers of deaths. We have analyzed the Duffy and Carroll data, but present only our 1960 estimates. There was little qualitative difference between these results and those from the Duffy and Carroll figures.

We begin by analyzing the total mortality rate, adjusted for age, sex, and race. This adjusted total mortality rate is contrasted with the unadjusted total mortality rate in table 4.2. Regressions 4.2-1 and 4.2-5 represent identical specifications for the two total mortality rates. The relatively low explanatory power of regression 4.2-5 ($R^2 = 0.285$) results in part from adjusting the death rate for age, sex, and race; the explanatory power of age (≥ 65) and race (NW) are lost.[4] In addition, the drop in explanatory power stems from the fact that the standard deviation of the adjusted mortality rate was about half as large as that for the unadjusted mortality rate (78.0 versus 153.3). This means that the inherent variability (or stochastic element) discussed earlier in terms of the Poisson distribution, will be (in relative terms) approximately twice as large.

Comparison of the two mortality rates is easier when four air pollution variables are dropped (regressions 4.2-2 and 4.2-6). It is striking that the estimated coefficients of the air pollution variables are virtually the same for the two regressions. Another way to compare regressions 4.2-1, 4.2-2, 4.2-5, and 4.2-6 is to examine the effect on total mortality associated with a 10 percent decrease in the air pollution and socioeconomic variables. A 10 percent decrease in the sulfate measures was associated with 0.50,

---

[4] The low R^2 also indicates that omitted factors are very important in explaining variations in the mortality rate across SMSAs.

TABLE 4.2. Comparison of Unadjusted and Age–Sex–Race-adjusted Total Mortality Rates, 1960

	Unadjusted				Age–sex–race-adjusted			
	4.2-1	4.2-2	4.2-3	4.2-4	4.2-5	4.2-6	4.2-7	4.2-8
R^2	.831	.828	.882	.878	.285	.272	.437	.422
Constant	343.381	301.205	1195.582	1201.452	901.196	857.665	1584.490	1574.692
Air pollution variables								
Min S	.473 (1.67)	.631 (2.71)	.181 (.72)	.357 (1.72)	.678 (2.29)	.825 (3.38)	.388 (1.39)	.580 (2.52)
Mean S	.173 (.53)		.290 (.99)		.085 (.25)		.172 (.53)	
Max S	.028 (.25)		−.060 (−.60)		.076 (.66)		.029 (.26)	
Sum S elasticities	5.04	3.27	2.60	1.85	5.70	3.84	4.16	2.69
Min P	.199 (.32)		.533 (.98)		.199 (.31)		.385 (.64)	
Mean P	.303 (.71)	.452 (2.67)	.136 (.36)	.382 (2.48)	.332 (.75)	.465 (2.61)	.354 (.84)	.444 (2.59)
Max P	−.018 (−.19)		−.013 (−.15)		−.030 (−.29)		−.068 (−.69)	
Sum P elasticities	4.37	5.85	4.03	4.95	3.96	5.40	4.05	5.17
Socioeconomic variables								
P/M²	.083 (1.54)	.089 (1.71)	.028 (.60)	.039 (.83)	.052 (.92)	.055 (1.01)	.007 (.14)	.014 (.26)
≥65	6.880 (16.63)	7.028 (18.09)	.682 (.35)	.678 (.35)	.265 (.61)	.411 (1.01)	−1.378 (−.64)	−1.622 (−.76)
NW	.396 (3.82)	.422 (4.32)	−1.201 (−.47)	−1.364 (−.54)	.145 (1.34)	.165 (1.61)	−2.819 (−1.00)	−2.807 (−1.01)
Poor	.038 (.26)	−.002 (−.02)	.037 (.23)	−.024 (−.15)	.139 (.89)	.098 (.65)	.127 (.71)	.049 (.28)
Sum SE elasticities	70.07	71.03	−9.20	−12.59	6.80	7.55	−43.69	−46.91
Log Pop	−.276 (−1.38)	−.212 (−1.12)	−.459 (−2.42)	−.417 (−2.30)	−.093 (−.44)	−.022 (−.11)	−.367 (−1.75)	−.286 (−1.42)

Demographic principal components

W_1	-112.463 (-.64)	-79.226 (-.46)	-361.392 (-1.86)	-332.498 (-1.74)
W_2	137.228 (4.89)	134.280 (4.91)	106.485 (3.42)	108.421 (3.57)
W_3	1.954 (.10)	7.474 (.40)	-32.126 (-1.50)	-26.101 (-1.25)
W_4	-11.889 (-1.44)	-9.452 (-1.18)	-13.918 (-1.52)	-11.807 (-1.33)
NW_1	-40.591 (-.20)	13.180 (.07)	-88.499 (-.39)	-61.337 (-.28)
NW_2	-13.976 (-.88)	-9.382 (-.62)	-1.429 (-.08)	-.775 (-.05)

Note: All regressions are based on data for 117 SMSAs. The numbers in parentheses below the regression coefficients are *t* statistics. Elasticities are not given for the principal components since by construction their means and elasticities are equal to zero.

Principal components:

Eighteen white demographic measures:
Cumulative proportion of variance explained by component:
$W_1 = 0.545$, $W_2 = 0.824$, $W_3 = 0.889$, $W_4 = 0.930$
Eigenvalues:
$1 = 9.8044$, $2 = 5.0350$, $3 = 1.166$, $4 = 0.7278$
Eigenvectors:

	1	2	3	4
Males, newborn–4 years	.5949	-.7424	.0804	-.2272
Males, 5–14 years	.7693	-.5555	.0293	-.2182
Males, 15–24 years	.1096	-.5422	.5114	.6000
Males, 25–34 years	.4902	-.7560	-.0912	.2165
Males, 35–44 years	.8578	-.1330	-.3876	.1610
Males, 45–54 years	.8773	.3000	-.2668	.1011
Males, 55–64 years	.8618	.4447	-.0510	.0354
Males, 65–74 years	.7963	.5126	.1867	-.0677
Males, 75 years and over	.7986	.4056	.3507	-.1174
Females, newborn–4 years	.6014	-.7335	.0854	-.0231
Females, 5–14 years	.7569	-.5635	.0322	-.2259
Females, 15–24 years	.5724	-.5970	.3283	.0830
Females, 25–34 years	.6383	-.6251	-.2692	.1508
Females, 35–44 years	.8930	.0769	-.3671	.0841
Females, 45–54 years	.8653	.4130	-.1633	.1278
Females, 55–64 years	.8103	.5391	.0676	.0570
Females, 65–74 years	.7823	.5569	.2170	-.0211
Females, 75 years and over	.7757	.4438	.3258	-.0545

Eighteen nonwhite demographic measures:
Cumulative proportion of variance explained by components:
$NW_1 = 0.951$, $NW_2 = 0.979$
Eigenvalues:
$1 = 17.125$, $2 = 0.503$
Eigenvectors:

	1	2
Males, newborn–4 years	.9857	.1037
Males, 5–14 years	.9870	.0674
Males, 15–24 years	.9719	.0945
Males, 25–34 years	.9556	.2320
Males, 35–44 years	.9683	.1954
Males, 45–54 years	.9907	.0594
Males, 55–64 years	.9759	-.0847
Males, 65–74 years	.9647	-.2497
Males, 75 years and over	.9226	-.3494
Females, newborn–4 years	.9863	.1037
Females, 5–14 years	.9878	.0731
Females, 15–24 years	.9856	.0704
Females, 25–34 years	.9827	.1534
Females, 35–44 years	.9870	.1154
Females, 45–54 years	.9929	-.0069
Females, 55–64 years	.9844	-.1224
Females, 65–74 years	.9717	-.2141
Females, 75 years and over	.9537	-.2701

0.33, 0.57, and 0.38 percent decreases, respectively, in the total mortality rate for the regressions above; a 10 percent decrease in the suspended particulate measures was associated with 0.44, 0.59, 0.40, and 0.54 percent decreases, respectively, in the total mortality rate; and 10 percent decreases in the socioeconomic variables were associated with 7.01, 7.10, 0.68, and 0.76 percent decreases, respectively, in the total mortality rate. Thus, for equivalent specifications, the air pollution elasticities were extremely close. As expected from the adjustment procedure, the socioeconomic elasticities were much smaller in the regressions pertaining to the adjusted mortality rate.

The age–sex–race-adjusted total mortality rate for 1961 was analyzed with similar results (not reported). To test whether the structures of coefficients for the two years were statistically equivalent we calculated F statistics. The value for the age–sex–race-adjusted mortality rate was $F = 1.27$, with 8 and 218 degrees of freedom. Thus, neither for the unadjusted total mortality rate nor for the age–sex–race-adjusted total mortality rate can one reject the null hypothesis of identical structures in the two years.

An additional examination was suggested to us by John Tukey. Regression 4.2-1 contains only two controls for the composition of the population at risk—the proportion of the nonwhite population and the proportion of the population aged sixty-five and older. These two variables are not sufficient, at least conceptually, to account for the age, sex, and racial mix of the population. One way to handle this is by directly adjusting the total mortality rate, as was done in regressions 4.2-5 through 4.2-8. Another way is to account explicitly for the detailed age, sex, and racial compositions of the populations at risk. Specifically, we divided the populations into thirty-six groups (nine age groups for each sex and racial combination). We then computed the proportion of the total population in each of these thirty-six categories for each SMSA. Finally, we performed a principal components analysis for the eighteen categories that described whites and the eighteen that described nonwhites.[5] The percentages of the variation explained by the first five principal components for whites were 54.5, 27.9, 6.5, 4.0, and 2.3, respectively; for nonwhites, they were 95.1, 2.8, 0.9, 0.4, and 0.3, respectively. We then entered the first four principal components for whites and the first two principal components for nonwhites as independent variables (regressions 4.2-3, 4.2-4, 4.2-7, and 4.2-8). These demographic principal components contributed significantly to the explanatory power of the regression in all cases; F statistics for the four regressions were 7.16, 7.10, 4.47, and 4.48, with 6 degrees and 99 or 103 degrees of freedom, respectively. As can be seen by comparing regressions 4.2-2 and 4.2-4 and regressions 4.2-6 and 4.2-8, the principal

---

[5] The weights for the vectors are shown in the note to table 4.2.

components had only a limited effect on the estimated pollution coefficients (there was a drop in the sulfate coefficients, but the suspended particulate coefficients were much less affected). The estimated coefficients for all of the socioeconomic variables exhibited far more change than those for the air pollution variables.

The implication seems to be that the original specifications (regressions 4.2-1 and 4.2-2) exert sufficient control for the age, sex, and racial composition of the populations at risk. Neither direct adjustment of the total mortality rate nor addition of the principal components had a marked effect on the estimated air pollution coefficients.

AGE–SEX–RACE-SPECIFIC RATES

Table 4.3 presents analyses of age–sex–race-specific (age-adjusted) mortality rates. Regression 4.3-1 reproduces the adjusted total mortality rate equation with two air pollution variables, regression 4.2-6, for comparison. The same specification is shown for each of the other dependent variables analyzed in table 4.3.[6] For each age group (all ages, newborn–fourteen, fifteen–forty-four, forty-five–sixty-four, and sixty-five years and over), five mortality rates were analyzed: the total age–sex–race-adjusted rate, and age-adjusted rates for male whites, female whites, male nonwhites, and female nonwhites (the infant mortality rates were analyzed in table 4.1).

In disaggregating the mortality rates, sample size becomes a greater problem. For all ages, the population of the sex–race groups—male whites, female whites, male nonwhites, and female nonwhites—would be approximately 350,000, 350,000, 50,000, and 50,000, respectively, in the average SMSA. Given the inherent variation in mortality (see chapter 3 for discussion), the reduction in the underlying population from 800,000 to 50,000 can be expected to increase the inherent stochastic factor fourfold, which impairs our ability to estimate the effect of air pollution. The further disaggregation by age reduces the underlying population by a factor of four and further impairs our ability to estimate the association between air pollution and mortality. As a consequence, we should expect that statistical significance will occur less often and that the estimated coefficients will be somewhat dispersed.[7]

Regressions 4.3-2, 4.3-3, 4.3-4, and 4.3-5 represent the four sex–race-specific mortality rates for all ages. Between 18 and 31 percent of the variation in the mortality rates is explained by the regressions; small samples and failure to include important explanatory variables are probable

[6] The specification contains the socioeconomic and two air pollution variables, as determined for the total mortality rate.

[7] Additional dispersion may result from the fact that the four demographic groupings may have systematically different air pollution-exposure histories that are not well represented by the air pollution variables.

TABLE 4.3.   Age–Sex–Race-specific Mortality Rates, 1960

	All ages				
	4.3-1 *Total*	*4.3-2* *MW*	*4.3-3* *FW*	*4.3-4* *MNW*	*4.3-5* *FNW*
R^2	.272	.181	.311	.222	.281
Constant	857.665	1059.749	770.168	517.434	446.520
Air pollution variables					
Min S	.825	.481	.935	1.405	1.795
	(3.38)	(1.78)	(3.81)	(1.51)	(2.70)
Min S elasticities	3.84	1.99	4.91	5.92	9.70
Mean P	.465	.300	.274	2.059	1.366
	(2.61)	(1.52)	(1.53)	(3.03)	(2.81)
Mean P elasticities	5.40	3.09	3.60	21.70	18.45
Socioeconomic variables					
P/M^2	.055	.090	.055	−.059	−.063
	(1.01)	(1.49)	(1.01)	(−.28)	(−.42)
≥ 65	.411	.189	.413	2.110	.277
	(1.01)	(.42)	(1.01)	(1.35)	(.25)
NW	.165	.221	−.015	.636	.592
	(1.61)	(1.95)	(−.15)	(1.63)	(2.12)
Poor	.098	.115	−.137	1.069	.711
	(.65)	(.69)	(−.91)	(1.87)	(1.74)
Sum SE elasticities	7.55	6.17	1.31	39.77	25.32
Log Pop	−.022	−.078	.073	−.268	−.070
	(−.11)	(−.35)	(.37)	(−.35)	(−.13)

factors. *F* tests indicated that Min S and Mean P added significantly to the explanatory power of all regressions. Air pollution appears to be more closely associated with nonwhite mortality in this group. The estimated elasticities for the air pollution variables are somewhat erratic; the estimated effect of a 10 percent abatement in both minimum sulfates and mean suspended particulates ranges from a 0.51 percent to a 2.82 percent decrease in mortality.

Regressions 4.3-6 through 4.3-10 analyze the mortality rate for children (under fifteen years of age). For the aggregated children's mortality rate, *F* tests indicated that Min S and Mean P made a significant contribution. Suspended particulates were more significant than sulfates. Air pollution did not contribute significantly in explaining the two white mortality rates. Mean P was statistically significant for male nonwhites, and Min S approached statistical significance for female nonwhites. For the aggregated children's mortality rate, a 10 percent abatement in air pollution (Min S and Mean P) was estimated to be associated with a decrease in mortality of 1.39 percent; the elasticities for nonwhite children were much larger.

TABLE 4.3. (*Continued*)

	Newborn to 14 years				
	4.3-6 Total	4.3-7 MW	4.3-8 FW	4.3-9 MNW	4.3-10 FNW
R^2	.248	.090	.234	.120	.121
Constant	181.386	217.084	201.504	72.275	−22.800
Air pollution variables					
Min S	.077 (.77)	−.043 (−.36)	−.032 (−.42)	.667 (.78)	.757 (1.49)
Min S elasticities	1.69	−.95	−.93	7.90	11.40
Mean P	.222 (3.04)	.028 (.31)	.080 (1.43)	1.886 (3.01)	.427 (1.15)
Mean P elasticities	12.19	1.51	5.79	55.88	16.09
Socioeconomic variables					
P/M²	.017 (.77)	.018 (.67)	.030 (1.74)	−.060 (−.31)	.027 (.24)
≥65	−.228 (−1.36)	−.357 (−1.76)	−.378 (−2.96)	1.064 (.74)	.028 (.03)
NW	−.085 (−2.02)	−.138 (−2.72)	−.078 (−2.43)	.281 (.78)	−.197 (−.92)
Poor	.249 (4.04)	.181 (2.44)	.167 (3.55)	.462 (.87)	.872 (2.79)
Sum SE elasticities	7.74	−6.04	−5.59	51.11	43.86
Log Pop	−.022 (−.27)	.019 (.19)	−.066 (−1.06)	−.233 (−.33)	.199 (.48)

(*Continued*)

The interpretation of the other regressions is straightforward. Air pollution was not closely associated with the mortality rate for young adults but was closely associated with the rates for those forty-five through sixty-four, and with the rates for those sixty-five and older. *F* tests indicated statistical significance for air pollution in one of the five regressions for those fifteen to forty-four, three of the five regressions for those forty-five to sixty-four, and all of the regressions for those sixty-five and older. The estimated elasticities of air pollution tend to rise with age, suggesting that air pollution has less effect on the young than on the old.[8]

As noted above, a comparison of these 1960 mortality rates with those for 1959–61 revealed little qualitative difference. As one might expect, there was less inherent variation with three-year mortality rates and the explanatory power was generally higher. For five of the twenty-five mortality rates, an additional air pollution variable became significant in analyzing the three-year rates (Mean P for total ≥ 65, white males 15–

[8] The estimated elasticities for infants (see table 4.1) were generally larger than those for children newborn to age fourteen; hence, this positive relation must be qualified to exclude infants.

TABLE 4.3.   (*Continued*)

	15 to 44 years				
	4.3-11 *Total*	4.3-12 *MW*	4.3-13 *FW*	4.3-14 *MNW*	4.3-15 *FNW*
R^2	.238	.123	.082	.202	.265
Constant	141.823	208.712	103.119	96.744	8.185
Air pollution variables Min S	−.041 (−.56)	.004 (.04)	−.025 (−.46)	−.424 (−.88)	−.074 (−.23)
Min S elasticities	−1.16	.09	−1.15	−5.60	−1.41
Mean P	.124 (2.33)	.072 (1.06)	.102 (2.57)	.364 (1.04)	.363 (1.57)
Mean P elasticities	8.81	4.45	11.83	12.00	17.37
Socioeconomic variables P/M²	.009 (.54)	.005 (.22)	.002 (.20)	.042 (.39)	.048 (.68)
≥ 65	−.079 (−.65)	−.163 (−1.04)	−.010 (−.11)	.023 (.03)	−.034 (−.06)
NW	.025 (.82)	−.039 (−1.00)	−.017 (−.73)	.460 (2.28)	.331 (2.49)
Poor	.127 (2.84)	.147 (2.54)	.035 (1.04)	.378 (1.28)	.372 (1.91)
Sum SE elasticities	12.12	4.35	3.54	36.46	44.25
Log Pop	−.015 (−.26)	−.059 (−.77)	−.028 (−.64)	.191 (.49)	.159 (.62)

44, all white females, white females ≥ 65, and nonwhite females 45–64).
For two mortality rates, an air pollution variable lost significance (Mean
P for white females 15–44 and 45–64). By comparison, sixteen additional
socioeconomic variables were significant, and one lost significance.

LIFE EXPECTANCY

If a causal link between both sulfates and suspended particulates and
mortality exists, one crucial question is whether abating such pollution
would merely add a few days to the life expectancy of those who would
die, or whether a significant increase in life expectancy would result. If
one makes the assumption that those individuals "saved" by improving
air quality would have the life expectancy of others in their age cohort,
one can use the results presented in the preceding sections to calculate the
increase in life expectancy for the general population.

The life expectancy for a cohort is defined as the time period during
which exactly half of that cohort survive and half die. It is calculated by
applying the age-specific death rate to the survivors in each age group.
For example, a 50 percent reduction in suspended particulates and sul-

TABLE 4.3. (*Continued*)

	45 to 64 years				
	4.3-16 Total	4.3-17 MW	4.3-18 FW	4.3-19 MNW	4.3-20 FNW
R^2	.359	.316	.318	.291	.290
Constant	783.222	1105.829	609.141	−76.296	465.717
Air pollution variables					
Min S	.927 (2.39)	.441 (.85)	.810 (2.70)	2.582 (1.08)	4.434 (2.36)
Min S elasticities	3.58	1.32	5.13	5.38	12.81
Mean P	.676 (2.39)	.546 (1.43)	.599 (2.74)	1.687 (.97)	1.512 (1.10)
Mean P elasticities	6.53	4.08	9.50	8.80	10.93
Socioeconomic variables					
P/M²	.174 (2.00)	.274 (2.34)	.096 (1.43)	.346 (.65)	−.085 (−.20)
≥65	.444 (.69)	.513 (.59)	.469 (.94)	.374 (.09)	−.227 (−.07)
NW	.271 (1.67)	.415 (1.90)	−.156 (−1.24)	1.297 (1.30)	1.982 (2.52)
Poor	.800 (3.36)	1.006 (3.13)	−.012 (−.07)	5.351 (3.65)	2.304 (1.99)
Sum SE elasticities	18.66	18.75	3.27	52.36	39.12
Log Pop	.156 (.49)	.163 (.38)	.005 (.02)	1.475 (.76)	.250 (.16)

(*Continued*)

fates was associated with a reduction in the adjusted infant mortality rate of 6.51 percent.[9] Those saved would have a life expectancy of approximately sixty-nine years. For the group aged newborn to fourteen, a 50 percent reduction in suspended particulates and sulfates was associated with a decrease in that mortality rate of 6.94 percent (regression 4.3-6); those saved would have a life expectancy of about sixty-four years. The reductions in the mortality rates for the other age groups were as follows: fifteen to forty-four, 3.83 percent (regression 4.3-11); forty-five to sixty-four, 5.06 percent (regression 4.3-16); and those aged sixty-five and older, 4.31 percent (regression 4.3-21).

The change-in-life-expectancy calculation was made by starting with 1,000 newborns and applying the current age-specific mortality rates to a control group and a lower age-specific mortality rate (associated with improved air quality) to a second "experimental" group. Life expectancy was then calculated for both groups by summing the number of individuals alive at each age breakdown (through age 100) and dividing by

[9] This percentage was derived from the elasticities in regression 4.1-5. The calculation is $0.50 \times (3.31 + 9.71) = 6.51$.

TABLE 4.3. *(Continued)*

	65 years and older				
	4.3-21 Total	4.3-22 MW	4.3-23 FW	4.3-24 MNW	4.3-25 FNW
R^2	.250	.156	.268	.148	.155
Constant	5938.553	7717.364	4636.457	7330.808	5119.192
Air pollution variables					
Min S	6.373 (3.56)	4.530 (2.22)	6.641 (3.70)	14.627 (1.72)	11.484 (2.19)
Min S elasticities	4.68	2.80	5.62	9.36	10.05
Mean P	2.137 (1.64)	1.687 (1.13)	.706 (.54)	15.038 (2.42)	11.249 (2.94)
Mean P elasticities	3.93	2.61	1.49	24.06	24.62
Socioeconomic variables					
P/M²	.110 (.27)	.290 (.63)	.221 (.55)	−1.736 (−.91)	−1.082 (−.92)
≥65	4.199 (1.40)	2.877 (.84)	3.542 (1.18)	26.157 (1.84)	4.427 (.51)
NW	1.242 (1.65)	2.169 (2.54)	.392 (.52)	2.173 (.61)	2.564 (1.17)
Poor	−1.919 (−1.74)	−2.356 (−1.88)	−1.644 (−1.49)	−1.709 (−.33)	−1.660 (−.51)
Sum SE elasticities	2.60	1.38	1.14	27.54	5.84
Log Pop	−.408 (−.28)	−1.049 (−.63)	.861 (.59)	−7.862 (−1.13)	−3.371 (−.79)

Note: All regressions are based on data for 117 SMSAs. The numbers in parentheses below the regression coefficients are *t* statistics.

Abbreviations: FNW, nonwhite females; *FW*, white females; *MNW*, nonwhite males; *MW*, white males; *Total*, males and females, whites and nonwhites.

the number of age categories included to derive the average number of people alive at each age. The difference between the life expectancies of the control group and the "experimental" group then indicates the change in life expectancy (assuming the air pollution–mortality association is causal) that is associated with a 50 percent reduction in ambient levels of sulfates and suspended particulates. This difference was equal to 0.72 years.

While keeping in mind that the above calculation is crude, there is an alternative method for examining the magnitude of the result.[10] Preston, Keyfitz, and Schoen (1972) provide a data base presenting mortality-rate calculations that estimate the number of persons surviving to age X if specific causes of death are eliminated.[11]

[10] We are indebted to Richard C. Schwing for providing the basis for this examination. The reader is referred to Schwing (1976).

[11] These calculations embody the very stringent assumption that the tolls due to the remaining risk categories are independent of the cause which has been eliminated in each case.

Schwing (1976) has found that plots of the unadjusted mortality rates (*crude rate*) per 100,000 across several populations versus increased longevity (Δ *years*) in those populations, fall reasonably close to the linear equation:

$$\Delta \text{ years} = 0.02 \times \text{crude rate} \qquad\qquad 4.1$$

One can use Equation 4.1, together with the air pollution elasticities we have previously estimated, to obtain a separate calculation of the implications of improved air quality on longevity. Specifically, from the elasticities derived in our basic result (see regression 3.2-1, page 34), a 50 percent reduction in sulfates and suspended particulates was associated with a 4.7 percent decrease in the unadjusted total mortality rate. This translates to a change in the unadjusted total mortality rate of 42.9 per 100,000. Substituting this figure in Equation 4.1 for the crude rate, we obtain a change in longevity of 0.86 years. Although we note that this estimate agrees quite closely with the above estimate, we stress that these estimates are presented primarily to illustrate the approximate magnitude of the change in life expectancy relating to our results. As we have done in other sections, we caution the reader against taking such estimates out of context.

DISEASE-SPECIFIC RATES

The accuracy of the disease-specific death rates depends on how accurately the cause of death is determined. Unfortunately, only a small and varying proportion of deaths are verified by autopsy, and not all physicians determine the cause of death with equal skill. Furthermore, where the cause of death is a relatively rare disease, the variability inherent in a small sample confounds the analysis, impeding our ability to isolate the factors associated with the death rate.

To illustrate the problem, consider a disease-specific mortality rate averaging one death per 10,000 persons per year. In a population of 10,000, there might be no deaths from this disease in one year, two deaths in another year, and one death in a third year. Assume that the occurrence of such deaths is modeled as a Poisson process whose mean is the mortality rate. Observing the annual number of deaths from this disease in many different populations of 10,000, one would find that in approximately 36.8 percent of the populations no deaths occurred during the year, in 36.8 percent one death occurred, in 18.4 percent two deaths occurred, in 6.1 percent three deaths occurred, and so on. There is a great deal of variability in the number of deaths among the populations, since the standard deviation is one death. For a larger population, the variation in observed deaths would be much smaller: in a population of 100,000, the average number of deaths from the disease would be 10, and the standard deviation would be 3.16;

for a population of one million, the average number of deaths would be 100, and the standard deviation would be 10.

A further difficulty stems from the fact that we do not have measures of many important factors affecting the incidence of disease and hence, disease-specific mortality (see table 1.2, page 10). Thus, an unknown amount of variation occurs with respect to personal characteristics and other uncontrolled factors. Having no measures of these factors is more crucial for disease-specific than for aggregate mortality rates. For example, variation in cigarette smoking across areas should have a greater effect on the death rates for lung cancer than on the total mortality rates, since lung cancer deaths make up only a small portion of total deaths. If these factors are uncorrelated with the air pollution variables, our inability to measure them will not bias the air pollution estimates, but it will hamper our ability to explain the variation in the disease rates across areas. Respiratory diseases are particularly subject to this problem because of our inability to observe smoking habits.

These two problems are confounded; together they imply that much less than half of the variation across SMSAs in the mortality rate for many diseases will be accounted for in the regression. Particularly, for diseases with low incidence that are also sensitive to unmeasured factors (such as smoking habits), the confounding of the two factors will mean that we cannot have great confidence in the estimated effects of air pollution.

Another way of examining the amount of inherent variation in mortality rates is to use the assumption of an underlying Poisson process to calculate the expected standard deviation for each disease-specific mortality rate, and then to compare it with the observed standard deviation. For example, in 1960 the mean mortality rate from all cardiovascular diseases was 482.3 per 100,000 for the 117 SMSAs. Since the mean population of an SMSA was 800,000, the average number of expected deaths due to cardiovascular diseases was about 3,858.4. Under a Poisson process, the standard deviation of the mortality rate would have been approximately 62.1 deaths per 800,000 (or approximately 7.8 per 100,000). The actual standard deviation observed among the 117 SMSAs was 114.6 per 100,000. Thus, an underlying Poisson process would have led to about 6.8 percent of the observed variation in the cardiovascular mortality rate.

Similar calculations were performed for the mean total cancer mortality rate (143.4 per 100,000) and the mean bronchitis mortality rate (2.3 per 100,000). Under a Poisson process, the corresponding standard deviations are 4.2 per 100,000 and 0.5 per 100,000, respectively, indicating that the "inherent" variation would account for 12.8 percent and 49.0 percent of the observed standard deviations (32.9 and 1.1 per 100,000, respectively). Thus, there is a high enough incidence of death from all cardiovascular diseases for a reasonable analysis of the factors associated with these diseases to be undertaken. However, the lower prevalence of cancer deaths makes it more difficult to analyze the factors associated with cancer. Finally, the fact that only about eighteen bronchitis deaths are expected to occur within the average SMSA makes it extremely difficult to analyze the factors associated with this mortality rate. In general, one expects that as the mortality rates for specific diseases become smaller, the difficulty of performing a satisfactory analysis of the factors associated with the diseases becomes greater.

In the following discussion, the diseases are grouped by categories— cancers, cardiovascular diseases, and respiratory diseases—which are based on *International Classifications of Diseases* (ICDA, 1962) and come from vital statistics. Regressions on the 1960 data, found in table 4.4, were derived in the same manner as the results for the previous mortality rates. Results of a 1961 replication of the same specification are also presented.

Cancer mortality

Death from total cancers $(143.4)^{12}$ had an R^2 of 0.887 in regression 4.4-1. In 1960 both the minimum levels of sulfate pollution and suspended particulate pollution were used in explaining cancer mortality (the latter was statistically nonsignificant). It would appear from the negative and significant coefficient of Poor that cancers are diseases related to higher-income levels. Population density, the percentage of nonwhites in the population, the percentage of those aged sixty-five and older in the population, and the size of the SMSA were all related positively to the cancer mortality rate. Regression 4.4-2 reports the 1961 results for all cancer mortality. The R^2 dropped from 0.887 to 0.854, and all variables lost some significance, but the relationship appeared quite stable (the sulfate measure remained statistically significant).

The cancer category is subclassified into buccal and pharyngeal $(344.5)^*$, digestive $(472.1)^\dagger$, respiratory $(222.4)^\dagger$, and breast cancers $(126.0)^\dagger$. The coefficient of determination for regression 4.4-3 on cancer of the buccal cavity and pharynx $(R^2 = 0.356)$ was considerably lower than that for total cancers. No pollution variable was statistically significant. (Min P was retained in accordance with our general procedure.) All socioeconomic variables were positively associated with mortality, but only the percentage of old persons in the population was statistically significant. The 1961 result (regression 4.4-4) reflected a decrease in R^2 to 0.248; its implications were similar to the 1960 regression.

Cancer of the digestive system (regression 4.4-5) had an R^2 of 0.784. The minimum levels of both sulfate and suspended particulate pollution

---

[12] The number in parentheses following each disease is the 1960 mortality rate per 100,000 (those with * are per 10 million and those with † are per 1 million). We do not report the 1961 rate here, since there was little difference between the 1960 and 1961 rates; it is, however, reported in table D.3 (pages 327–328).

TABLE 4.4.   Disease-specific Mortality Rates, 1960 and 1961

	Total cancers		Buccal and pharyngeal cancers		Digestive cancers	
	1960	1961	1960	1961	1960	1961
	4.4-1	4.4-2	4.4-3	4.4-4	4.4-5	4.4-6
R^2	.887	.854	.356	.248	.784	.756
Constant	−5.249	21.248	−370.570	−157.434	−195.267	−92.428
Air pollution variables						
Min S	.130	.097			.770	.362
	(3.21)	(2.15)			(3.01)	(1.39)
Mean S						
Max S						
Sum S elasticities	4.28	3.17			7.71	3.65
Min P	.072	.069	.619	.249	.448	−.038
	(1.11)	(.96)	(.93)	(.38)	(1.08)	(−.09)
Mean P						
Max P						
Sum P elasticities	2.30	2.13	8.17	3.18	4.31	−.36
Socioeconomic variables						
P/M²	.029	.030	.131	.165	.178	.196
	(3.18)	(2.96)	(1.41)	(1.82)	(3.09)	(3.33)
≥65	1.350	1.386	4.317	2.952	4.920	5.322
	(20.80)	(18.91)	(6.49)	(4.48)	(11.98)	(12.55)
NW	.048	.047	.301	.103	−.031	.076
	(2.97)	(2.54)	(1.73)	(.60)	(−.30)	(.70)
Poor	−.094	−.079	.262	.211	−.242	−.353
	(−3.78)	(−2.69)	(.99)	(.77)	(−1.55)	(−2.07)
Sum SE elasticities	72.78	76.57	132.42	88.89	79.92	87.23
Log Pop	.062	.009	.408	.327	.412	.242
	(1.87)	(.24)	(1.19)	(.95)	(1.98)	(1.13)

were positively associated with mortality, although only the former was statistically significant. Population density, the proportion of old people in the population, and SMSA size appeared to be related positively and, for the most part, significantly to this mortality rate, the proportion of poor families was again related negatively. For 1961, the coefficient of determination decreased to 0.756 in regression 4.4-6, and minimum sulfates lost statistical significance.

Regression 4.4-7 reports the results for cancer of the respiratory system. The only air pollution variable that approached significance was the mean level of sulfate pollution. Population density, the proportion of the population which was nonwhite, and the percentage of the population aged sixty-five and older were positively and significantly related to the death rate. The percentage of poor families was inversely related to the death rate. The corresponding 1961 result (regression 4.4-8) again exhibited a reduction in the coefficient of determination (from 0.609 to 0.560). The

TABLE 4.4. *(Continued)*

Respiratory cancers		Breast cancers		Total cardiovascular disease		Heart disease	
1960	1961	1960	1961	1960	1961	1960	1961
4.4-7	4.4-8	4.4-9	4.4-10	4.4-11	4.4-12	4.4-13	4.4-14
.609	.560	.709	.658	.829	.820	.549	.768
8.763	17.777	−13.269	73.392	109.795	176.704	32.875	55.133
				.691	.612	.842	.554
				(4.15)	(3.55)	(3.07)	(3.56)
.117	.106						
(1.41)	(1.26)						
		.022	.059				
		(1.34)	(3.17)				
5.24	4.67	4.02	10.46	6.77	6.11	11.39	7.77
				.071	.056		
				(1.94)	(1.49)		
				3.95	3.09		
.102	.076	.027	.030	.032	.065	.039	.091
(3.30)	(2.29)	(1.76)	(1.79)	(.83)	(1.65)	(.60)	(2.50)
2.193	2.311	1.149	1.221	5.086	4.967	3.707	3.535
(10.01)	(9.48)	(10.46)	(9.65)	(17.59)	(16.64)	(8.07)	(13.53)
.198	.236	.058	.027	.282	.203	.187	.083
(3.53)	(3.79)	(2.01)	(.82)	(3.91)	(2.83)	(1.61)	(1.25)
−.165	−.196	−.216	−.142	−.199	−.189	−.309	−.136
(−1.93)	(−1.97)	(−4.96)	(−2.72)	(−1.87)	(−1.64)	(−1.75)	(−1.29)
83.56	84.43	52.66	63.19	88.72	87.33	80.46	85.97
.029	.013	.120	−.068	−.189	−.283	−.008	−.060
(.26)	(.11)	(2.13)	(−1.04)	(−1.38)	(−2.04)	(−.03)	(−.47)

(Continued)

air pollution variable lost statistical significance, but the estimated relationships were similar.

Breast cancer followed the same pattern (regression 4.4-9). The most closely related air pollution variable was the maximum level of sulfates, which approached statistical significance. The socioeconomic variables had the same signs as those for total cancers. For 1961, regression 4.4-10 indicates that the air pollution variable became highly significant, while two socioeconomic variables lost statistical significance.

Cardiovascular disease mortality

The results relating to the aggregate category of cardiovascular diseases (482.3) are reported in regression 4.4-11. Both the minimum sulfate and maximum suspended particulate levels of pollution were closely associated with cardiovascular deaths. (The sulfate measure was statistically significant, while the particulate measure approached statistical significance.)

TABLE 4.4. *(Continued)*

	Endocarditis		Hypertensive disease		Total respiratory disease	
	1960	1961	1960	1961	1960	1961
	4.4-15	4.4-16	4.4-17	4.4-18	4.4-19	4.4-20
R^2	.346	.286	.434	.459	.227	.307
Constant	−152.565	−94.800	105.738	257.208	−52.675	−158.384
Air pollution variables						
Min S	1.160	.970				
	(2.24)	(1.92)				
Mean S					•	
Max S			.353	.455		
			(4.15)	(5.71)		
Sum S elasticities	19.56	17.62	22.86	32.31		
Min P	1.168	1.528			.763	.623
	(1.40)	(1.88)			(1.52)	(1.38)
Mean P						
Max P						
Sum P elasticities	18.97	26.03			7.65	7.48
Socioeconomic variables						
P/M²	.268	.038	.033	.014	.089	.157
	(2.30)	(.33)	(.42)	(.19)	(1.27)	(2.51)
≥65	3.308	3.501	2.864	2.044	1.517	1.431
	(3.98)	(4.26)	(5.09)	(3.76)	(3.01)	(3.14)
NW	.071	.219	.920	.818	−.055	−.198
	(.34)	(1.05)	(6.24)	(5.83)	(−.42)	(−1.66)
Poor	.409	.019	.038	.042	.666	.600
	(1.29)	(.06)	(.17)	(.19)	(3.33)	(3.16)
Sum SE elasticities	135.36	125.56	103.35	84.75	54.50	56.60
Log Pop	−.906	−.153	−.350	−.555	.397	.516
	(−.23)	(−.37)	(−1.21)	(−1.98)	(1.52)	(2.17)

The percentage of nonwhites in the population and the percentage of old persons were the most significant socioeconomic variables. The 1961 results corresponded closely to the 1960 results (regression 4.4-12), although the t statistics corresponding to the pollution variables dropped a bit; Min S remained significant.

Under the general heading of cardiovascular disease, the subclassifications include diseases of the heart (349.2), nonrheumatic chronic endocarditis and other myocardial degeneration (280.0)[†], and hypertensive heart disease (352.4)[†]. Regression 4.4-13 reports the results for diseases of the heart. The minimum sulfate pollution level was statistically significant. The only significant socioeconomic factor was the percentage of old persons in the population. Regression 4.4-14 relates the corresponding 1961 results. Min S remained significant and population density became statistically significant, as R^2 increased from 0.549 to 0.768.

Mortality from nonrheumatic chronic endocarditis and other myocardial degeneration is the dependent variable in regression 4.4-15. The minimum levels of sulfates and suspended particulates were positively related to this death rate although only the former was statistically significant.

TABLE 4.4. (*Continued*)

	Tuberculosis		Asthma		Influenza	
	1960	1961	1960	1961	1960	1961
	4.4-21	4.4-22	4.4-23	4.4-24	4.4-25	4.4-26
	.283	.319	.087	.058	.341	.094
	−1137.744	−1248.492	85.616	320.910	258.772	58.294
					.593	.441
					(1.29)	(1.86)
					17.39	51.50
	1.735	2.105	.732	.521		
	(3.01)	(3.43)	(2.34)	(1.42)		
	37.47	47.36	29.82	22.73		
	.331	.312	.025	−.092	−.158	.097
	(1.87)	(1.67)	(.26)	(−.83)	(−.92)	(−1.04)
	2.050	3.091	.956	.198	−1.595	−.524
	(1.57)	(2.22)	(1.34)	(.24)	(−1.31)	(−.76)
	.041	−.152	−.100	−.221	−.514	.046
	(.12)	(−.41)	(−.53)	(−1.01)	(−1.64)	(.26)
	1.927	2.455	.309	−.008	2.593	.459
	(3.79)	(4.29)	(1.12)	(−.02)	(5.43)	(1.64)
	100.41	135.96	43.26	−7.29	76.68	38.69
	1.645	1.460	−.013	−.177	−.422	−.088
	(2.49)	(2.10)	(−.04)	(−.43)	(−.68)	(−.25)

(*Continued*)

Population density and the percentage of old persons were the significant socioeconomic variables. Regression 4.4-16 presents the 1961 results. The *t* statistic for minimum sulfates became slightly smaller (decreasing from 2.24 to 1.92), while that for minimum suspended particulates became slightly larger (increasing from 1.40 to 1.88); of the socioeconomic variables, only the percentage of old persons retained significance (R^2 dropped from 0.346 to 0.286).

Regression 4.4-17 reports the results on hypertensive heart disease. The maximum sulfate measure was statistically significant; the percentage of older persons in the population and the percentage of nonwhites were the significant socioeconomic variables. The 1961 results (regression 4.4-18) were in close agreement with the 1960 regression.

Respiratory disease mortality

The mortality rates for tuberculosis, asthma, influenza, pneumonia, and bronchitis were aggregated to obtain a category of total respiratory disease deaths excluding cancer (453.7)[†]. Regression 4.4-19 reports the results for this category. The minimum level of suspended particulates was posi-

TABLE 4.4. *(Continued)*

	Pneumonia		Bronchitis	
	1960	1961	1960	1961
	4.4-27	4.4-28	4.4-29	4.4-30
R^2	.140	.233	.082	.117
Constant	4.841	−94.706	162.781	38.006
Air pollution variables				
Min S				
Mean S				
Max S				
Sum S elasticities				
Min P	.319	.039		
	(.71)	(.10)		
Mean P				
Max P			.079	.022
			(.99)	(.28)
Sum P elasticities	4.64	.65	9.23	2.88
Socioeconomic variables				
P/M²	.062	.133	.010	.087
	(.99)	(2.42)	(.12)	(1.06)
≥65	1.387	1.139	.826	1.075
	(3.06)	(2.84)	(1.36)	(1.71)
NW	.039	−.121	.003	−.162
	(.33)	(−1.15)	(.02)	(−.99)
Poor	.189	.283	−.307	−.012
	(1.05)	(1.69)	(−1.32)	(−.05)
Sum SE elasticities	51.00	52.32	6.44	36.01
Log Pop	.237	.388	.053	.156
	(1.01)	(1.86)	(.18)	(.51)

Note: All regressions are based on data for 117 SMSAs. The numbers in parentheses below the regression coefficients are *t* statistics.

tively related to the death rate, although not statistically significant. The percentages of older persons and of poor families were positively and significantly related to the death rate. The 1961 results (regression 4.4-20) were similar; the *t* statistic for the pollution variable decreased, while those corresponding to the socioeconomic variables increased (R^2 rose from 0.227 to 0.307).

For tuberculosis (547.0)*, the mean level of suspended particulate pollution was significant in regression 4.4-21. In addition, tuberculosis was significantly associated with the proportion of poor families in the population and the size of the SMSA. The 1960 results were corroborated closely by the results for 1961 in regression 4.4-22 (R^2 rose from 0.283 to 0.319).

As shown in regression 4.4-23, R^2 was only 0.087 in the regression related to asthma mortality (290.0)*. We presume that this was due largely to sampling variation. Again, the mean level of suspended particulate pollution was significant. No socioeconomic variables were statistically significant. For 1961 (regression 4.4-24), R^2 dropped to 0.058, and the pollution variable became statistically nonsignificant.

Mortality from influenza (340.0)* is examined in regression 4.4-25. The only statistically significant variable was the proportion of poor families in the population, with influenza deaths positively related to this variable. The 1961 results (regression 4.4-26) displayed a much smaller coefficient of determination (R^2 decreased from 0.341 to 0.094). This may have been an artifact of the influenza epidemic that occurred in 1960. (The mean influenza mortality rate was only 87.7 per 10 million in 1961.) However, our measures of air pollution were not closely related to influenza deaths.

In regression 4.4-27, the coefficient of determination was only 0.140 in explaining deaths due to pneumonia (313.1)†. Again, this was probably due to sampling variation. No air pollution variable was statistically significant, and the only significant socioeconomic variable was the proportion of older persons in the population. For 1961 (regression 4.4-28), R^2 increased from 0.140 to 0.233, and population density became significant.

The last disease covered is bronchitis (228.3)*. Once more, the poor results seem indicative of sampling variation (R^2 was 0.082 in regression 4.4-29). Neither air pollution variables nor socioeconomic variables were statistically significant. The 1961 results (regression 4.4-30) were quite similar to the 1960 results.[13]

CONCLUSION

Infant mortality, age–sex–race-adjusted and age–sex–race-specific mortality, and disease-specific mortality were investigated to determine their association with our measures of air pollution in a cross-sectional analysis of 117 SMSAs in the United States for 1960. The method was similar to that employed for total mortality in chapter 3.

For infant mortality, suspended particulates were more important than sulfates. The importance of suspended particulates and sulfates was enhanced when the infant mortality rate was adjusted for race. The 1961 replication corroborated the 1960 findings.

Air pollution (as measured by sulfates and suspended particulates) remained a significant factor in explaining the variation in the age–sex–race-adjusted total mortality rates across SMSAs. For the age–sex–race-specific rates, air pollution was more closely associated with mortality among nonwhites than among whites. Furthermore, the analysis of individual age–sex–race-specific mortality rates corroborated the estimated relationship for the age–sex–race-adjusted mortality rates. Finally, replications involving mortality rates averaged over the period 1959–61 corroborated the 1960 results.

---

[13] We have reviewed a number of studies that show a close association between air pollution and both bronchitis mortality and morbidity. The relationship seems to be weaker in the United States than in Great Britain because of differences in the definition of the disease, as discussed in appendix A (p. 273).

It is interesting to note that the estimated effect of the air pollution variables on mortality increased with age. The implication is that abating air pollution would benefit primarily the very old. However, one should be cautious since we are examining mortality, not morbidity, rates. One interpretation of the results is that the primary effect of air pollution is cumulative; thus, the very old will experience the greatest effect, although younger groups are likely to experience increased morbidity. Furthermore, if one assumes that a causal link exists between mortality and both sulfates and suspended particulates, and that those individuals "saved" by improving air quality have the life expectancy of others in their age cohort, the increase in life expectancy corresponding to a 50 percent reduction in ambient levels of these pollutants is estimated to be between 0.72 and 0.86 years at birth.

Fifteen disease-specific mortality rates were examined for both 1960 and 1961. For the five cancer mortality rates, suspended particulates never made a significant contribution, while sulfates made a consistent contribution for the total cancer mortality rate only.[14] Deaths from cardiovascular disease and its subcategories showed a close association with sulfate pollution in 1960, and in this case, the 1961 results further strengthened the relationship. For the total and five specific diseases of the respiratory system, only the tuberculosis mortality rate exhibited a close association with suspended particulates in both 1960 and 1961. We attribute this to the variability inherent in the small mortality rates.

Several important problems (in addition to the general methodological ones discussed in chapter 2) tend to obfuscate the association between air pollution and the disaggregated mortality rates: the inaccurate diagnosis of cause of death, and, perhaps more serious, the sampling variability when the mortality rate for a disease is small, or the population at risk is not very large. These problems are especially important in considering the age–sex–race-specific mortality rates for nonwhites and the disease-specific mortality rates. A further difficulty in analyzing these results is our lack of information on personal characteristics and other factors affecting mortality. Even slight variations in such factors may impede our ability to explain certain mortality rates. The respiratory disease death rates are characterized both by low incidence and by susceptibility to the problem of unmeasured factors, such as smoking. Thus, the disappointing results for these diseases are not entirely unexpected.

Given the difficulties with both the data and the estimation techniques, we conclude that these results support those of chapter 3. Air pollution (as measured by suspended particulates and sulfates) is closely associated with mortality, even after the total death rate is disaggregated. Again, these results must be interpreted with caution.

---

[14] See the discussion of cancer mortality in chapter 5; our later results suggested some difficulty with this original formulation.

Effects of occupation mix, climate, and home-heating characteristics, 1960

Across 117 SMSAs in the United States we have established a statistical association between the 1960 total mortality rate and sulfates and suspended particulates. We have elaborated this relationship by consideration of infant, age–sex–race-adjusted, age–sex–race-specific, and disease-specific mortality rates. The association between the two air pollutants and mortality was subjected to a number of tests, but the possibility remains that another factor, or a set of factors, was the cause of the observed association.

To test this possibility, we investigated a number of factors that had been suggested as the "true" causes of these relationships. We obtained measures of several of these factors and inserted them into the previously estimated regressions. If one (or more) of the new variables is the so-called true cause of the association between mortality and both sulfates and suspended particulates, it should be statistically significant when entered and should cause the estimated effect of the two air pollutants to diminish substantially in both magnitude and significance.

This test, however, is not entirely straightforward. As discussed earlier, the factors associated with increased mortality may be highly correlated— for example, income and occupation mix, or air pollution and climate—in which case the additional variables can give rise to multicollinearity problems in the estimation. If a variable is correlated with sulfates or suspended particulates, adding it to the equation is likely to change the previously estimated coefficients corresponding to those two air pollutants and lower their statistical significance. Primary emphasis, therefore, will be placed on the estimated air pollution coefficients, with less credence given to their statistical significance.[1] Secondary consideration will be given to discussions of the additional variables that seemed of interest.

---

[1] Blalock (1964) gives examples, as well as a general argument, to show that the

OCCUPATIONAL CATEGORIES AS EXPLANATORY VARIABLES

Occupational accidents and diseases are important factors influencing the mortality rate among workers. Since occupation is associated with both air pollution and mortality, it may be the source of spurious correlation. We began by looking at measures from the 1960 census representing the occupational mix in each SMSA. The data are answers to census questions concerning type of work; the variables used in the analysis are the percentage of workers in each group, and results are reported in table 5.1. First, the original 1960 regression for each mortality rate is presented. Then each even-numbered regression presents the results of adding the occupation variables.

Unadjusted total mortality

When the occupation-mix variables were added to regression 3.1-2 (reproduced here as regression 5.1-1) for the total unadjusted death rate, the coefficients of the air pollution variables and their t statistics decreased, with Min S losing statistical significance (regression 5.1-2). An F test showed that Min S and Mean P jointly contributed significantly to regression 5.1-2 ($F = 4.52$). The coefficients of the socioeconomic variables were also affected slightly.

Looking at the significant occupation variables, we note that the unemployed percentage of the working force was, as we had expected, positively associated with the total mortality rate. The percentages of agricultural and construction workers were negatively related to the death rate. The percentage of people working in transportation, communication, and other public utilities was associated positively with the total death rate, as was that for those employed in public administration. When the types of occupations were aggregated, we found that the percentage of white-collar workers was negatively related to total mortality. Finally, a related variable—the percentage of people utilizing public transportation to and from work—was positively related to the total death rate, suggesting that this was a relatively high-risk group of workers, or possibly reflecting their relatively low incomes.

Age–sex–race-adjusted total mortality

The results of adding the occupational variables for the age–sex–race-adjusted mortality rate (regression 5.1-4) were similar to those for the unadjusted total mortality rate; Mean P retained its statistical significance while Min S lost significance when the occupation variables were added. The two air pollution variables together contributed significantly to the regression ($F = 5.27$). R^2 increased substantially (from 0.272 to 0.624).

---

partial correlation (or t statistic for a coefficient) is expected to change, although the estimated coefficient should be approximately constant.

The estimated coefficients of the significant occupation variables were generally similar to those shown previously for the unadjusted total mortality rate.

Race-adjusted infant mortality

In regression 5.1-6, the occupation variables were added to the equation explaining the race-adjusted mortality rate for infants under one year of age. There was little change in the coefficients of the air pollution and socioeconomic variables. Min S and Mean P together contributed significantly to the regression ($F = 5.38$). Considering the significant occupation variables, one notes that the percentages of those employed in agriculture, in the manufacture of nondurable goods, and in education were all negatively related to this infant death rate.[2]

Cancer mortality

The occupation variables were added to the analysis of total cancer deaths in regression 5.1-8. The coefficients and t statistics of both air pollution variables dropped substantially. [Min S became statistically nonsignificant and both variables together failed to contribute significantly to the regression ($F = 1.53$).] Of the socioeconomic variables, P/M^2 and Log Pop lost statistical significance. Two occupation variables were statistically significant and positively related to the cancer mortality rate: the percentage of unemployment and the percentage of workers traveling to and from their jobs on public transportation. Employment in the construction industry was negatively related to cancer mortality.

The four specific cancer mortality rates were analyzed next. The previously estimated associations of air pollution with buccal and pharyngeal, respiratory, and breast cancers remained nonsignificant when the occupation variables were added (regressions 5.1-10, 5.1-14, and 5.1-16); while the previously significant association with cancer of the digestive system became nonsignificant (regression 5.1-12). There was also considerable change in the socioeconomic coefficients, especially for population density. No specific pattern was discernible among the employment variables; the magnitude and significance of the coefficients varied with the particular category of cancer.

In the presence of the occupation-mix variables, the air pollution measures did not make a significant contribution for any of the cancer mortality rates. (The corresponding F statistics were 1.53, 1.28, 1.61, 0.17, and 0.28, respectively.) Evidently, our original formulations of factors affecting cancer mortality were not satisfactory (see table 4.4), since

[2] The statistically significant coefficient for nondurable manufacturing reveals the possibility of spurious correlation in this analysis. Although the regressions provide a crude look at the associations between occupation mix and mortality, one should not overinterpret particular regression coefficients, since this analysis was not replicated.

80

TABLE 5.1. Mortality Rates (the Effects of Occupation Variables), 1960

	Unadjusted total mortality		Age-sex-race-adjusted total mortality		Race-adjusted infant mortality		Total cancers		Buccal and pharyngeal cancers		Digestive cancers	
	5.1-1	5.1-2	5.1-3	5.1-4	5.1-5	5.1-6	5.1-7	5.1-8	5.1-9	5.1-10	5.1-11	5.1-12
R^2	.828	.922	.272	.624	.180	.366	.887	.932	.356	.459	.784	.879
Constant	301.205	964.802	857.665	1394.106	196.098	379.967	−5.249	31.606	−370.570	807.716	−195.267	608.007
Air pollution variables												
Min S	.631 (2.71)	.236 (1.17)	.825 (3.38)	.376 (1.68)	.176 (1.72)	.164 (1.42)	.130 (3.21)	.067 (1.65)			.770 (3.01)	.352 (1.41)
Mean S												
Max S												
Sum S elasticities	3.27	1.22	3.84	1.75	3.31	3.07	4.28	2.21			3.53	
Min P							.072 (1.11)	.004 (.06)	.619 (.93)	.785 (1.13)	.447 (1.08)	.221 (.63)
Mean P	.452 (2.67)	.319 (2.38)	.465 (2.61)	.337 (2.26)	.207 (2.76)	.192 (2.50)						
Max P												
Sum P elasticities	5.85	4.13	5.41	3.92	9.71	9.04	2.30	.12	8.17	10.37	4.31	2.13
Socioeconomic variables												
P/M²	.089 (1.71)	−.052 (−1.09)	.055 (1.01)	−.059 (−1.11)	−.004 (−.19)	.000 (.00)	.029 (3.18)	.004 (.38)	.131 (1.41)	.098 (.84)	.178 (3.09)	.007 (.13)
≥65	7.028 (18.09)	6.295 (20.00)	.411 (1.01)	−.182 (−.52)	−.005 (−.03)	−.134 (−.74)	1.350 (20.80)	1.277 (20.97)	4.317 (6.49)	3.578 (4.81)	4.920 (11.98)	4.264 (11.42)
NW	.422 (4.32)	.332 (3.96)	.165 (1.61)	.093 (.99)	.034 (.80)	−.031 (−.65)	.048 (2.97)	.047 (2.85)	.301 (1.73)	.306 (1.48)	−.031 (−.30)	−.088 (−.88)
Poor	−.002 (−.02)	−.290 (−1.88)	.098 (.65)	−.127 (−.74)	.111 (1.77)	.169 (1.90)	−.094 (−3.78)	−.121 (−3.95)	.262 (.99)	−.270 (−.70)	−.242 (−1.55)	−.519 (−2.78)

	71.02	56.25	7.55	−3.04	9.43	6.14	72.78	63.72	132.42	86.00	79.92	53.61
Sum SE elasticities												
Log Pop	−.212 (−1.12)	−.260 (−1.38)	−.022 (−.11)	−.014 (−.07)	−.002 (−.02)	−.095 (−.88)	.062 (1.87)	.007 (.18)	.408 (1.19)	.493 (1.04)	.412 (1.98)	.128 (.55)
Occupation variables[a]												
Unemployed		1.577 (3.89)		1.721 (3.81)		−.081 (−.35)		.230 (2.83)		1.952 (1.90)		2.113 (4.25)
Males		−.429 (−1.52)		−.372 (−1.18)		−.141 (−.87)		.060 (1.10)		−1.462 (−2.11)		−.438 (−1.31)
Agriculture		−.592 (−2.08)		−.780 (−2.47)		−.358 (−2.19)		−.056 (−.99)		−.708 (−.99)		−.319 (−.92)
Construction		−1.081 (−2.18)		−.645 (−1.17)		.238 (.84)		−.220 (−2.22)		−1.340 (−1.07)		−.791 (−1.30)
Manufacturing (durables)		−.132 (−1.32)		−.053 (−.48)		.047 (.81)		−.032 (−1.60)		−.215 (−.88)		−.145 (−1.19)
Manufacturing (nondurables)		.138 (1.26)		.218 (1.79)		−.132 (−2.10)		.014 (.66)		.009 (.03)		−.026 (−.20)
Transportation		.719 (2.19)		.672 (1.83)		−.121 (−.64)		.036 (.56)		−.832 (−1.01)		.202 (.51)
Trade		−.153 (−.52)		−.288 (−.87)		.148 (.87)		−.076 (−1.28)		.792 (1.05)		−.703 (−1.93)
Finance		.642 (1.06)		.887 (1.32)		.041 (.12)		.170 (1.41)		−.677 (−.44)		1.191 (1.61)
Education		.063 (.16)		.068 (.16)		−.588 (−2.63)		−.017 (−.22)		.756 (.79)		.450 (.96)
Public administration		.372 (2.00)		.372 (2.14)		.009 (.09)		.031 (1.00)		−.264 (−.67)		−.031 (−.16)
White collar		−.654 (−2.84)		−.633 (−2.46)		−.031 (−.23)		−.059 (−1.27)		−.380 (−.66)		−.551 (−1.95)
Use of transit		.256 (1.99)		.151 (1.06)		.010 (.14)		.070 (2.72)		−.008 (−.03)		.469 (2.99)

(*Continued*)

TABLE 5.1. (Continued)

	Respiratory cancers		Breast cancers		Total cardiovascular disease		Heart disease		Endocarditis		Hypertensive disease	
	5.1-13	5.1-14	5.1-15	5.1-16	5.1-17	5.1-18	5.1-19	5.1-20	5.1-21	5.1-22	5.1-23	5.1-24
R^2	.609	.693	.709	.774	.829	.926	.549	.624	.346	.463	.434	.593
Constant	8.763	−359.066	−13.269	127.247	109.795	450.743	32.875	425.851	−152.565	−558.351	105.738	245.526
Air pollution variables												
Min S	.117 (1.41)	.039 (.41)			.691 (4.15)	.296 (2.10)	.842 (3.07)	.562 (1.72)	1.160 (2.24)	.936 (1.54)		
Mean S												
Max S			.022 (1.34)	.010 (.53)							.353 (4.15)	.245 (2.74)
Sum S elasticities	5.24	1.73	4.02	1.75	6.77	2.90	11.39	7.60	19.56	15.80	22.85	15.90
Min P									1.168 (1.40)	1.237 (1.44)		
Mean P					.071 (1.94)							
Max P						.017 (.58)						
Sum P elasticities					3.95	.92			18.97	20.08		
Socioeconomic variables												
P/M²	.102 (3.30)	.108 (2.94)	.027 (1.76)	−.006 (−.30)	.032 (.83)	−.064 (−1.86)	.039 (.60)	−.070 (−.88)	.268 (2.30)	.289 (2.04)	.033 (.42)	−.110 (−1.20)
≥65	2.193 (10.01)	2.351 (9.92)	1.149 (10.46)	1.015 (8.61)	5.086 (17.59)	4.616 (20.48)	3.707 (8.07)	3.433 (6.75)	3.308 (3.98)	3.584 (3.92)	2.864 (5.09)	2.544 (4.38)
NW	.198 (3.53)	.256 (3.96)	.058 (2.01)	.022 (.66)	.282 (3.91)	.237 (3.93)	1.87 (1.61)	.107 (.78)	.071 (.34)	.309 (1.26)	.920 (6.24)	.897 (5.54)
Poor	−.165 (−1.93)	−.208 (−1.72)	−.216 (−4.96)	−.214 (−3.50)	−.199 (−1.87)	−.374 (−3.35)	−.309 (−1.75)	−.371 (−1.45)	.409 (1.29)	−.259 (−.57)	.038 (.17)	−.082 (−.27)

	83.57	89.49	52.66	38.66	88.72	71.43	80.46	65.63	135.36	111.56	103.35	85.90
Sum SE elasticities												
Log Pop	.029	.041	.120	.075	−.189	−.219	−.008	−.399	−.096	.408	−.350	−.116
	(.26)	(.28)	(2.13)	(1.01)	(−1.38)	(−1.60)	(−.03)	(−1.26)	(−.23)	(.72)	(−1.21)	(−.31)
Occupation variables[a]												
Unemployed		−.198		−.024		.916		.824		2.592		1.786
		(−.62)		(−.14)		(3.11)		(1.21)		(2.13)		(2.23)
Males		.657		−.073		−.065		−.178		.142		−.271
		(2.91)		(−.64)		(−.31)		(−.39)		(.17)		(−.48)
Agriculture		−.234		.229		−.466		−.213		−.288		−.100
		(−1.03)		(2.02)		(−2.26)		(−.45)		(−.34)		(−.18)
Construction		−.241		−.141		−.913		.756		.263		−1.114
		(−.62)		(−.71)		(−2.54)		(.91)		(.18)		(−1.13)
Manufacturing (durables)		−.140		−.022		−.124		−.037		−.194		.039
		(−1.83)		(−.58)		(−1.72)		(−.22)		(−.65)		(.20)
Manufacturing (nondurables)		−.034		.016		.200		.184		.670		.521
		(−.40)		(.38)		(2.54)		(1.02)		(2.08)		(2.41)
Transportation		.288		−.178		.211		−.387		.738		.867
		(1.11)		(−1.35)		(.89)		(−.71)		(.76)		(1.34)
Trade		.003		−.138		−.100		−.520		.201		−.714
		(.01)		(−1.16)		(−.47)		(−1.04)		(.23)		(−1.21)
Finance		.248		.195		.301		−.586		.148		.643
		(.52)		(.81)		(.69)		(−.58)		(·08)		(.54)
Education		−.267		−.132		.214		−.569		.859		.849
		(−.90)		(−.88)		(.78)		(−.90)		(.75)		(1.14)
Public administration		.040		.018		.215		−.105		.931		.861
		(.33)		(.29)		(1.88)		(−.40)		(1.99)		(2.81)
White collar		−.086		−.046		−.477		.095		−.540		−.365
		(−.49)		(−.50)		(−2.90)		(.25)		(−.78)		(−.81)
Use of transit		−.057		.118		.211		.480		−.364		.119
		(−.56)		(2.28)		(2.27)		(2.25)		(−.95)		(.47)

(Continued)

TABLE 5.1. (Continued)

	Total respiratory disease		Tuberculosis		Asthma		Influenza		Pneumonia		Bronchitis	
	5.1-25	5.1-26	5.1-27	5.1-28	5.1-29	5.1-30	5.1-31	5.1-32	5.1-33	5.1-34	5.1-35	5.1-36
R^2	.227	.375	.283	.451	.087	.236	.341	.484	.140	.282	.082	.206
Constant	−52.675	579.479	−1137.744	728.439	85.616	921.969	258.772	−1598.276	4.841	504.105	162.781	1429.276
Air pollution variables												
Min S												
Mean S							.593 (1.29)	.288 (.55)				
Max S												
Sum S elasticities							17.39	8.44				
Min P	.763 (1.52)	.585 (1.14)							.319 (.71)	.220 (.47)	.079 (.99)	.171 (1.94)
Mean P			1.735 (3.01)	1.417 (2.36)	.732 (2.34)							
Max P						.884 (2.58)						
Sum P elasticities	7.65	5.86	37.47	30.60	29.82	36.01			4.64	3.20	9.23	20.11
Socioeconomic variables												
P/M²	.089 (1.27)	−.064 (−.73)	.331 (1.87)	−.095 (−.44)	.025 (.26)	.038 (.31)	−.158 (−.92)	−.266 (−1.30)	.062 (.99)	−.035 (−.44)	.010 (.12)	.049 (.47)
≥65	1.517 (3.01)	.618 (1.12)	2.050 (1.57)	.707 (.51)	.956 (1.34)	.422 (.53)	−1.595 (−1.31)	−1.175 (−.89)	1.387 (3.06)	.682 (1.35)	.826 (1.36)	.522 (.77)
NW	−.055 (−.42)	−.237 (−1.54)	.041 (.12)	−.333 (−.86)	−.100 (−.53)	−.201 (−.91)	−.514 (−1.64)	−.404 (−1.12)	.039 (.33)	−.103 (−.73)	.003 (.02)	−.069 (−.37)
Poor	.666 (3.33)	.500 (1.74)	1.927 (3.79)	1.190 (1.66)	.309 (1.12)	−.109 (−.27)	2.593 (5.43)	3.724 (5.56)	.189 (1.05)	.038 (.15)	−.307 (−1.32)	−.660 (−1.90)

	(1)	(2)	(3)	(4)	(5)	(6)	(7)	(8)	(9)	(10)	(11)	(12)
Sum SE elasticities	54.50	23.86	100.41	41.42	43.26	−2.38	76.69	149.13	51.00	15.60	6.44	−35.41
Log Pop	.397 (1.52)	.259 (.74)	1.645 (2.49)	1.436 (1.66)	−.013 (−.04)	.550 (1.12)	−.422 (−.68)	−.390 (−.47)	.237 (1.01)	.081 (.25)	.053 (.18)	.248 (.59)
Occupation variables[a]												
Unemployed		.798 (1.05)		4.362 (2.32)		−.290 (−.27)		−.629 (−.35)		.453 (.65)		.054 (.06)
Males		−.661 (−1.28)		−1.190 (−.91)		−.508 (−.68)		2.167 (1.72)		−.710 (−1.51)		−1.412 (−2.20)
Agriculture		−.064 (−.12)		−2.003 (−1.52)		−.601 (−.80)		−1.007 (−.80)		.374 (.77)		−.513 (−.80)
Construction		−.293 (−.32)		2.216 (.97)		.483 (.37)		−4.877 (−2.24)		.015 (.02)		−.716 (−.64)
Manufacturing (durables)		.006 (.03)		−.337 (−.75)		−.374 (−1.46)		.370 (.87)		.059 (.36)		−.169 (−.77)
Manufacturing (nondurables)		.218 (1.08)		−.230 (−.45)		−.448 (−1.55)		.438 (.92)		.289 (1.56)		−.827 (−3.38)
Transportation		.761 (1.25)		1.077 (.71)		.228 (.26)		3.440 (2.38)		.362 (.65)		.264 (.36)
Trade		.075 (.13)		−1.927 (−1.40)		−.094 (−.12)		−1.820 (−1.39)		.390 (.76)		.572 (.85)
Finance		1.482 (1.31)		2.897 (1.04)		3.945 (2.49)		5.925 (2.25)		.159 (.15)		.157 (.12)
Education		−.693 (−.98)		1.338 (.75)		−.313 (−.31)		2.033 (1.24)		−.941 (−1.45)		.656 (.77)
Public administration		.032 (.11)		1.228 (1.70)		−.110 (−.27)		−.061 (−.09)		−.076 (−.28)		−.307 (−.87)
White collar		−.337 (−.79)		−2.133 (−2.03)		−1.614 (−2.70)		.520 (.53)		.042 (.11)		−.767 (−1.51)
Use of transit		.250 (1.05)		.998 (1.70)		−.447 (−1.34)		−.566 (−1.00)		.242 (1.11)		−.170 (−.60)

Note: All regressions are based on data for 117 SMSAs. The numbers in parentheses below the regression coefficients are t statistics.

[a] Some occupational classifications are abbreviated from the full composition of category. Complete information appears in table D.4, page 329.

both the 1961 replication and the introduction of additional explanatory variables resulted in significant variations in the associations with the air pollution variables and the socioeconomic factors. One cannot have confidence in the estimated coefficients of the air pollution variables and their importance in explaining the cancer mortality rates. The relatively high R^2 suggests that some occupational factor such as occupational exposure or the emissions from the related industries are associated with cancer mortality.

Cardiovascular disease mortality

In regression 5.1-18, the variables representing occupation mix were added to the original regression for total cardiovascular disease mortality. The magnitude and significance of the estimated associations with the two air pollution measures were reduced considerably, although Min S remained statistically significant. Together, Min S and Max P failed to make a significant contribution to this regression ($F = 2.38$). Of the socioeconomic variables, population density switched "sign," and the percentage of poor families became statistically significant; the other socioeconomic coefficients exhibited little change. The coefficients of the statistically significant occupation-mix variables indicated that unemployment was again associated with higher mortality. In addition, employment in agriculture, construction, and white-collar jobs was negatively related to cardiovascular mortality, while employment in manufacturing (nondurable goods) as well as the proportion of workers riding to and from work on public transit were positively related to this death rate.

For the three subclassifications under cardiovascular diseases, the coefficients for the sulfate measures were reduced when the occupation variables were added (regressions 5.1-20, 5.1-22, and 5.1-24). Nevertheless, the air pollution variables made a significant contribution to the regressions for endocarditis and hypertensive heart disease (the F statistics were 3.16 and 7.50, respectively). (For diseases of the heart, the F statistic was equal to 2.96.) The estimated coefficients of the socioeconomic variables displayed mixed results when the occupation-mix variables were added. As before, the magnitude and significance of the coefficients for the specific occupation variables varied with the specific disease in question.

Respiratory disease mortality

Adding the occupation variables to the mortality rate for total noncancerous respiratory diseases (regression 5.1-26) had only a slight effect on Min P (it remained statistically nonsignificant) but had a major effect on the socioeconomic variables. Population density switched signs (remaining nonsignificant), the percentage of older people and the percentage of poor families lost statistical significance, the percentage of nonwhites increased in magnitude, and the population variable decreased in magnitude (the latter two variables remained nonsignificant). None of the occupation variables was statistically significant.

For the five subcategories of respiratory disease, the results were mixed with the addition of the occupation-mix variables (regressions 5.1-28, 5.1-30, 5.1-32, 5.1-34, and 5.1-36). For tuberculosis and asthma, the statistical significance of Mean P was retained. For influenza and pneumonia, the magnitudes of the (nonsignificant) air pollution coefficients were reduced. Finally, for bronchitis, the pollution variable approached statistical significance. The socioeconomic variables displayed mixed results. Again, the importance of the specific occupation variables varied with the specific respiratory disease in question.

With few exceptions, the addition of the occupation variables lowered the statistical significance of the air pollution measures. Often the magnitude of the coefficients fell by 50 percent or more. In four of the eleven regressions, where the sulfate and suspended particulate variables had previously made a significant contribution, the addition of the occupation-mix variables resulted in their losing statistical significance. The effect on the socioeconomic coefficients was even more marked. Their coefficients often exhibited substantial changes in magnitude and significance, as well as in sign. These results, if somewhat disappointing, are consistent with our expectations. Occupation mix is closely associated with the socioeconomic structure of an area, helping to determine income, unemployment, and working conditions. In addition, occupation mix is directly related to occupational accidents and occupational exposures to noxious substances. Finally, occupation mix is itself one way of "measuring" air pollution emissions; for example, the manufacture of primary metals can indicate the presence of sulfate and suspended particulate pollution.[3] Thus, occupation mix might be a surrogate for air quality. Because of all these characteristics, we would expect the inclusion of the occupation variables to diminish the magnitude and significance of the estimated effects of air pollution.

HOME-HEATING CHARACTERISTICS AND CLIMATE AS EXPLANATORY VARIABLES

In addition to examining the effect of occupation mix on the observed relationship between air pollution and mortality, we studied how indoor and outdoor environmental characteristics influenced this association by adding sets of heating and weather variables to our previous results.

Heating variables (derived from census data) were grouped according to the type of heating equipment, home-heating fuel, and water-heating fuel, and a measure of the proportion of air-conditioned homes was included. The specific variables used were the proportion of homes in each category.[4]

[3] Given the poor quality of available air pollution data, in some cases occupation mix may be a better indication of the air quality in an area than direct measurement of ambient pollution levels.

[4] Strictly speaking, the heating-equipment variables were defined as a percentage of total housing units, while the home-heating and water-heating fuels were defined as a percentage of *occupied* housing units.

We added each group, as well as a group of climate variables, and tested the results to see if the explanatory power (R^2) of the regression was increased significantly. When an F test showed that a group contributed significantly to the explanatory power of the regression, that regression is reported. In addition, we investigated whether two or more groups jointly made a contribution. First, we added the water-heating fuel variables, since in general they added the most explanatory power to the basic regressions. If the contribution of this category was statistically significant, we continued to add the remaining sets of variables (in the order of home-heating fuel, home-heating equipment, and climate) until there was no longer a significant increase in R^2. When water-heating fuels did not prove to be a significant factor in the first instance, we tried the other groups of heating variables and the climate variables, following the same procedure.

This method of sequential estimation provides a number of estimated coefficients for the air pollution and socioeconomic variables. Even if air pollution increases mortality (as hypothesized), the introduction of these additional sets of variables would result in some changes in the estimated air pollution coefficients due to correlations between the air pollution variables and the new sets of variables. However, if either home-heating characteristics or climate factors were the "true" causes of increased mortality and also "caused" air pollution (so that the effects we measured were spurious), the estimation procedure would highlight this, since the estimated coefficients of the pollution variables would approach zero.[5] We believe that this approach will enhance our knowledge of the true association between the air pollution measures and the mortality rates; the range of estimated coefficients gives some indication of the range of uncertainty.

Tables 5.2 through 5.5 present the results of adding the heating and climate variables to the total mortality and disease-specific mortality rate regressions reported in chapter 4. Because the heating variables were defined as the percentage of all homes in an area heated by a particular method (for example, steam), the sum of all variables within each set is 100 percent. Adding all the variables in a particular class of heating characteristics would preclude inverting the matrix of cross products and make it impossible to derive estimates for the regression coefficients. The solution is to exclude one of the variables. However, in reporting the results, we have added the excluded variable and constrained the sum of the

---

[5] Since only significant variables were added, and since the resulting parameter estimates were not checked by reestimating the relations with data from another year, care must be taken in using these results to estimate the effect of either home-heating characteristics or climate on mortality rates. However, the reported coefficients can be used to gain some notion of the possible *range* of the estimated effects of these variables. For some of the heating and climate variables, the parameter estimates exhibit little change as the specification is altered, which suggests that these estimates are unlikely to vary greatly if the relations were reestimated with new data. For other variables, the parameter estimates fluctuate to a greater degree and one can have little confidence in the exact estimates.

coefficients to be zero. This rescaling means that the magnitude of each coefficient is relative to all the others and that the previously estimated standard errors are no longer applicable; they are not reported.[6]

Total mortality

For the unadjusted total mortality rate, we ran a complete set of regressions (see table 5.2), including each set of heating variables alone. No other group increased the explanatory power significantly when the water-heating fuels were present. Our primary concern is with the effect of the heating and climate variables on the Min S and Mean P coefficients. If regression 5.2-1 is compared with the original 1960 result (see regression 5.1-1), one notes that both the magnitude and significance of the air pollution coefficients decreased, although both remained statistically significant. Together the two variables contributed significantly to the regression, $F = 6.10$. In the presence of home-heating fuels (regression 5.2-2), both air pollution variables lost statistical significance ($F = 1.15$). In the remaining three regressions, the air pollution variables again contributed significantly ($F = 8.42$, 8.93, and 4.27, respectively).

One explanation for the nonsignificance of the pollution variables in regression 5.2-2 may lie in the association between home-heating fuels and our air pollution measures. For example, the simple correlation between Min S and Coal was 0.42. It seems likely that the type of fuel used for home heating contributes substantially to the air pollution level in the city. Note that this interpretation does not mean the previous association between air pollution and mortality is disproved, but rather that it is made more specific by directing the association to home-heating fuels, rather than to all sources of air pollution. As noted previously, our measures of air pollution exposure are crude and may only approximate the true exposure. Specifying which fuels were used for home heating may provide better approximations of the exposure than our measures of ambient air quality. It is also possible that home-heating fuels are measuring life-style or some other factor. This would also tend to weaken the estimated air pollution–mortality relationship.

The socioeconomic variables displayed mixed results across the five specifications; the coefficients for population density and the percentage of poor families showed considerable fluctuations as the sets of variables were added.

Homes with coal and "other" water-heating fuels (see table D.5, page 330)—as well as those having no water-heating fuels ("none"), and presumably no hot water—were positively associated with the mortality rate (regression 5.2-1). Coal and "none" were also positively associated with the mortality rate in the home-heating fuel category (regression 5.2-2). The estimated coefficients suggested that steam heat was the

---

[6] In the discussion that follows, we will focus on the largest coefficients (in absolute value) for these additional variables.

TABLE 5.2. Unadjusted and Age-Sex-Race-adjusted Total Mortality Rates (the Effects of Home-heating Characteristics and Climate), 1960

	Unadjusted					Age-sex-race-adjusted				
	5.2-1	5.2-2	5.2-3	5.2-4	5.2-5	5.2-6	5.2-7	5.2-8	5.2-9	5.2-10
R^2	.901	.881	.872	.840	.872	.540	.467	.457	.327	.450
Constant	630.245	311.870	381.611	144.405	−1115.186	1146.517	816.783	926.245	681.896	−629.203
Air pollution variables										
Min S	.408 (2.18)	.184 (.85)	.523 (2.40)	.506 (2.20)	.409 (1.60)	.610 (2.97)	.372 (1.60)	.699 (3.07)	.685 (2.85)	.485 (1.80)
Sum S elasticities	2.11	.95	2.71	2.62	2.12	2.84	1.73	3.25	3.19	2.26
Mean P	.298 (2.10)	.171 (1.08)	.418 (2.57)	.452 (2.75)	.378 (2.04)	.326 (2.09)	.225 (1.31)	.459 (2.70)	.465 (2.71)	.411 (2.11)
Sum P elasticities	3.85	2.22	5.41	5.86	4.89	3.79	2.61	5.34	5.41	4.78
Socioeconomic variables										
P/M^2	.031 (.72)	.111 (2.44)	.017 (.35)	.099 (1.94)	.087 (1.72)	−.005 (−.11)	.069 (1.42)	−.022 (−.43)	.066 (1.24)	.057 (1.08)
≥65	6.589 (19.62)	6.625 (18.56)	6.168 (15.91)	6.862 (17.98)	6.226 (14.42)	−.067 (−.18)	−.107 (−.28)	−.479 (−1.18)	.226 (.57)	−.498 (−1.09)
NW	.417 (5.26)	.483 (5.48)	.391 (4.44)	.468 (4.87)	3.97 (3.59)	.164 (1.89)	.213 (2.24)	.128 (1.38)	.216 (2.16)	.084 (.73)
Poor	−.470 (−2.87)	−.063 (−.41)	.093 (.52)	.063 (.45)	.483 (2.58)	−.314 (−1.75)	.146 (.88)	.175 (.94)	.171 (1.16)	.605 (3.06)
Sum SE elasticities	57.19	67.10	64.04	71.49	72.93	−4.17	4.83	.57	8.02	8.10
Log Pop	−.126 (−.78)	−.123 (−.73)	−.254 (−1.43)	−.189 (−1.02)	−.125 (−.63)	.046 (.26)	.060 (.33)	−.061 (−.33)	.004 (.02)	.021 (.10)
Variables added	WHF	HHF	HHE	AC	CL	WHF	HHF	HHE	AC	CL

Note: All regressions are based on data for 117 SMSAs. The numbers in parentheses below the regression coefficients are t statistics.
Abbreviations: AC, without air conditioning; CL, climate; HHE, home-heating equipment; HHF, home-heating fuels; WHF, water-heating fuels.

Scaled regression coefficients for home-heating characteristics and coefficients and t statistics for air-conditioning and climate variables:

Water-heating fuel

Type	Regression 5.2-1	Regression 5.2-6
Gas	−.278	−.234
Electricity	−.290	−.245
Coal	.174	.209
Bottled gas	−.653	−.550
Oil	−.181	−.121
Other	.921	.656
None	.307	.285

Home-heating fuel

Type	Regression 5.2-2	Regression 5.2-7
Gas	.010	.056
Oil	.028	.097
Coal	.249	.270
Electricity	.022	.002
Bottled gas	−.426	−.413
Other	−.014	−.198
None	.130	.185

Heating equipment

Type	Regression 5.2-3	Regression 5.2-8
Steam	.157	.173
Floor	−.062	−.054
Electric	.073	−.016
With flue	.040	.082
Without flue	−.011	.008
Warm-air furnace	−.032	−.024
None	−.165	−.169

Without air conditioning

Regression 5.2-4	Regression 5.2-9
.172 (2.77)	.193 (2.98)

Climate

Variable	Regression 5.2-5	Regression 5.2-10
Min temp.	.750 (1.23)	.734 (1.14)
Max temp.	1.256 (1.27)	1.391 (1.33)
Degree days	1.419 (2.10)	1.487 (2.09)
Precipitation	.054 (.58)	.097 (.99)
1:00 A.M. humidity	.205 (.10)	1.031 (.48)
1:00 P.M. humidity	−2.142 (−1.05)	−3.070 (−1.43)
Wind	−.038 (−.10)	.042 (.10)
.01 in. rain	−.758 (−1.40)	−.840 (−1.47)
1 in. snow	−.425 (−.22)	−.173 (−.08)
Fog	−.221 (−.56)	−.372 (−.90)
Max temp. ≥ 90° F.	−1.715 (−2.41)	−1.864 (−2.49)
Max temp. ≤ 32° F.	−.626 (−.91)	−.189 (−.26)
Min temp. ≤ 32° F.	−1.961 (−2.05)	−2.248 (−2.23)
Min temp. ≤ 0° F.	−3.657 (−2.13)	−5.010 (−2.77)

most unhealthful type of home-heating equipment, possibly because it represents the burning of such fuels as coal (regression 5.2-3). The percentage of homes without air conditioning was added in regression 5.2-4. The coefficient of the variable suggested that air conditioning was associated with lower mortality rates.[7] The statistically significant climate variables were measures of extreme temperature (regression 5.2-5).

Similar results were apparent in the analysis of the age–sex–race-adjusted total mortality rate in regressions 5.2-6 through 5.2-10. In fact, the air pollution coefficients were even more stable (both in magnitude and statistical significance) than in the results for the unadjusted total mortality rate. (The F statistics for the contribution of the two air pollution variables were 8.72, 2.62, 11.32, 11.23, and 4.90, respectively.)

Race-adjusted infant mortality

None of the heating groups or climate variables contributed significantly to the explanatory power of the basic regression for the race-adjusted infant mortality rate. Thus, we report no results in the tables.

Cancer mortality

Cancer mortality is analyzed in table 5.3. Water-heating fuels, home-heating fuels, home-heating equipment, and water- and home-heating fuels each made significant contributions to the explanatory power of the basic regression for total cancer mortality (regressions 5.3-1 through 5.3-4). The coefficient for minimum sulfates remained relatively stable while that for minimum suspended particulates evidenced instability as the sets of variables were added. [Min S and Min P contributed significantly to the regression when either water-heating fuels or home-heating equipment were present ($F = 5.56$ and 5.97, respectively), but not when home-heating fuels or the combination of water-heating and home-heating fuels were present ($F = 1.20$ and 1.95, respectively).] The socioeconomic coefficients showed little effect. As with total mortality, the lack of heating fuel ("none"), as well as the presence of steam equipment, were positively associated with higher mortality rates. (The category of "other" fuels displayed mixed signs, depending on the purpose for which it was used.) The climate variables did not contribute significantly to these regressions.

The only "improvement" in the explanatory power of the basic regression for buccal and pharyngeal cancer took place when the air-conditioning variable was added in regression 5.3-5 (Min P remained nonsignificant). The presence of air conditioning was associated with lower death rates for this category of cancers.

---

[7] This result may be an artifact of the relationship between air conditioning and climate or possibly between air conditioning and income. When the air-conditioning variable was included in a regression with climate variables (not reported), it became statistically nonsignificant.

The pattern for digestive cancer (regressions 5.3-6 through 5.3-10) was similar to that of total cancers, although air conditioning, as well as the combination of water-heating fuels, home-heating equipment, and air conditioning were important. Again, the sulfate coefficient was more stable than the suspended particulate coefficient. Min S and Min P contributed significantly to regressions containing water-heating fuels, home-heating equipment, air conditioning, and the combination of these three groups ($F = 5.93$, 5.14, 5.02, and 3.21, respectively); they did not contribute in the presence of home-heating fuels alone ($F = 1.03$). Most of the socioeconomic coefficients exhibited relatively little variation. The signs of the heating variables followed patterns similar to those in the previous regressions.

For respiratory cancer (regressions 5.3-11 through 5.3-15), home-heating fuels, home-heating equipment, air conditioning, climate, and the combination of home-heating fuels and home-heating equipment contributed significantly to the basic regression. The coefficient of the air pollution variable (Mean S) was relatively stable throughout, as were coefficients for three of the five socioeconomic variables. Mean S contributed significantly when home-heating equipment was present ($F = 5.45$) but not in the other regressions ($F = 2.36$, 3.37, 2.65, and 2.13, respectively). Although the individual heating-fuel and equipment variables displayed different associations than they had in the previous regressions, it is difficult to disentangle the individual effects, since both home-heating equipment and fuels were simultaneously included in regression 5.3-15. Among the weather variables, measures of temperature and precipitation displayed significant coefficients; however, the directions of the associations were mixed, and no clear pattern was discernible.

For breast cancer (regression 5.3-16), only water-heating fuels contributed significantly to the basic regression (see regression 5.1-15). The air pollution variable remained statistically nonsignificant and, in general, the coefficients for the socioeconomic variables had diminished magnitudes and statistical significance. The variable representing the absence of water-heating fuel was positively related to this cancer rate.

Cardiovascular disease mortality

Each individual set of heating variables (and the combined set of water-heating and home-heating fuels), as well as the climate variables, contributed to the explanatory power of the basic regression for total cardiovascular disease deaths (regressions 5.4-1 through 5.4-6) in table 5.4. It is noteworthy that the Min S and Max P coefficients did not exhibit great change across the various specifications. Min S and Max P made significant contributions in all specifications, except in regression 5.4-2 which contained home-heating fuels alone ($F = 8.75$, 2.83, 9.53, 9.05, 5.29,

TABLE 5.3. Cancer Mortality Rates (the Effects of Home-heating Characteristics and Climate), 1960

	Total cancers				Buccal and pharyngeal	Digestive	
	5.3-1	5.3-2	5.3-3	5.3-4	5.3-5	5.3-6	5.3-7
R^2	.913	.905	.909	.925	.382	.877	.825
Constant	44.172	−11.560	1.891	59.322	−616.606	331.485	−139.576
Air pollution variables							
Min S	.104	.063	.101	.074		.575	.348
	(2.74)	(1.53)	(2.58)	(1.91)		(2.78)	(1.35)
Mean S							
Max S							
Sum S elasticities	3.43	2.07	3.32	2.43		5.76	3.48
Min P	.066	−.000	.108	.015	.445	.396	.094
	(1.08)	(−.00)	(1.65)	(.25)	(.68)	(1.20)	(.23)
Sum P elasticities	2.08	−.00	3.42	.48	5.88	3.82	.91
Socioeconomic variables							
P/M²	.020	.031	.018	.019	.133	.116	.195
	(2.23)	(3.56)	(2.04)	(2.15)	(1.46)	(2.42)	(3.59)
≥65	1.278	1.295	1.233	1.240	3.987	4.136	4.424
	(19.09)	(19.43)	(18.17)	(18.62)	(5.94)	(11.34)	(10.65)
NW	.050	.067	.041	.062	.362	.019	.039
	(3.24)	(4.03)	(2.70)	(3.88)	(2.08)	(.22)	(.38)
Poor	−.128	−.076	−.097	−.100	.362	−.435	−.291
	(−3.87)	(−2.57)	(−3.07)	(−2.65)	(1.37)	(−2.42)	(−1.58)
Sum SE elasticities	63.88	73.50	64.36	66.23	131.93	59.01	71.34
Log Pop	.058	.054	.044	0.38	.486	.335	.440
	(1.79)	(1.67)	(1.35)	(1.18)	(1.43)	(1.90)	(2.20)
Variables added	WHF	HHF	HHE	WHF, HHF	AC	WHF	HHF

Note: All regressions are based on data for 117 SMSAs. The numbers in parentheses below the regression coefficients are *t* statistics.

Abbreviations: *AC*, without air conditioning; *CL*, climate; *HHE*, home-heating equipment; *HHF*, home-heating fuels; *WHF*, water-heating fuels.

Scaled regression coefficients for home-heating characteristics and coefficients and *t* statistics for air-conditioning and climate variables:

Water-heating fuel

	Regression				
Type	5.3-1	5.3-4	5.3-6	5.3-10	5.3-16
Gas	−.038	−.047	−.414	−.145	.007
Electricity	−.049	−.077	−.469	−.305	.001
Coal	.011	−.022	.059	.133	.038
Bottled gas	−.050	−.176	−.381	−.271	−.128
Oil	−.020	−.049	−.269	−.221	.056
Other	.133	.359	1.692	1.149	−.095
None	.013	.012	−.218	−.341	.122

Home-heating fuel

	Regression				
Type	5.3-2	5.3-4	5.3-7	5.3-11	5.3-15
Gas	.017	.008	−.025	.089	.503
Oil	.023	.030	.023	.101	.524
Coal	.041	.029	.193	.052	.530
Electricity	−.001	.033	−.164	.071	.643
Bottled gas	−.049	.050	−.134	.222	.295
Other	−.122	−.195	−.227	−.690	−.174
None	.093	.043	.334	.156	−2.322

Heating equipment

	Regression				
Type	5.3-3	5.3-8	5.3-10	5.3-12	5.3-15
Steam	.020	.173	.044	−.073	−.447
Floor	−.022	−.148	−.301	−.062	−.368
Electric	−.016	−.149	.036	−.079	−.594
With flue	.003	−.003	.119	−.002	−.322
Without flue	.012	.018	.021	.052	−.290
Warm-air furnace	−.007	−.059	−.149	−.036	−.354
None	.010	.168	.230	.200	2.375

94

TABLE 5.3. *(Continued)*

Digestive			Respiratory					Breast
5.3-8	5.3-9	5.3-10	5.3-11	5.3-12	5.3-13	5.3-14	5.3-15	5.3-16
.855	.795	.901	.687	.669	.623	.759	.756	.760
−19.008	−348.234	177.520	−39.629	64.051	88.523	−1729.702	−86.326	−18.255
.530	.662	.369						
(2.35)	(2.60)	(1.82)						
			.130	.199	.153	.136	.116	
			(1.53)	(2.33)	(1.83)	(1.63)	(1.46)	
								.001
								(.05)
5.30	6.62	3.70	5.84	8.93	6.84	6.11	5.18	.16
.602	.387	.438						
(1.59)	(.96)	(1.33)						
5.80	3.73	4.22						
.091	.187	.100	.097	.108	.098	.109	.129	.002
(1.76)	(3.31)	(2.15)	(3.41)	(3.56)	(3.24)	(4.11)	(4.61)	(.15)
3.816	4.753	3.923	2.155	2.391	2.274	2.075	2.268	1.057
(9.73)	(11.65)	(10.87)	(9.71)	(10.17)	(10.36)	(8.88)	(10.29)	(9.09)
−.082	.012	.086	.243	.193	.178	.161	.227	.037
(−.92)	(.12)	(1.03)	(4.36)	(3.57)	(3.16)	(2.67)	(4.39)	(1.33)
−.148	−.180	−.402	−.035	−.340	−.193	−.202	−.196	−.264
(−.81)	(−1.16)	(−1.87)	(−.35)	(−3.14)	(−2.26)	(−1.98)	(−1.49)	(−4.51)
61.28	80.61	58.02	95.08	76.70	83.08	74.24	86.40	36.23
.273	.443	.125	−.068	−.007	.001	−.115	.096	.150
(1.47)	(2.17)	(.69)	(−.64)	(−.06)	(.00)	(−1.08)	(.91)	(2.58)
HHE	AC	WHF, HHE, AC	HHF	HHE	AC	CL	HHF, HHE	WHF

Without air conditioning					Climate	
Regression						Regression
5.3-5	5.3-9	5.3-10	5.3-13		Variable	5.3-14
.251	.166	.192	−.079		Min temp.	1.075
(2.17)	(2.40)	(2.70)	(−2.07)			(3.23)
					Max temp.	1.462
						(2.68)
					Degree days	.818
						(2.22)
					Precipitation	−.125
						(−2.45)
					1:00 A.M. humidity	.217
						(.20)
					1:00 P.M. humidity	1.971
						(1.79)
					Wind	.283
						(1.36)
					.01 in. rain	−.116
						(−.40)
					1 in. snow	.692
						(.66)
					Fog	.073
						(.35)
					Max temp. ≥ 90° F.	−1.334
						(−3.42)
					Max temp. ≤ 32° F.	−.518
						(−1.41)
					Min temp. ≤ 32° F.	−.362
						(−.70)
					Min temp. ≤ 0° F.	−.243
						(−.26)

TABLE 5.4. Cardiovascular Disease Mortality Rates (the Effects of Home-heating Characteristics and Climate), 1960

	Total cardiovascular disease					
	5.4-1	5.4-2	5.4-3	5.4-4	5.4-5	5.4-6
R^2	.894	.886	.880	.844	.881	.909
Constant	290.354	78.934	126.861	−25.091	−777.225	302.650
Air pollution variables						
Min S	.534	.317	.565	.590	.494	.352
	(3.79)	(2.03)	(3.70)	(3.63)	(2.75)	(2.39)
Max S						
Sum S elasticities	5.23	3.10	5.53	5.78	4.84	3.45
Min P						
Max P	.044	.037	.060	.061	.059	.031
	(1.42)	(1.14)	(1.87)	(1.73)	(1.62)	(1.02)
Sum P elasticities	2.45	2.05	3.34	3.38	3.28	1.71
Socioeconomic variables						
P/M²	−.023	.040	−.022	.040	.031	−.003
	(.69)	(1.19)	(−.62)	(1.07)	(.85)	(−.10)
≥65	4.759	4.772	4.392	4.917	4.513	4.601
	(18.22)	(18.29)	(15.79)	(17.45)	(14.50)	(17.76)
NW	.261	.316	.247	.317	.246	.319
	(4.27)	(4.89)	(3.92)	(4.53)	(3.09)	(5.11)
Poor	−.517	−.174	−.084	−.139	.086	−.433
	(−4.08)	(−1.53)	(−.67)	(−1.33)	(.64)	(−3.01)
Sum SE elasticities	69.76	85.20	79.30	89.08	88.51	71.94
Log Pop	−.124	−.142	−.189	−.163	−.105	−.092
	(−1.02)	(−1.19)	(−1.53)	(−1.24)	(−.76)	(−.74)
Variables added	WHF	HHF	HHE	AC	CL	WHF, HHF

Note: All regressions are based on data for 117 SMSAs. The numbers in parentheses below the regression coefficients are t statistics.

Abbreviations: AC, without air conditioning; CL, climate; HHE, home-heating equipment; HHF, home-heating fuels; WHF, water-heating fuels.

Scaled regression coefficients for home-heating characteristics and coefficients and t statistics for air-conditioning and climate variables:

Water-heating fuel

	Regression				
Type	5.4-1	5.4-6	5.4-7	5.4-9	5.4-12
Gas	−.150	−.279	−.167	−.148	−.468
Electricity	−.148	−.235	−.175	−.148	−.502
Coal	.121	−.167	.079	.684	.169
Bottled gas	−.541	−.289	−.306	.380	−.367
Oil	−.052	−.106	.064	−.143	−.449
Other	.474	.996	.489	−1.043	.689
None	.296	.080	.017	.418	.928

Home-heating fuel

	Regression			
Type	5.4-2	5.4-6	5.4-10	5.4-13
Gas	.037	.097	.016	−.057
Oil	.064	.038	.015	−.028
Coal	.190	.212	.550	.289
Electricity	.010	.041	−.034	−.396
Bottled gas	−.390	−.143	.233	−.089
Other	.001	−.149	−.518	.290
None	.087	−.098	−.262	−.010

TABLE 5.4. (*Continued*)

	Heart disease		Endocarditis			Hypertensive disease			
	5.4-7	5.4-8	5.4-9	5.4-10	5.4-11	5.4-12	5.4-13	5.4-14	5.4-15
	.646	.642	.483	.483	.434	.632	.588	.536	.479
	251.977	178.756	46.448	−87.459	11.289	445.678	118.970	4.216	−191.391
	.777 (2.96)	.781 (2.90)	.639 (1.30)	.231 (.45)	1.172 (2.26)				
						.273 (3.68)	.270 (3.39)	.268 (3.18)	.302 (3.62)
	10.51	10.57	10.78 .861 (1.09)	3.87 .152 (.19)	19.77 1.023 (1.18)	17.68	17.50	17.38	19.60
			13.99	2.47	16.61				
	−.052 (−.82)	−.052 (−.83)	.269 (2.35)	.338 (3.13)	.180 (1.53)	−.037 (−.54)	.015 (.22)	−.038 (−.50)	.037 (.49)
	2.871 (5.97)	2.851 (6.01)	3.093 (3.57)	2.922 (3.52)	2.487 (2.76)	2.626 (4.95)	2.085 (3.80)	1.724 (2.84)	2.511 (4.53)
	.165 (1.49)	.161 (1.48)	.208 (1.04)	.358 (1.73)	.109 (.53)	.887 (6.91)	.969 (6.94)	.838 (5.96)	.986 (6.86)
	−.355 (−1.50)	−.328 (−1.50)	−.259 (−.60)	.029 (.08)	.718 (1.71)	−1.009 (−3.78)	−.135 (−.54)	.428 (1.53)	.153 (.70)
	55.41 −.008 (−.04)	56.16 −.133 (−.61)	91.89 −.057 (−.14)	113.82 −.064 (−.16)	130.30 −.380 (−.89)	41.30 .059 (.22)	76.97 −.157 (−.59)	91.95 −.228 (−.80)	103.27 −.246 (−.88)
	WHF	HHE	WHF	HHF	HHE	WHF	HHF	HHE	AC

	Heating equipment				Without air conditioning		Climate	
	Regression				Regression			Regression
Type	5.4-3	5.4-8	5.4-11	5.4-14	5.4-4	5.4-15	Variable	5.4-5
Steam	.145	.176	.268	.240	.149 (3.26)	.297 (3.06)	Min temp.	.687 (1.57)
Floor	−.043	−.044	.203	.027			Max temp.	.501 (.70)
Electric	.045	.013	.266	−.275			Degree days	.914 (1.87)
With flue	.066	.031	−.195	.120			Precipitation	−.041 (−.61)
Without flue	.019	.024	−.128	−.020			1:00 A.M. humidity	1.970 (1.38)
Warm-air furnace	.007	−.064	−.030	.085			1:00 P.M. humidity	−2.800 (−1.92)
None	−.239	−.135	−.384	−.177			Wind	−.019 (−.07)
							.01 in. rain	−.205 (−.51)
							1 in. snow	−.877 (−.63)
							Days fog	.077 (.27)
							Max temp. ≥ 90° F.	−.888 (−1.73)
							Max temp. ≤ 32° F.	−.881 (−1.78)
							Min temp. ≤ 32° F.	−1.062 (−1.54)
							Min temp. ≤ 0° F.	−2.313 (−1.88)

and 3.45, respectively). Of the socioeconomic variables, considerable variation was exhibited in the coefficients for both population density and the percentage of poor families. As has generally been true in the above results, coal and "other" heating fuels, as well as steam-heating equipment, were again associated with higher mortality rates. The presence of air conditioning was associated with lower mortality rates. In regression 5.4-5, the climate variables were added to the original regression. There is evidence in the literature that the daily average temperature is related inversely to mortality from cardiovascular disease (Rogot and Blackwelder, 1970). This was borne out by regression 5.4-5. It also appears that lower cardiovascular mortality rates are found in areas having damp climates with extreme temperatures.

For diseases of the heart, both water-heating fuels and home-heating equipment contributed significantly to the explanatory power of the basic regression (regressions 5.4-7 and 5.4-8). The air pollution (Min S) and socioeconomic coefficients exhibited little change from the basic results (see regression 5.1-19); Min S remained statistically significant in both regressions. Again, coal and "other" water-heating fuels were most positively associated with this mortality rate; steam equipment was also positively related.

In regressions 5.4-9, 5.4-10, and 5.4-11, water-heating fuels, home-heating fuels, and home-heating equipment were added to the basic results for nonrheumatic chronic endocarditis and other myocardial degeneration. In general, the addition of the two fuel groups diminished the importance of Min S and Min P; Min S and Min P did not make a significant contribution in the first two regressions but did so in the third ($F = 1.98$, 0.14, and 4.07, respectively). The addition of home-heating equipment had little effect. The socioeconomic coefficients experienced some fluctuations. The most positively related fuel was coal, and the most positively related equipment was steam.

Hypertensive heart disease is examined in regressions 5.4-12 through 5.4-15. The same heating groups that were significant for endocarditis were important for this category. In addition, the air-conditioning variable was significant. In this case, the Max S coefficient remained stable and statistically significant. Only the coefficient representing the proportion of poor families experienced significant change. The same general pattern as that observed for the other cardiovascular disease categories held for the sets of heating variables.

Respiratory disease mortality

Analysis of the respiratory disease mortality rates is presented in table 5.5. The first set of regressions relates to the category of total respiratory diseases (regressions 5.5-1 through 5.5-3). The coefficient of Min P decreased slightly with the addition of the sets of water-heating fuels, climate variables, and water-heating fuels and climate variables together. However, the socioeconomic variables displayed considerably more variation. "Other" water-heating fuels and the absence of water-heating fuels (and presumably hot water) were associated positively with respiratory disease deaths. Measures of rain, snow, and fog were the climate variables of greatest significance; however, their implication was not clear.

Several sets and combinations of sets of heating variables contributed significantly to the regressions pertaining to tuberculosis mortality (regressions 5.5-4 through 5.5-8) The air pollution (Mean P) coefficient remained relatively stable except in the presence of the home-heating fuels; it then lost statistical significance. In the presence of the combination of water-heating fuels and home-heating equipment, Mean P approached statistical significance. At the same time, the socioeconomic variables displayed minor fluctuations across specifications. The same general pattern for the heating variables was seen, although additional variables displayed relatively large, if somewhat unstable, positive coefficients.

Only home-heating fuels contributed significantly to the explanatory power of the regression for asthma (regression 5.5-9); neither the air pollution nor the socioeconomic coefficients exhibited much change from the original results (regression 5.1-29); Mean P remained significant. The lack of home-heating fuel (and presumably home heating) was positively related to the asthma mortality rate. Only the home-heating fuels made a significant contribution to explaining influenza mortality (regression 5.5-10). The air pollution (Mean S) and socioeconomic coefficients were similar to those in the original specification (regression 5.1-31). Coal and "other" fuels were again positively associated with this mortality rate.

For the pneumonia mortality rate, water-heating fuels and the climate variables made significant contributions (regressions 5.5-11 and 5.5-12). The coefficient of the air pollution variable (Min P) remained stable (and nonsignificant), while the socioeconomic coefficients displayed mixed results. "Other" water-heating fuel and the lack of any water-heating fuel were the heating variables most positively associated with pneumonia mortality. In addition, measures of precipitation were significantly related to the mortality rate.

No set of additional variables contributed significantly to the explanatory power of the bronchitis mortality rate equation.

Thus, in general, the additional variables significantly increased the explanatory power of the previous regressions, and their estimated effects had plausible interpretations. The group of home-heating fuels had the most substantial effect in lowering the estimated air pollution elasticities. This may have been because they represented specific air pollution exposures. Nevertheless, taken together, we believe that the air pollution coefficients continue to suggest that air pollution is an important factor to consider in explaining variation among most of these mortality rates.

TABLE 5.5. Respiratory Disease Mortality Rates (the Effects of Home-heating Characteristics and Climate), 1960

	Total respiratory disease			Tuberculosis	
	5.5-1	5.5-2	5.5-3	5.5-4	5.5-5·
R^2	.357	.428	.509	.453	.375
Constant	221.990	637.701	−1269.908	−528.849	−1357.226
Air pollution variables Mean S					
Sum S elasticities Min P	.762 (1.55)	.669 (1.23)	.514 (.97)		
Mean P				1.155 (2.04)	.682 (1.09)
Sum P elasticities	7.64	6.71	5.15	24.95	14.70
Socioeconomic variables P/M²	.007 (.09)	.073 (1.08)	.062 (.89)	.141 (.83)	.327 (1.90)
≥ 65	1.138 (2.12)	1.453 (2.42)	1.738 (2.89)	.779 (.60)	1.545 (1.11)
NW	−.172 (−1.33)	.120 (.77)	.048 (.30)	.159 (.49)	.359 (1.04)
Poor	.196 (.72)	.862 (3.28)	.061 (.18)	1.689 (2.57)	2.210 (3.41)
Sum SE elasticities	24.26	65.68	36.84	73.32	105.95
Log Pop	.657 (2.44)	.596 (2.19)	.863 (3.05)	1.259 (1.91)	1.646 (2.50)
Variables added	WHF	CL	WHF, CL	WHF	HHF

Note: All regressions are based on data for 117 SMSAs. The numbers in parentheses below the regressions coefficients are t statistics.

Abbreviations: AC, without air conditioning; CL, climate; HHE, home-heating equipment; HHF, home-heating fuels; WHF, water-heating fuels.

Scaled regression coefficients for home-heating characteristics and coefficients and t statistics for climate variables:

Water-heating fuel

	Regression					
Type	5.5-1	5.5-3	5.5-4	5.5-7	5.5-8	5.5-11
Gas	−.359	−.409	−.138	−.871	−.167	−.223
Electricity	−.394	−.395	−.359	−1.539	−.757	−.233
Coal	−.258	−.201	.985	.674	1.022	−.261
Bottled gas	−.648	−.495	−1.320	−3.232	−1.375	−.363
Oil	−.228	−.461	.099	−1.051	−.108	−.073
Other	1.344	1.296	.799	5.731	1.313	.680
None	.543	.665	−.066	.288	.071	.473

Home-heating fuel

	Regression			
Type	5.5-5	5.5-7	5.5-9	5.5-10
Gas	−.373	.264	−.096	−.189
Oil	.748	.613	−.043	−.318
Coal	.691	.022	−.132	.213
Electricity	−.673	1.755	.231	−.422
Bottled gas	.311	.608	−.164	.569
Other	−2.127	−3.455	−.870	2.117
None	.676	.193	1.074	−1.971

TABLE 5.5. (Continued)

	Tuberculosis			Asthma	Influenza	Pneumonia	
5.5-6	5.5-7	5.5-8		5.5-9	5.5-10	5.5-11	5.5-12
.400	.573	.550		.193	.420	.277	.375
−589.508	85.693	194.701		253.992	325.927	127.923	−188.527
					.480 (.97) 14.07		
						.466 (1.05)	.499 (1.03)
1.767 (2.98)	.683 (1.23)	1.042 (1.86)		.811 (2.36)			
38.16	14.76	22.52		33.02		6.77	7.24
.162 (.92)	.093 (.58)	.073 (.44)		.015 (.16)	−.116 (−.70)	−.010 (−.15)	.042 (.71)
1.168 (.81)	.873 (.68)	1.568 (1.17)		.876 (1.15)	−1.372 (−1.06)	1.012 (2.08)	1.199 (2.25)
.107 (.32)	.283 (.90)	.309 (1.00)		−.003 (−.01)	−.507 (−1.56)	−.090 (−.77)	.149 (1.07)
1.675 (2.49)	1.695 (2.33)	.567 (.71)		.359 (1.06)	1.814 (3.12)	−.089 (−.36)	.307 (1.31)
77.89	77.17	50.82		47.98	41.75	18.19.	56.76
1.017 (1.53)	1.083 (1.72)	.961 (1.44)		−.197 (−.55)	−.085 (−.14)	.470 (1.93)	.368 (1.51)
HHE	WHF, HHF	WHF, HHE		HHF	HHF	WHF	CL

Home-heating equipment			Climate			
	Regression				Regression	
Type	5.5-6	5.5-8	Variable	5.5-2	5.5-3	5.5-12
Steam	.303	−.361	Min temp.	.638 (.75)	.899 (1.05)	.191 (.25)
Floor	.014	−.547				
Electric	.721	1.261	Max temp.	.171 (.12)	1.075 (.75)	.064 (.05)
With flue	−.353	.070				
Without flue	.054	−.223	Degree days	1.134 (1.20)	1.515 (1.58)	.809 (.96)
Warm-air furnace	−.237	−.512				
None	−.503	.312	Precipitation	.228 (1.73)	.191 (1.30)	.302 (2.57)
			1:00 A.M. humidity	−.199 (−.07)	−.439 (−.16)	−.485 (−.20)
			1:00 P.M. humidity	−4.020 (−1.41)	−1.337 (−.44)	−3.278 (−1.29)
			Wind	.075 (.14)	.322 (.60)	.193 (.40)
			.01 in. rain	−1.972 (−2.63)	−2.557 (−3.13)	−1.783 (−2.67)
			1 in. snow	3.628 (1.35)	5.765 (2.15)	2.576 (1.07)
			Days of fog	1.316 (2.44)	1.133 (2.01)	1.314 (2.74)
			Max temp. ≥ 90° F.	.191 (.19)	−.265 (−.26)	.186 (.21)
			Max temp. ≤ 32° F.	−.516 (−.55)	−.928 (−.83)	−.341 (−.40)
			Min temp. ≤ 32° F.	−2.017 (−1.52)	−2.181 (−1.64)	−1.833 (−1.55)
			Min temp. ≤ 0° F.	−2.826 (−1.18)	−3.868 (−1.49)	−1.985 (−.93)

TABLE 5.6.   The Effects of Adding Air Pollution Measures to Alternative Specifications
Explaining Unadjusted Total Mortality Rates, 1960

Specification	F statistic[a]	Degrees of freedom
Socioeconomic variables	10.58	2 and 109
Socioeconomic and climate variables	4.27	2 and 95
Socioeconomic and occupation-mix variables	4.52	2 and 96
Socioeconomic and home-heating equipment variables	8.42	2 and 103
Socioeconomic and home-heating fuel variables	1.15	2 and 103
Socioeconomic and water-heating fuel variables	6.10	2 and 103
Socioeconomic and air-conditioning variables	8.93	2 and 108

[a] $F_{0.05} = 3.07$, with 2 and 120 degrees of freedom.

THE CONTRIBUTION OF AIR POLLUTION

Adding sets of variables representing occupation mix, climate, home-heating equipment, home-heating fuels, and water-heating fuels to the original regressions (containing air pollution and socioeconomic variables) raises analytical problems. For example, if all the variables were added simultaneously, multicollinearity is certain to reduce the precision of the estimate. Even when only one subset is added, interpreting the results is difficult because the variables tend to reflect many of the same aspects of the underlying socioeconomic structure of the areas. In an attempt to investigate these problems, further analysis was undertaken. The questions to be answered are, Under what conditions do the air pollution variables make significant contributions to the explanatory power of the regressions, and under what conditions do the additional sets of variables make significant contributions to the explanatory power of the regressions?

To test whether the air pollution variables or the other sets of variables made statistically significant contributions to the explanatory power of various specifications for the unadjusted total mortality rate, we performed a series of F tests. Tables 5.6 and 5.7 report the specific results of these tests. Table 5.6 displays the effects of combining the two air pollution measures (Min S and Mean P) with regressions containing (1) socioeconomic variables only; (2) socioeconomic and climate variables; (3) socioeconomic and occupation-mix variables; (4) socioeconomic and home-heating equipment variables; (5) socioeconomic and home-heating fuel variables; (6) socioeconomic and water-heating fuel variables; and (7) socioeconomic and air-conditioning variables. Since $F_{0.05} = 3.07$, with 2 and 120 degrees of freedom, it can be seen that the air-pollution variables made statistically significant contributions to all the specifications except for the one that included the home-heating fuel variables.

TABLE 5.7.   The Effects of Adding Sets of Variables to a Basic Specification Explaining Unadjusted Total Mortality Rates, 1960

Additional set	F statistic	Degrees of freedom
Occupation-mix variables	8.82	13 and 96
Climate variables	2.30	14 and 95
Water-heating fuel variables	12.63	6 and 103
Home-heating equipment variables	5.83	6 and 103
Home-heating fuel variables	7.70	6 and 103

Note: The F statistics indicate that each additional set contributed significantly to the basic specification containing Min S, Mean P, and the five socioeconomic variables.

Table 5.7 presents analogous results for adding sets of variables to regressions containing the two air pollution measures and the five socioeconomic variables. The additional sets were (1) occupation-mix variables; (2) climate variables; (3) water-heating fuel variables; (4) home-heating equipment variables; and (5) home-heating fuel variables. Each set of variables made a statistically significant contribution to the basic regression.

More important than individual significance tests or the coefficients corresponding to the new variables is the change in the estimated coefficients of the air pollution measures when the new variables were added. Table 5.8 shows the summed elasticities of the three sulfate variables, the three suspended particulate variables, and four of the socioeconomic variables (excluding Log Pop). These elasticities are shown for a number of mortality rates, each with nine specifications. The first is with air pollution and socioeconomic variables only. Then the five sets of variables (climate, occupation, home-heating equipment, home-heating fuel, and water-heating fuels) were added, one at a time. Specification 7 adds climate and occupation variables to the basic regression; to this, specification 8 adds home-heating equipment. Finally, all of the groups, including the prevalence of air conditioning, are present in specification 9.

For the unadjusted total mortality rate, the sulfate elasticities (Sum S elasticities) dropped by two-thirds, going from specification 1 to 2, and then remained relatively stable through specification 6, finally losing all importance in specifications 7 through 9. Thus, the sulfate elasticities appeared to be sensitive to the specifications, implying either that an important variable was omitted in the original regression or that multicollinearity among the explanatory variables was a serious difficulty. The sum of suspended particulate elasticities (Sum P elasticities) were far more stable over the range of specifications, except for specification 5 in which the home-heating fuels were introduced. The robustness of these estimated elasticities across changing specifications lends confidence to our results.

TABLE 5.8. The Effects of Climate, Occupation, and Home-heating Characteristics on Mortality Rates (Alternative Specifications), 1960

Specification no.	1	2	3	4	5	6	7	8	9
Unadjusted total mortality									
Sum S elasticities	5.04	1.71	1.03	2.21	2.54	3.33	.32	-.29	-1.17
Sum P elasticities	4.37	5.24	4.34	6.03	.61	2.44	2.52	3.44	3.07
Sum SE elasticities	70.07	72.93	56.05	63.67	66.25	56.19	61.57	56.89	49.11
Age–sex–race-adjusted total mortality									
Sum S elasticities	5.71	2.22	2.10	3.10	3.08	4.10	1.23	.71	-.52
Sum P elasticities	3.97	5.07	4.08	5.80	1.37	2.57	2.13	2.88	2.56
Sum SE elasticities	6.80	8.21	-3.18	.34	4.36	-4.85	2.18	-3.00	-6.15
Race-adjusted infant mortality									
Sum S elasticities	1.70	1.90	2.27	1.48	2.00	1.74	3.58	2.53	2.53
Sum P elasticities	10.94	7.39	9.28	13.76	10.12	11.46	7.02	9.07	8.88
Sum SE elasticities	8.90	10.83	5.48	3.21	7.24	12.89	11.56	11.48	19.93
All cancers									
Sum S elasticities	6.02	2.64	1.47	3.04	3.75	4.47	.40	-.24	-1.15
Sum P elasticities	1.89	6.20	.86	5.21	-.42	1.80	3.58	5.00	3.18
Sum SE elasticities	73.51	70.35	64.35	65.76	73.60	64.61	56.80	51.90	54.60
Buccal and pharyngeal cancers									
Sum S elasticities	1.54	-5.23	-8.34	-4.00	-3.14	-5.70	-11.93	-12.49	-17.78
Sum P elasticities	-2.94	3.98	1.99	4.85	-3.20	3.12	5.00	9.09	15.01
Sum SE elasticities	117.92	107.88	80.24	93.04	108.23	76.05	72.33	67.30	42.38
Digestive cancers									
Sum S elasticities	10.14	5.24	1.97	2.59	5.67	6.70	1.66	.51	1.48
Sum P elasticities	5.11	8.96	6.01	12.22	2.58	5.77	6.57	10.04	7.05
Sum SE elasticities	82.24	81.16	56.31	64.62	73.19	61.82	52.31	47.40	56.19
Respiratory cancers									
Sum S elasticities	5.40	2.97	4.39	7.30	6.19	7.91	.87	-.10	-2.39
Sum P elasticities	-6.71	1.33	-12.47	-2.38	-6.86	-7.45	-3.37	-3.80	-2.96
Sum SE elasticities	79.63	77.22	82.58	75.64	90.77	95.53	62.72	54.33	77.19
Breast cancers									
Sum S elasticities	5.83	1.23	3.85	2.30	3.18	.20	.02	-.29	-2.43
Sum P elasticities	.54	8.95	.28	2.83	.94	4.58	9.68	11.29	11.11
Sum SE elasticities	51.70	44.90	37.73	43.06	55.20	37.97	24.97	21.65	.62
All cardiovascular disease									
Sum S elasticities	11.16	4.81	4.09	6.81	7.10	8.31	2.33	1.54	.78
Sum P elasticities	.87	4.90	1.69	2.70	-3.77	-.97	1.79	1.56	2.15
Sum SE elasticities	86.70	88.36	70.98	78.47	82.50	68.04	71.19	66.83	49.62
Heart disease									
Sum S elasticities	17.30	8.30	9.42	9.80	10.54	9.34	4.02	2.66	1.34
Sum P elasticities	-2.60	7.36	-3.25	5.16	-2.71	5.50	3.95	2.54	5.11
Sum SE elasticities	83.72	74.25	69.69	60.80	81.37	62.20	63.10	68.72	60.19

	1	2	3	4	5	6	7	8	9
Endocarditis									
Sum S elasticities	31.95	28.52	34.64	26.58	23.38	32.11	21.92	17.74	24.09
Sum P elasticities	25.26	31.42	27.29	24.50	.31	9.70	29.01	21.48	6.54
Sum SE elasticities	147.08	133.26	111.61	141.67	111.21	103.72	87.27	94.17	44.33
Hypertensive disease									
Sum S elasticities	26.01	14.67	16.47	18.51	17.94	20.79	12.07	11.19	7.66
Sum P elasticities	5.70	14.42	7.75	8.21	-3.19	-3.05	9.58	5.66	.00
Sum SE elasticities	99.71	92.34	86.58	88.47	78.19	38.09	72.57	70.65	23.08
All respiratory disease									
Sum S elasticities	1.04	.42	-1.75	-1.76	-1.33	-4.36	1.05	1.54	.50
Sum P elasticities	9.11	9.03	8.39	16.42	10.84	12.25	4.50	7.91	4.91
Sum SE elasticities	56.82	63.75	27.15	36.23	56.45	27.03	50.03	43.62	19.80
Tuberculosis									
Sum S elasticities	-8.93	-15.97	-26.16	-17.76	-16.78	-13.94	-27.13	-29.83	-25.70
Sum P elasticities	45.57	33.62	47.08	55.25	24.08	35.73	28.43	33.74	13.14
Sum SE elasticities	108.99	125.83	63.63	82.50	123.89	81.55	54.42	48.31	83.43
Asthma									
Sum S elasticities	-30.52	-34.90	-31.38	-32.63	-34.64	-32.17	-32.41	-28.37	-31.27
Sum P elasticities	59.14	65.64	64.07	64.64	64.72	68.02	61.80	56.53	39.85
Sum SE elasticities	64.42	61.86	23.04	50.68	76.27	64.53	43.51	71.59	76.72
Influenza									
Sum S elasticities	20.61	13.92	8.72	23.01	21.98	30.10	21.05	22.06	29.33
Sum P elasticities	-9.95	-8.23	-10.52	-31.59	-35.51	-32.13	-33.17	-44.86	-46.14
Sum SE elasticities	66.89	97.88	141.63	107.98	24.82	17.37	211.92	189.57	29.60
Pneumonia									
Sum S elasticities	5.32	6.60	5.39	2.86	3.90	-2.35	8.28	8.83	6.51
Sum P elasticities	-.52	1.48	-2.89	10.12	7.65	7.55	-2.37	2.98	5.42
Sum SE elasticities	48.51	50.26	12.26	20.40	48.05	17.68	35.44	29.07	5.85
Bronchitis									
Sum S elasticities	-22.92	-20.43	-19.58	-24.49	-28.64	-25.22	-18.39	-17.23	-22.25
Sum P elasticities	19.20	7.90	28.20	20.55	23.95	15.87	25.53	31.41	10.75
Sum SE elasticities	22.51	53.04	-19.84	18.65	34.10	-7.46	6.69	-21.17	-27.95

Note: All estimates are based on data for 117 SMSAs. Each specification included the six air pollution measures and the five socioeconomic variables. In addition, the following sets of variables were added:

Specification no.	Variables
1	None
2	14 Climate (CL)
3	13 Occupation (Occ)
4	6 Home-heating equipment (HHE)
5	6 Home-heating fuels (HHF)
6	6 Water-heating fuels (WHF)
7	CL and Occ
8	CL, Occ, HHE
9	CL, Occ, HHE, HHF, WHF, without air conditioning

Again, the population variable is excluded from the summed socioeconomic elasticities.

105

It should also be noted that the socioeconomic elasticities (Sum SE elasticities) were relatively stable across specifications.

For the age–sex–race-adjusted total mortality rate, the suspended particulate elasticities continued to remain stable across specifications, and the sulfate elasticities also displayed more stability. On the other hand, the elasticities for the four socioeconomic variables exhibited a great deal of variation. Presumably this was because the adjusted mortality rate directly incorporated specific socioeconomic characteristics.

Both sets of air pollution elasticities, as well as the socioeconomic elasticities, were relatively stable across specifications for the race-adjusted infant death rate. For the disease-specific mortality rates, the stability of the elasticities varied with the individual disease under consideration. We hypothesized that all of the air pollution elasticities in table 5.8 would be positive and of plausible magnitude. In addition, table 5.8 was designed to show the sensitivity of the elasticities under changing specifications. It is disturbing that some of the air pollution elasticities are almost consistently negative across specifications for certain disease-specific mortality rates.[8] This would imply that either air pollution (as measured by suspended particulates or sulfates) was beneficial for the disease in question or that uncontrolled factors (such as migration) were giving rise to spurious negative partial correlations between the air pollution variables and the individual disease-specific mortality rates. We reject the first possibility.

If the air pollution–mortality relationship were random, one would expect to see as many negative as positive elasticities. Instead, positive elasticities predominate. In addition, multicollinearity will give rise to large, standard errors for the estimated coefficients and lead one to distrust any single coefficient. The sum of sulfate and suspended particulate elasticities are nearly always positive, and negative elasticities are rarely significant. While there are individual contrary results, we believe that, taken as a whole, the results presented in table 5.8 support our previous findings.

CONCLUSION

To explore further the hypothesis that there is a causal relationship between our measures of air pollution and mortality, we added additional sets of explanatory variables to the original estimated relationships for each of the mortality rates. The new variables characterized the occupation mix (including its unemployment rate); distribution of home-heating equipment; home-heating and water-heating fuels; prevalence of air conditioning; and climate in the SMSA.

---

[8] We attribute the scattering of minus signs to sampling variability and problems of multicollinearity. The cases where the coefficients are almost consistently negative occur for mortality rates where sampling variability is high because of the low mortality rate.

Earlier we discussed the general problems associated with our attempt to prove causation and with the quality of available information on air pollution exposure rates, causes of death, and other relevant factors. Adding a large number of additional explanatory variables—particularly when they are correlated with air pollution (and other previously included variables)—is likely to change both the magnitude and statistical significance of some of the estimated coefficients. Thus, if the reestimated effects of air pollution on mortality were generally similar to the previous results, those results would be generally confirmed.

Although the additional sets of variables generally lowered the magnitudes of the air pollution coefficients and almost invariably decreased their statistical significance, this was not entirely unexpected since many of the variables were likely to represent specific types of air pollution exposure. At the same time, the results were not consistent with the hypothesis that occupation-mix or home-heating variables were the "true" causes of mortality and that our previously estimated associations were due to the air pollution variables acting as surrogates for these variables. If this were true, we would have expected that regressions incorporating the so-called true causes would have not only eliminated the statistical significance of the air pollution variables, but also reduced their estimated coefficients to approximately zero.[9] Thus, incorporating the additional variables did not disprove the previously estimated associations between our measures of air pollution and the various mortality rates we have examined. We view the results of this chapter as giving a *qualified* endorsement to the hypothesis of causality.

[9] This is not to argue that occupation mix and home-heating characteristics do not exert an important, independent influence.

CHAPTER 6

Suicides, venereal disease, and crime rates, 1960 and 1961

Like most scientists, epidemiologists are extremely suspicious of associations based on nonexperimental data. The price of tea in China may be highly correlated with the price of eggs in Paris, but they are obviously not causally related. Although caution is required in interpreting statistical estimates based on nonexperimental data, there is often no alternative to using such data, as we have argued in the introductory chapters.

We have found air pollution (as measured by sulfates and suspended particulates) to be an important determinant of mortality rates, even when we controlled statistically for many other factors thought to be related to health status. While this supports the view that air pollution is a significant factor affecting health, a critic might still reserve judgment on the grounds that some factors remain unmeasured and others are measured inadequately.

Another method for testing the validity of our observed relationship was suggested to us by Robert Dorfman. Some of the same factors that influence mortality also affect other social ills. Dorfman suggested that we analyze social ills affected by the same factors as mortality but not caused by air pollution. Consequently, we analyzed rates for suicide, venereal disease, and various crimes, hypothesizing that they were associated with urbanization in particular and thus with many of the same variables included in our original equation explaining the mortality rate. If unmeasured factors were responsible for the significance of the air pollution variables in explaining the previously analyzed mortality rates, it seems plausible that the same unmeasured factors might cause the air pollution variables to be significant in explaining suicides, venereal disease, and crime rates. Since we presume that air pollution does not cause these social ills, its significance in an estimated relation can be taken as an indication that it

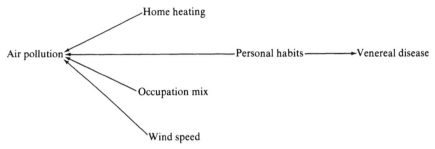

FIG. 6.1. Path analysis of the air pollution-venereal disease model.

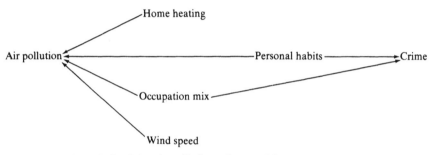

FIG. 6.2. Path analysis of the air pollution-crime model.

is acting as surrogate for omitted factors.[1] The essential question is whether air pollution will be a significant, consistent explanatory factor for these other social ills when we employ the methods previously used to relate air pollution to mortality.

A path analysis similar to figure 1.1 will help to clarify our hypothesis. Figures 6.1 and 6.2 represent path analyses for venereal disease and crime, respectively. The factors associated with air pollution in these two path analyses are the same as those shown in figure 1.1. Of these, the only one hypothesized to cause venereal disease, is the personal-habits factor; both personal habits and occupation mix are assumed to be causally related to crime.[2]

Personal habits and other factors are unmeasured or measured inadequately in our data. Since many of these factors may be systematically related to air pollution levels, measurement difficulties could give spurious significance to the estimated effects of air pollution on mortality, even

[1] We do admit the possibility that highly polluted days might have a depressing influence on people, which in turn could affect suicide rates. In this context, it should be noted that the most significant pollution variable associated with suicides was the maximum suspended particulate measure (table 6.1).

[2] The personal-habits category includes aspects of life-style (for example, apartment rather than a single-family dwelling), and occupation mix represents unemployment, income levels, and undesirable jobs. Many additional causal hypotheses can be offered; for simplicity, we have restricted the models.

when variables representing these factors are included explicitly in the analysis. The following analysis of these social ills should test this possibility.

SUICIDES

We first analyzed the suicide rate across the same 117 SMSAs in our study of air pollution and total mortality. Our method was the same as that used for the original regressions, estimating two equations for the 1960 suicide rates (the first containing all six air pollution measures, the second excluding nonsignificant pollution variables) and then reestimating the reduced equation with 1961 data. The results are presented in table 6.1; the three regressions pertaining to total mortality are included for comparison.

In regression 6.1-4, using all six pollution measures, the most significant pollution variable was maximum suspended particulates. In regression 6.1-5, the nonsignificant air pollution variables were dropped and the coefficient of Max P decreased and lost significance. If our measures of air pollution were associated with the suicide rate, their effects were probably not very important.[3] F tests showed that all six air pollution variables made statistically significant contributions to the regression in 1960 ($F = 2.31$) but not in 1961 ($F = 0.74$).[4] None of the socioeconomic variables was statistically significant. The 1961 reestimation (regression 6.1-6) showed similar results. The air pollution variable (Max P) became even less important, and the socioeconomic variables remained nonsignificant.

VENEREAL DISEASE

Next, we looked at rates for venereal disease. We obtained data from the Center for Disease Control (CDC) on three classifications of venereal disease for 1960 and 1961—primary and secondary syphilis, all stages of syphilis, and gonorrhea.

Several data problems were encountered. Some incidence data are reported by central city and some by county; some data are for fiscal years and some for calendar years. In addition, many cases go unreported.[5] The importance of the reporting unit is exemplified by the fact that incidence rates for counties are lower than those for central cities. To impose some consistency on the data, we assumed that all cases of venereal disease

---

[3] Before dismissing the association completely, one should note that suicides are a relatively rare cause of death (approximately 1 per 10,000 deaths); hence, sampling variability may contribute to the nonsignificance of the air pollution coefficients.

[4] The 1961 reestimation with six air pollution variables is not shown in table 6.1.

[5] Klarman (1965, p. 385) has estimated that only about 9–16 percent of primary and secondary cases of syphilis are reported each year and that the procedures utilized by the Center for Disease Control infer the remaining number of cases (probably only 40 to 60 percent of the actual number).

TABLE 6.1. Comparison of Unadjusted Total Mortality and Suicide Rates, 1960 and 1961

	Total			Suicide		
	1960		1961		1960	1961
	6.1-1	6.1-2	6.1-3	6.1-4	6.1-5	6.1-6
R^2	.831	.828	.823	.164	.066	.055
Constant	343.381	301.205	379.633	96.797	127.058	74.832
Air pollution variables						
Min S	.473 (1.67)	.631 (2.71)	.456 (1.87)	−.015 (−.11)		
Mean S	.173 (.53)			−.196 (−1.22)		
Max S	.028 (.25)			−.025 (−.45)		
Sum S elasticities	5.04	3.27	2.42	−24.31		
Min P	.199 (.32)			.305 (1.00)		
Mean P	.303 (.71)	.452 (2.67)	.516 (2.90)	−.266 (−1.27)		
Max P	−.018 (−.19)			.126 (2.58)	.031 (1.23)	.015 (.58)
Sum P elasticities	4.37	5.85	6.56	15.33	7.71	3.84
Socioeconomic variables						
P/M²	.083 (1.54)	.089 (1.71)	.125 (2.35)	.000 (.01)	−.026 (−1.03)	−.034 (−1.29)
≥65	6.880 (16.63)	7.028 (18.09)	7.057 (17.59)	.221 (1.08)	.016 (.08)	.070 (.35)
NW	.396 (3.82)	.422 (4.32)	.342 (3.40)	−.036 (−.70)	−.045 (−.91)	−.045 (−.89)
Poor	.038 (.26)	−.002 (−.02)	−.048 (−.31)	−.079 (−1.07)	−.044 (−.60)	−.030 (−.37)
Sum SE elasticities	70.07	71.03	71.39	−.16	−13.17	−7.21
Log Pop	−.276 (−1.38)	−.212 (−1.12)	−.360 (−1.90)	.034 (.35)	−.026 (−.28)	.055 (.57)

Note: All regressions are based on data for 117 SMSAs. The numbers in parentheses below the regression coefficients are t statistics.

111

occurred in the central city; consequently, we assumed that the population at risk was the city population (even where cases were reported for the county). This assumption made the rates more uniform. To account for the various inconsistencies in reporting, we defined dummy variables (DV) for the area reporting and the period reported. For example, dummy variable one (DV_1) assumed a value of one if the cases were reported for the county, and a value of zero if they were not. The dummy variables were inserted in all of the venereal disease regressions.[6]

The procedure for investigating the venereal disease rates was similar to that used in the previous analyses; all six air pollution variables were included in the first regression, and then the least significant ones and those with negative coefficients were excluded.

In table 6.2, regression 6.2-1 shows the 1960 results for primary and secondary syphilis. The air pollution variable with the most significant positive coefficient was the maximum sulfate measure (it was not quite statistically significant). The most statistically significant socioeconomic variable was the percentage of nonwhites in the population; it was positively associated with this syphilis rate. After we eliminated the least significant air pollution variables, the maximum sulfate measure became statistically nonsignificant, but the percentage of nonwhites in the SMSA remained statistically significant (regression 6.2-2). In the 1961 reestimation (regression 6.2-3), the air pollution variable continued to be statistically nonsignificant; two additional socioeconomic variables, the proportion of poor families in the area and Log Pop, were statistically significant in explaining the 1961 primary and secondary syphilis rates. The most statistically significant dummy variables indicated that incidence rates by counties were higher than rates reported by cities (DV_1) and that areas reporting county data in 1960 and city data in 1961 had relatively lower rates (DV_3). F tests indicated that the addition of the six air pollution variables did not contribute significantly to the regressions in either 1960 ($F = 1.06$) or 1961 ($F = 0.65$).

The estimates for all stages of syphilis follow a pattern similar to those for primary and secondary stages. For 1960 (regression 6.2-4), the minimum sulfate reading was the most important air pollution variable (it was not statistically significant); the most statistically significant socioeconomic variable was again the percentage of nonwhites in the population, and DV_1 and DV_3 were again the most statistically significant dummy variables. In the second-round estimation (regression 6.2-5), minimum sulfates and Log Pop attained statistical significance; the previously significant coefficients remained so. However, in the 1961 replication (regression 6.2-6), the minimum sulfate measure was statistically nonsignificant while the two

---

[6] For definitions of the remaining dummy variables, see table D.7, page 332. Note that some of the dummy variables, particularly DV_4 and DV_6, represent few observations.

socioeconomic variables and DV_1 retained their significance. The addition of all six pollution variables did not contribute significantly to either the 1960 ($F = 1.22$) or 1961 ($F = 1.40$) regressions.

Regression 6.2-7 reports the initial 1960 results for gonorrhea. The most significant (positively related) air pollution variable was the mean sulfate reading (it was not statistically significant). The percentage of nonwhites and Log Pop were the significant socioeconomic variables. When the other air pollution variables were dropped in regression 6.2-8, the coefficient for Mean S became negative and remained statistically nonsignificant; both socioeconomic variables remained significant. In the 1961 reestimation (regression 6.2-9), the air pollution variable remained negative and statistically nonsignificant, while both socioeconomic variables remained significant. None of the dummy variables ever attained statistical significance in these regressions. The addition of all six air pollution variables did not contribute significantly to either the 1960 ($F = 1.68$) or 1961 ($F = 0.90$) regressions.

Thus, no air pollution variable was statistically significant in both the second-round 1960 regression and its 1961 replication. In addition, the six air pollution measures taken together never contributed significantly to explaining any of the venereal disease rates. The socioeconomic variables, however, displayed more consistent results. Note that the 1961 replication played an important role in ruling out some of the ad hoc results found for the 1960 data. This result would tend to lend confidence to the 1961 replications of the 1960 mortality-rate analyses.

CRIME RATES

Finally, we examined rates for criminal offenses occurring in 114 SMSAs,[7] hypothesizing that air pollution would not be associated with these rates across areas of the country. The approach used for these rates was similar to that used above, except that a replication using 1961 data was not undertaken.

The only crime rate we discuss in detail is for total offenses in the SMSA. The initial result of regressing the total crime rate on all the air pollution and socioeconomic variables is shown in regression 6.3-1. The most significant, positively related pollution variable was the maximum suspended particulate level (it was statistically nonsignificant). When four of the six air pollution measures were eliminated in regression 6.3-2, the coefficient of Max P became negative and continued to be nonsignificant. Log Pop was statistically significant in both regressions, indicating that crime rates were higher in more populated SMSAs. In addition, the coefficient for the variable representing the percentage of those sixty-five and older was negative and significant in the second regression. This would suggest

[7] Crime rate data were unavailable for Bridgeport, Orlando, and Salt Lake City.

TABLE 6.2. Venereal Disease Rates, 1960 and 1961

| | Primary- and secondary-stage syphilis | | | All stages of syphilis | | | Gonorrhea | | |
| | 1960 | | 1961 | 1960 | | 1961 | 1960 | | 1961 |
	6.2-1	6.2-2	6.2-3	6.2-4	6.2-5	6.2-6	6.2-7	6.2-8	6.2-9
R^2	.380	.341	.423	.433	.419	.413	.478	.432	.395
Constant	−405.265	−448.571	−1006.996	−153.474	−190.163	−342.143	−602.157	−648.560	−848.634
Air pollution variables									
Min S	1.163 (1.35)			.418 (1.32)	.545 (2.22)	.339 (1.36)			
Mean S	−1.731 (−1.79)			−.014 (−.04)			1.180 (1.23)	−.460 (−1.10)	−.305 (−.79)
Max S	.615 (1.83)	−.020 (−.12)	−.044 (−.25)	.071 (.57)			−.755 (−2.26)		
Sum S elasticities	15.92	−3.20	−5.20	32.45	24.21	14.04	−44.05	−17.37	−11.29
Min P	1.058 (.56)			.609 (.88)			1.495 (.79)		
Mean P	−.645 (−.49)			−.237 (−.49)			−.102 (−.08)		
Max P	−.152 (−.51)			.038 (.35)			.102 (.35)		
Sum P elasticities	−47.69			9.35			31.49		
Socioeconomic variables									
P/M²	−.023 (−.15)	−.044 (−.30)	−.059 (−.37)	−.073 (−1.26)	−.072 (−1.28)	.004 (.01)	−.064 (−.40)	−.052 (−.34)	−.112 (−.75)
≥65	−.508 (−.38)	−.402 (−.32)	.154 (.11)	.495 (1.00)	.487 (1.07)	.376 (.80)	−.363 (−.27)	−.250 (−.20)	.330 (.26)

NW	1.095 (3.41)	1.075 (3.54)	1.381 (4.13)	.553 (4.68)	.550 (5.04)	.523 (4.62)	1.333 (4.17)	1.467 (4.81)	1.423 (4.67)
Poor	.725 (1.48)	.716 (1.48)	1.105 (1.97)	.098 (.54)	.078 (.45)	.169 (.89)	.052 (.11)	−.016 (−.03)	−.379 (−.74)
Sum SE elasticities	155.30	157.53	186.13	115.77	111.66	110.26	53.31	58.89	48.31
Log Pop	1.016 (1.67)	.691 (1.24)	1.255 (2.01)	.328 (1.47)	.420 (2.09)	.457 (2.25)	1.301 (2.16)	1.650 (2.92)	1.797 (3.16)
Dummy variables[a]									
DV_1	−95.939 (−1.78)	−107.723 (−2.07)	−129.645 (−2.29)	−52.629 (−2.66)	−52.958 (−2.77)	−50.983 (−2.64)	−4.647 (−.09)	3.901 (.07)	32.863 (.64)
DV_2	188.442 (1.50)	152.831 (1.23)	141.242 (1.05)	−5.207 (−.11)	.889 (.02)	37.351 (.82)	−1.593 (−.01)	50.401 (.40)	70.724 (.58)
DV_3	−195.949 (−1.77)	−204.693 (−1.88)		−88.036 (−2.16)	−86.743 (−2.21)		−137.144 (−1.24)	−85.239 (−.78)	
DV_4	−174.229 (−.75)	14.957 (.07)		−75.252 (−.88)	−67.217 (−.88)		28.912 (.12)	−131.344 (−.62)	
DV_5			175.062 (1.48)			72.052 (1.81)			−7.693 (−.07)
DV_6			−24.385 (−.11)			32.150 (.42)			66.456 (.32)

Note: All regressions are based on data for 117 SMSAs. The numbers in parentheses below the regression coefficients are *t* statistics.

[a] The dummy variables are defined in table D.7, page 332.

that areas with a high percentage of older persons had relatively low crime rates.

Seven subclassifications of crimes were examined: murder and nonnegligent manslaughter (regressions 6.3-3 and 6.3-4), forcible rape (regressions 6.3-5 and 6.3-6), robbery (regressions 6.3-7 and 6.3-8), aggravated assault (regressions 6.3-9 and 6.3-10), burglary (regressions 6.3-11 and 6.3-12), larceny—fifty dollars and over (regressions 6.3-13 and 6.3-14), and auto theft (regressions 6.3-15 and 6.3-16). The results for these crime rates were similar to the results for the aggregate category. In no regression was there a positive, statistically significant air pollution coefficient.[8] The socioeconomic variable had consistent, often significant coefficients. Population density was never statistically significant; the percentage of persons sixty-five and older was almost invariably negative and often statistically significant; the nonwhite variable was positive for seven of the eight categories and often statistically significant; the percentage of poor families was often positive (and particularly significant in explaining manslaughter and homicides); while Log Pop was always positive and often statistically significant. To test the contributions of the air pollution variables, we performed a series of F tests. The F statistics for testing the addition of the six pollution variables to crime rate regressions in which only the five socioeconomic variables were initially included, were as follows: total, 2.11; murder and nonnegligent manslaughter, 1.11; forcible rape, 1.05; robbery, 1.27; aggravated assault, 0.36; burglary, 2.37; larceny (fifty dollars and over), 0.88; auto theft, 2.51; all with 6 and 102 degrees of freedom. Since $F_{0.05} = 2.18$, with 6 and 120 degrees of freedom, it can be seen that in the only cases for which the contribution of the air pollution variables was significant (burglary and auto theft), the relationship was negative.

CONCLUSION

In a further effort to determine whether omitted factors or other difficulties with the data may have been responsible for the observed association between both sulfates and suspended particulates, and mortality, we examined the variation in suicide rates, three venereal disease rates, and eight crime rates across the SMSAs. It was hypothesized that such ills are associated with many of the urban factors considered earlier and that they should be amenable to the type of analysis performed for the mortality rates. Since it can be reasonably assumed that sulfates and suspended particulates do not cause these social ills, we further hypothesized that air pollution would not be an important explanatory factor.

This type of analysis is not conclusive. Errors of observation charac-

---

[8] Mean P approached statistical significance in regression 6.3-3; however, it became totally nonsignificant in regression 6.3-4.

TABLE 6.3. Crime Rates, 1960

	Total offenses		Murder and nonnegligent manslaughter		Forcible rape		Robbery	
	6.3-1	6.3-2	6.3-3	6.3-4	6.3-5	6.3-6	6.3-7	6.3-8
R^2	.372	.295	.717	.699	.248	.203	.407	.365
Constant	−11897.610	−11844.237	−21.230	−20.565	−72.704	−80.170	−2747.103	−2509.140
Air pollution variables								
Min S	−30.661 (−1.69)		−.095 (−.96)		−.245 (−1.17)		.579 (.40)	
Mean S	4.318 (.21)		.008 (.07)		−.020 (−.08)		−1.102 (−.65)	
Max S	−11.542 (−1.60)		−.030 (−.74)		−.068 (−.81)		−.513 (−.88)	
Sum S elasticities	−31.12		−18.61		−35.19		−41.55	
Min P	9.914 (.26)		−.329 (−1.55)		.142 (.32)		.857 (.28)	
Mean P	4.338 (.16)		.262 (1.80)	.030 (.52)	.219 (.71)	.045 (.38)	1.992 (.94)	.500 (.60)
Max P	3.061 (.49)		−.023 (−.67)		−.017 (−.24)		−.128 (−.26)	
Sum P elasticities	15.30		17.75	6.29	33.64	6.42	50.02	12.31
Socioeconomic variables								
P/M²	.537 (.16)	−2.327 (−.73)	.002 (.10)	−.007 (−.41)	−.038 (−.98)	−.058 (−1.61)	−.255 (−.95)	−.307 (−1.21)
≥65	−30.164 (−1.16)	−60.245 (−2.47)	−.289 (−2.02)	−.403 (−3.14)	−.308 (−1.02)	−.522 (−1.93)	.340 (.16)	−.835 (−.44)
NW	10.933 (1.68)	9.182 (1.45)	.213 (5.96)	.194 (5.73)	.124 (1.64)	.110 (1.55)	1.369 (2.61)	1.267 (2.55)
Poor	4.845 (.52)	8.790 (.94)	.167 (3.25)	.192 (3.85)	−.084 (−.78)	−.060 (−.57)	−.705 (−.94)	−.484 (−.66)
Sum SE elasticities	−1.96	−20.94	59.57	44.85	−34.08	−54.22	11.36	−4.13
Log Pop	45.456 (3.63)	46.834 (3.97)	.078 (1.14)	.085 (1.32)	.327 (2.26)	.358 (2.64)	5.538 (5.52)	5.217 (5.53)

(Continued)

117

TABLE 6.3. (Continued)

	Aggravated assault		Burglary		Larceny ($50 and over)		Auto theft	
	6.3-9	6.3-10	6.3-11	6.3-12	6.3-13	6.3-14	6.3-15	6.3-16
R^2	.358	.344	.308	.217	.173	.130	.383	.297
Constant	−945.463	−1059.022	−3528.735	−2981.914	−877.180	−1163.207	−3706.590	−4153.409
Air pollution variables								
Min S	−.696 (−.26)		−14.369 (−1.51)		−6.951 (−1.22)		−8.886 (−2.31)	
Mean S	3.360 (1.07)	−.084 (−.06)	−2.717 (−.25)		1.873 (.28)		2.915 (.65)	
Max S	−1.362 (−1.25)		−4.709 (−1.24)		−2.118 (−.93)		−2.744 (−1.79)	
Sum S elasticities	−.84	−1.09	−37.40		−21.63		−37.01	
Min P	−2.063 (−.35)		−3.562 (−.17)		11.224 (.92)	−.549 (−.08)	3.626 (.44)	
Mean P	.838 (.21)		3.445 (.25)		−6.818 (−.82)		4.411 (.79)	1.971 (.87)
Max P	−.225 (−.24)		1.460 (.45)	−1.382 (−.83)	1.778 (.91)		.214 (.16)	
Sum P elasticities	−7.17		11.81	−6.88	6.37	−.87	36.71	11.49
Socioeconomic variables								
P/M²	−.051 (−.10)	.086 (.18)	.067 (.04)	−1.811 (−1.07)	−.137 (−.13)	−.714 (−.73)	.949 (1.33)	.398 (.58)
≥65	−9.333 (−2.39)	−8.392 (−2.44)	−3.806 (−.28)	−21.873 (−1.70)	−7.752 (−.95)	−11.559 (−1.62)	−9.016 (−1.63)	−14.658 (−2.85)
NW	1.927 (1.97)	2.199 (2.50)	6.143 (1.79)	4.663 (1.39)	1.413 (.69)	1.741 (.94)	−.255 (−.18)	−.437 (−.32)
Poor	2.079 (1.48)	1.880 (1.40)	2.956 (.60)	5.833 (1.18)	−.532 (−.18)	−.399 (−.14)	.964 (.48)	1.481 (.74)
Sum SE elasticities	−21.29	−10.11	18.42	−5.75	−20.03	−30.24	−26.82	−48.46
Log Pop	3.439 (1.83)	3.392 (1.97)	16.501 (2.51)	16.057 (2.57)	8.449 (2.15)	8.741 (2.39)	11.126 (4.19)	12.270 (4.77)

Note: All regressions are based on data for 114 SMSAs (see table C.1, pp. 317–320). The numbers in parentheses below the regression coefficients are t statistics.

118

terize all of the dependent variables, especially those for venereal disease.[9] Furthermore, as noted above, the suicide rate was quite small and subject to considerable sampling variability. Nevertheless, following a procedure similar to that used for the mortality rates, we found that the sulfate and suspended particulate measures were not consistent, significant explanatory variables for these social ills; whereas, in general, the socioeconomic variables were. We conclude that air pollution was not acting as a surrogate for other variables in explaining these rates. This conclusion lends confidence to previous evidence that the estimated relationship between our measures of air pollution and mortality was not spurious.

[9] The fact that the regressions for venereal disease and crime had relatively high explanatory power (due to the socioeconomic variables) suggests that errors of observation did not dominate the analysis.

CHAPTER 7

1969 Replication, further verification, and summary

Throughout our cross-sectional analyses, we have been testing our basic findings pertaining to the 1960 unadjusted total mortality rate. We have addressed such questions as: Do the results replicate with 1961 data? Do analyses of other mortality rates support the results? Are there plausible alternative explanations for the results (other than a causal relationship between air pollution and mortality)?

We begin this chapter with a further replication of the association, using 1969 air pollution, total mortality (unadjusted and adjusted), and socio-economic data.[1] This replication is designed to show whether the association is stable over time. In addition to this direct replication, by using jackknife techniques, we will again examine the effects of extreme observations on our estimates; we also will reexamine alternative functional forms, analyze the residuals (the differences between the predicted and actual mortality rates) from both the 1960 and 1969 regressions for evidence of misspecification, and examine cross-lagged cross-sectional tests as another means of focusing on the interrelationships over time. Following this, we will replicate chapter 4's analyses of the infant and age–sex–race-specific mortality rates. We will then investigate the association between mortality rates and additional air pollutants (nitrates, nitrogen dioxide, and sulfur dioxide), as well as that between mortality rates and interactions between air pollutants. Finally, we will present a summary of the complete cross-sectional work.

TOTAL MORTALITY

In table 7.1, 112 SMSAs, for which 1969 air pollution data were available, are used to estimate regressions comparable to the 1960 specifica-

[1] The 1969 mortality data were the most recent available at the time of the analysis. The 1969 socioeconomic data (including population figures) were derived by linear interpolation of 1960 and 1970 census data, using the 1960 geographical definitions for both years.

TABLE 7.1. Unadjusted and Age–Sex–Race-adjusted Total Mortality Rates (Comparison of the Largest 1960 and 1969 Data Sets)

| | Unadjusted | | | | | Age–sex–race-adjusted | | | | |
| | 1960 | | 1969 | | | 1960 | | 1969 | | |
	7.1-1	7.1-2	7.1-3	7.1-4	7.1-5	7.1-6	7.1-7	7.1-8	7.1-9	7.1-10
R^2	.831	.828	.817	.805	.789	.285	.272	.390	.348	.281
Constant	343.381	301.205	386.858	330.647	302.293	901.196	857.665	975.700	918.657	874.958
Air pollution variables										
Min S	.473 (1.67)	.631 (2.71)	−.038 (−.07)	.774 (2.11)		.678 (2.29)	.825 (3.38)	.049 (.11)	.784 (2.48)	
Mean S	.173 (.53)		.633 (1.81)			.085 (.25)		.618 (2.05)		
Max S	.028 (.25)		−.053 (−.67)			.076 (.66)		−.077 (−1.15)		
Sum S elasticities	5.04	3.27	5.92	2.97	5.20	5.70	3.84	5.02	2.83	4.21
S index[a]					1.093 (2.74)					.752 (2.85)
Min P	.199 (.32)		.434 (.69)			.199 (.31)		.329 (.61)		
Mean P	.303 (.71)	.452 (2.67)	.056 (.13)	.818 (3.39)		.332 (.75)	.465 (2.61)	.113 (.31)	.723 (3.48)	
Max P	−.018 (−.19)		.130 (1.83)			−.030 (−.29)		.109 (1.79)		
Sum P elasticities	4.37	5.85	5.59	8.66	5.30	3.96	5.40	4.99	7.21	3.70
P index[a]					1.563 (1.97)					1.158 (1.80)
Socioeconomic variables										
P/M²	.083 (1.54)	.089 (1.71)	.130 (2.51)	.131 (2.54)		.052 (.92)	.055 (1.01)	.093 (2.08)	.092 (2.07)	
≥65	6.880 (16.63)	7.028 (18.09)	6.403 (17.11)	6.568 (18.09)		.265 (.61)	.411 (1.01)	.164 (.51)	.315 (1.00)	
NW	.396 (3.82)	.422 (4.32)	.204 (2.24)	.204 (2.27)		.145 (1.34)	.165 (1.61)	.107 (1.37)	.109 (1.40)	
Poor	.038 (.26)	−.002 (−.02)	.511 (2.13)	.557 (2.29)		.139 (.89)	.098 (.65)	.599 (2.89)	.640 (3.06)	
Sum SE elasticities	70.07	71.03	72.88	74.99		6.80	7.55	9.34	11.14	
Log Pop	−.276 (−1.38)	−.212 (−1.12)	−.427 (−2.22)	−.365 (−1.94)		−.093 (−.44)	−.022 (−.11)	−.351 (−2.12)	−.283 (−1.74)	
SE index[a]					.972 (18.91)					1.495 (4.76)

Note: 1960 regressions are based on data for 117 SMSAs, while 1969 regressions are based on data for 112 SMSAs (see table C.1, pp. 317–320). The numbers in parentheses are the regression coefficients are *t* statistics.
[a] The indexes are defined in table D.10, page 335.

121

tions for the unadjusted total and the age–sex–race-adjusted total mortality rates. Regressions 7.1-1 and 7.1-2 reproduce the basic 1960 results (regressions 3.1-1 and 3.1-2) and regressions 7.1-3 and 7.1-4 are the 1969 replications. In both cases, the independent variables explain more than 80 percent of the variation in the 1969 mortality rates across SMSAs. If one compares regression 7.1-4 with regression 7.1-2 (dropping four of the six air pollution variables), one notes that the 1969 estimated coefficient of Min S was similar to that for 1960, while the magnitude of the coefficient of Mean P was considerably higher in 1969.[2]

The elasticities given in table 7.1 provide another comparison of the regressions. For example, if the mean values of the sulfate variables in 1960 (1969) were to decrease by 10 percent, the associated reduction in the unadjusted total mortality rate, from regression 7.1-1 (7.1-3), would be 0.50 (0.59) percent for the first specification and 0.33 (0.30) percent for the second specification, regression 7.1-2 (7.1-4). Similarly, if the mean values of the suspended particulate variables were to decrease by 10 percent, the corresponding reductions in the unadjusted total mortality rate would be 0.44 (0.56) percent and 0.59 (0.87) percent, respectively. Finally, if the mean value of each of the socioeconomic variables (excluding Log Pop) experienced a 10 percent reduction, the combined effect on the unadjusted total mortality rate would be a decrease of 7.01 (7.29) percent and 7.10 (7.50) percent, respectively.

A more homogeneous comparison is that between the adjusted total mortality rates for 1960 and 1969, since additional demographic factors are controlled. The implications of regressions 7.1-6 and 7.1-8 were generally comparable, as were regressions 7.1-7 and 7.1-9. In 1969, sulfates became somewhat less important and suspended particulates became somewhat more important, but the differences were small. If the mean values of the sulfate variables in 1960 (1969) were to decrease by 10 percent, the associated reduction in the adjusted total mortality rate, from regression 7.1-6 (7.1-8), would be 0.57 (0.50) percent for the first specification and 0.38 (0.28) percent for the second specification, regression 7.1-7 (7.1-9). If the mean values of the suspended particulate variables were to decrease by 10 percent, the corresponding reductions in the adjusted total mortality rate would be 0.40 (0.50) percent and 0.54 (0.72) percent, respectively. Finally, if the mean value of each of the socioeconomic variables (excluding Log Pop) were to decrease by 10 percent, the combined effect on the adjusted total mortality rate would be a decrease of 0.68 (0.93) percent and 0.76 (1.11) percent, respectively.

[2] The 1969 analysis was intended to provide a replication of the 1960 analysis. If we looked at only the 1969 results, it would appear that Mean S and Max P were the most important air pollution variables. Nevertheless, rather than analyzing non-comparable specifications for the two years, we will restrict our attention to the specifications given in regressions 7.1-3 and 7.1-4.

F tests indicated that the air pollution variables made a significant contribution to relevant regressions in table 7.1. Specifically, F statistics for the 1969 unadjusted total mortality rates (regressions 7.1-3 and 7.1-4) were 4.75 and 10.61, respectively, with 6 and 100 degrees of freedom; and those for the 1969 age–sex–race-adjusted total mortality rates (regressions 7.1-8 and 7.1-9) were 5.35 and 12.26, respectively, with 2 and 104 degrees of freedom.

Is the structure of the air pollution effects on mortality consistent for the two time periods? Specifically, are the estimated effects of sulfates and suspended particulates on the mortality rates essentially the same for the two sets of data? We have already compared the estimated coefficients and the associated elasticities and found a great deal of similarity. Another means of comparison was suggested to us by John Tukey. We constructed indexes for sulfates, suspended particulates, and the socioeconomic variables based on the estimated 1960 coefficients from the relevant regressions. For example, using regression 7.1-1, the sulfate index was defined as (0.473 Min S) + (0.173 Mean S) + (0.028 Max S); when 1969 sulfate data are inserted, this formula gives a 1969 sulfate index (using 1960 weights). Similar indexes were computed for the suspended particulate and the socioeconomic variables.

These three indexes were then used to explain the 1969 unadjusted total mortality rate in regression 7.1-5 and the 1969 adjusted total mortality rate in regression 7.1-10.[3] If the structure were precisely the same in the two periods, the coefficients would be 1.0. In regression 7.1-5 both air pollution coefficients are greater than 1.0, indicating that the measures of air pollution had a greater effect on the unadjusted total mortality rate in 1969 than they did in 1960. Regression 7.1-10 indicates that sulfates had a smaller effect and suspended particulates a larger effect on the adjusted total mortality rate than they did on the corresponding 1960 death rate. For the 1969 unadjusted total mortality rate, the coefficient of the socioeconomic index was slightly less than 1.0. For the 1969 adjusted total mortality rate, the coefficient was greater than unity, indicating that the socioeconomic variables had more effect in 1969 than in 1960. A formal test of the hypothesis that regression 7.1-5 explained as much of the variation in the adjusted total mortality rates across SMSAs as regression 7.1-3 (after accounting for degrees of freedom) can be made by computing an F statistic. ($F = 1.93$, with 8 and 100 degrees of freedom.) Since $F_{0.05} = 2.02$, with 8 and 120 degrees of freedom, we concluded that there was not a statistically significant difference in explanatory power of the two regressions. Thus, the structure from regression 7.1-1, for 1960, successfully described the relationship between unadjusted total mortality and both air pollution and

[3] Reestimation of the 1960 regression using these indexes is not shown, since we know that R^2 and the constant term will remain unchanged and that the coefficients of all three indexes will be unity.

socioeconomic factors in 1969. A similar comparison was made for the adjusted total mortality rate (regressions 7.1-8 and 7.1-10). The computed F statistic (with 8 and 100 degrees of freedom) was 2.24. This indicates that there was a statistically significant difference in the explanatory power of the two regressions; apparently the underlying structure explaining the adjusted total mortality rate differed for the two years.

In comparing the replications to earlier results, it is important to control for other confounding factors. Each of the data sets for 1960 and 1969 contains SMSAs that do not appear in the other data set. Consequently, an additional analysis is presented in which the SMSAs in the two years are identical.[4] Table 7.2 presents 1960 and 1969 regressions for the eighty-one SMSAs for which data were available in both years. In comparing table 7.2 with table 7.1, one notes that the estimated coefficients and elasticities for the air pollution variables are generally smaller for the smaller data sets. However, if one concentrates on the specifications that include only one sulfate and one suspended particulate variable, (regressions 7.2-3, 7.2-4, 7.2-8, and 7.2-9), the implications are comparable.[5] Finally, regressions 7.2-5 and 7.2-10 displayed mixed results compared with their counterparts in table 7.1, although the coefficients of the sulfate index were approximately equal to 1.0 and were statistically significant, the coefficients of the suspended particulate index were considerably less than 1.0 and were not statistically significant.

JACKKNIFE ANALYSIS

Previously (see table 3.4, page 39), the jackknife technique showed that the 1960 results were not sensitive to "extreme" observations or to the omission of individual observations.

The results of applying the jackknife technique to the 1969 data for both the unadjusted total and age–sex–race-adjusted total mortality rates are shown in table 7.3. The data were first sorted by the mean level of suspended particulates (Mean P), and then fourteen groups of 104 observations each were constructed by omitting the first eight observations, the second eight, and so on.[6] As shown in table 7.3, the jackknife estimates were similar to the estimates based on the entire sample. This was true for both the unadjusted total mortality rate and the adjusted total mortality

---

[4] It should be noted that these SMSAs are not necessarily typical of the total samples for the two years. See appendix C for a list of the eighty-one SMSAs. Appendix D can be used to compare the means of the variables for the different sets of SMSAs.

[5] When F statistics were computed to test the significance of the contribution of the air pollution variables to the explanatory power of regressions 7.2-1 through 7.2-4 and 7.2-6 through 7.2-9, they indicated that the contribution was statistically significant in each case except for regression 7.2-1. (F statistics were not computed for regressions 7.2-5 and 7.2-10 since they were not thought to be meaningful.)

[6] The observations were also sorted by the percentage of poor families (Poor) and then by the mortality rate, as in chapter 3. These additional results are unreported since they were generally similar to the sorting by suspended particulates.

TABLE 7.2. Unadjusted and Age-Sex-Race-adjusted Total Mortality Rates (Comparison of Identical 1960 and 1969 Data Sets)

| | Unadjusted | | | | | Age–sex–race-adjusted | | | | |
| | 1960 | | 1969 | | | 1960 | | 1969 | | |
	7.2-1	7.2-2	7.2-3	7.2-4	7.2-5	7.2-6	7.2-7	7.2-8	7.2-9	7.2-10
R^2	.850	.847	.872	.864	.846	.354	.336	.507	.479	.434
Constant	200.428	177.908	493.900	432.269	180.504	896.362	851.387	1097.551	1038.081	863.269
Air pollution variables										
Min S	.401 (1.32)		.091 (.19)			.444 (1.35)		.129 (.28)		
Mean S	.025 (.07)	.430 (1.82)	.386 (1.15)	.589 (1.74)		.166 (.45)	.559 (2.18)	.466 (1.47)	.682 (2.14)	
Max S	.050 (.42)		-.030 (-.40)			.035 (.28)		-.052 (-.72)		
Sum S elasticities	3.62	2.17	4.14	2.26	3.90	4.51	2.50	4.31	2.45	4.35
S index[a]					1.163 (2.35)					.969 (3.00)
Min P	-.555 (-.88)		-.008 (-.01)			-.640 (-.94)		-.034 (-.06)		
Mean P	.696 (1.64)	.389 (2.35)	.167 (.41)	.659 (2.89)		.714 (1.55)	.399 (2.22)	.183 (.48)	.613 (2.84)	
Max P	-.081 (-.70)		.113 (1.29)			-.100 (-.81)		.088 (1.06)		
Sum P elasticities	4.08	5.28	4.74	7.00	1.92	2.89	4.81	3.88	6.09	.96
P index[a]					.581 (1.07)					.382 (.75)
Socioeconomic variables										
P/M²	.092 (1.98)	.096 (2.13)	.103 (2.36)	.099 (2.30)		.061 (1.22)	.069 (1.41)	.084 (2.03)	.080 (1.97)	
≥65	7.737 (13.59)	7.827 (15.14)	7.791 (17.16)	7.918 (19.22)		.917 (1.49)	1.098 (1.96)	.917 (2.13)	1.086 (2.79)	
NW	.496 (4.44)	.488 (4.91)	.523 (5.10)	.512 (5.20)		.239 (1.98)	.247 (2.28)	.314 (3.24)	.313 (3.37)	
Poor	.138 (.94)	.143 (1.04)	-.011 (-.04)	.050 (.21)		.166 (1.05)	.157 (1.05)	.172 (.74)	.215 (.94)	
Sum SE elasticities	80.77	81.62	84.60	86.27		13.58	15.05	15.16	17.04	
Log Pop	-.167 (-.82)	-.138 (-.72)	-.748 (-3.91)	-.674 (-3.69)		-.159 (-.72)	-.106 (-.51)	-.612 (-3.38)	-.547 (-3.17)	
SE index[a]					.999 (19.19)					1.292 (6.10)

Note: All regressions are based on data for eighty-one SMSAs (see table C.1, pp. 317–320). The numbers in parentheses below the regression coefficients are t statistics.
[a] The indexes are defined in table D.10, page 335.

TABLE 7.3. Jackknife Analysis of Total Mortality Rates, 1969

| | Unadjusted | | | Age–sex–race–adjusted | | |
| | | Jackknife | | | Jackknife | |
	Whole sample[a]	Estimate[b]	95 percent confidence interval	Whole sample[c]	Estimate[b]	95 percent confidence interval
Constant	330.647	333.295	(−26.636, 693.225)	918.657	920.463	(686.529, 1154.398)
Air pollution variables						
Min S	.774	.857	(.417, 1.296)	.784	.831	(.346, 1.315)
Mean P	.818	.623	(−.391, 1.636)	.723	.564	(−.195, 1.323)
Socioeconomic variables						
P/M²	.131	.130	(.050, .210)	.092	.115	(.054, .175)
≥65	6.568	6.208	(4.068, 8.348)	.315	.144	(−.792, 1.080)
NW	.204	.105	(−.143, .353)	.109	.036	(−.126, .198)
Poor	.557	.711	(.278, 1.143)	.640	.775	(.356, 1.193)
Log Pop	−.365	−.293	(−.682, .097)	−.283	−.247	(−.557, .063)

[a] Estimates correspond to those for regression 7.1-4.
[b] Estimates based on fourteen groups of 104 observations sorted on Mean P.
[c] Estimates correspond to those for regression 7.1-9.

rate. Specifically, the jackknife estimates evidenced a greater effect for sulfates and a smaller effect for suspended particulates than did our basic results; the 95 percent confidence interval for Min S did not include zero, while the 95 percent confidence interval for Mean P did.[7] Several of the jackknife estimates associated with the socioeconomic variables indicated sensitivity to particular data points. Thus, as in the original jackknife analysis, the findings indicated that the air pollution coefficients were not very sensitive to particular data points or "extreme" observations. The socioeconomic coefficients were less stable.

ALTERNATIVE SPECIFICATIONS

A number of specifications of the relationship between our measures of air pollution and total mortality were analyzed in chapter 3 (see table 3.5, page 42). Although the linear form was adopted, statistical analyses indicated that it did not dominate all alternative functional forms. Table 7.4 shows a partial replication of this earlier analysis using 1969 data; both the unadjusted and age–sex–race-adjusted total mortality rates were analyzed.

The basic 1969 result for the unadjusted total mortality with one sulfate and one suspended particulate variable, regression 7.1-4, is reproduced as regression 7.4-1 for comparison. Regression 7.1-9 is reproduced as regression 7.4-7 for the adjusted total mortality rate. Regression 7.4-2 replicates the original log-log formulation (regression 3.5-3). Comparing regressions 7.4-1 and 7.4-2, one notes that R^2 rose slightly (from 0.805 to 0.827); the implications of the regressions are quite similar. This is apparent if one remembers that the coefficients in the log-log formulation can be interpreted as elasticities in the linear specification. A comparison of the coefficients in regression 7.4-2 (0.023 and 0.088) with scaled elasticities in regression 7.4-1 (0.030 and 0.087) shows them to be nearly identical for both sulfates and suspended particulates, respectively. The same is true for the analysis of the adjusted total mortality rate, comparing the air pollution coefficients in regression 7.4-8 (0.021 and 0.082) with scaled elasticities in regression 7.4-7 (0.028 and 0.072).

In regression 7.4-3 quadratic air pollution variables and an interaction term were added to regression 7.4-1. The results of an F test indicated that the quadratic terms did not make a significant contribution to the linear specification. $F = 1.13$, with 3 and 101 degrees of freedom. The implication of the negative coefficients for $(Min S)^2$ and $(Mean P)^2$ is that the effect of air pollution on mortality rises less than linearly with the level of air pollution.[8] Similar conclusions held for the adjusted total mortality rate (regression 7.3-9); $F = 0.88$.

[7] This occurred only for the sorting by Mean P. None of the other five jackknife confidence intervals for Mean P included zero.

[8] It is noteworthy that the 1960 quadratic specification (regression 3.5-4, page 42) also displayed a negative coefficient for $(Min S)^2$; it was statistically significant.

TABLE 7.4. Alternative Specifications of Total Mortality Rates, 1969

	Unadjusted						Age–sex–race-adjusted					
	Basic regression	Log-log	Quadratic	Dummy variable[a]	Linear spline[b]	Outliers deleted[c]	Basic regression	Log-log	Quadratic	Dummy variable[a]	Linear spline[b]	Outliers deleted[c]
	7.4-1	7.4-2	7.4-3	7.4-4	7.4-5	7.4-6	7.4-7	7.4-8	7.4-9	7.4-10	7.4-11	7.4-12
R^2	.805	.827	.811	.807	.814	.820	.348	.373	.365	.322	.380	.357
Constant	330.647	124.635	255.197	390.043	192.370	227.954	918.657	259.306	872.868	968.808	823.706	860.393
Air pollution variables												
Min S	.774 (2.11)	.023 (1.73)	.542 (.37)		.176 (.05)	.567 (1.54)	.784 (2.48)	.021 (1.89)	.428 (.34)		.304 (.09)	.617 (1.78)
(Min S)²			-.013 (-.08)						-.024 (-.18)			
Mean P	.818 (3.39)	.088 (3.34)	2.757 (2.51)		2.916 (1.46)	.655 (2.37)	.723 (3.48)	.082 (3.72)	2.128 (2.24)		2.210 (1.29)	.651 (2.51)
(Mean P)²			-.931 (-1.78)						-.732 (-1.61)			
Mean S × Mean P			.040 (.30)						.061 (.53)			
Sum AP elasticities	11.63	11.08	22.34	7.47	27.30	8.87	10.04	10.25	16.97	5.65	20.64	8.42
Socioeconomic variables												
P/M²	.131 (2.54)	.020 (1.97)	.127 (2.43)	.142 (2.62)	.127 (2.37)	.043 (.29)	.092 (2.07)	.016 (1.89)	.089 (1.98)	.102 (2.12)	.092 (2.01)	.003 (.02)
≥65	6.568 (18.09)	.694 (18.87)	6.532 (17.94)	6.426 (16.94)	6.526 (17.52)	7.812 (19.61)	.315 (1.00)	.041 (1.36)	.285 (.91)	.214 (.64)	.286 (.89)	.971 (2.59)
NW	.204 (2.27)	.021 (1.92)	.200 (2.20)	.186 (2.04)	.220 (2.31)	.502 (4.62)	.109 (1.40)	.011 (1.18)	.104 (1.31)	.086 (1.06)	.109 (1.33)	.315 (3.08)
Poor	.557 (2.29)	.092 (3.62)	.612 (2.50)	.658 (2.70)	.596 (2.39)	.191 (.70)	.640 (3.06)	.078 (3.71)	.679 (3.21)	.709 (3.29)	.676 (3.14)	.341 (1.33)
Sum SE elasticities	74.99	82.66	75.08	74.39	75.13	86.69	11.14	14.68	11.11	10.59	11.20	16.26
Log Pop	-.365 (-1.94)	.021 (-2.20)	-.403 (-2.10)	-.393 (-1.98)	-.373 (-1.93)	-.328 (-1.58)	-.283 (-1.74)	.017 (-2.15)	-.318 (-1.92)	-.288 (-1.64)	-.296 (-1.78)	-.243 (-1.25)

128

Note: Unless otherwise specified, the regressions are based on data for 112 SMSAs. The numbers in parentheses below the regression coefficients are *t* statistics.

[a] The air pollution dummy variables were defined as follows:

DS_1 = 1 if Min S ≤ 16 (μg per cubic meter × 10), 0 otherwise
DS_2 = 1 if 16 (μg per cubic meter × 10) < Min S ≤ 35 (μg per cubic meter × 10), 0 otherwise
DS_3 = 1 if 35 (μg per cubic meter × 10) < Min S ≤ 54 (μg per cubic meter × 10), 0 otherwise
DS_4 = 1 if 54 (μg per cubic meter × 10) < Min S, 0 otherwise
DP_1 = 1 if Mean P < 67 μg per cubic meter, 0 otherwise
DP_2 = 1 if 67 μg per cubic meter < Mean P ≤ 95 μg per cubic meter, 0 otherwise
DP_3 = 1 if 95 μg per cubic meter < Mean P ≤ 123 μg per cubic meter, 0 otherwise
DP_4 = 1 if 123 μg per cubic meter < Mean P, 0 otherwise.

For estimation purposes DS_1 and DP_1 were excluded.
The coefficients and *t* statistics for the remaining dummy variables were:

Variable	Regression 7.4-4	7.4-10
DS_2	3.874 (.19)	12.172 (.68)
DS_3	14.065 (.58)	21.916 (1.03)
DS_4	52.995 (2.01)	51.310 (2.20)

Variable	Regression 7.4-4	7.4-10
DP_2	42.730 (1.83)	24.386 (1.18)
DP_3	84.498 (3.30)	58.260 (2.58)
DP_4	82.844 (2.88)	63.247 (2.49)

[b] The air pollution linear spline variables were defined as follows:

Min S_1 = Min S − 16 (μg per cubic meter × 10) if Min S ≥ 16 (μg per cubic meter × 10), 0 otherwise
Min S_2 = Min S − 35 (μg per cubic meter × 10) if Min S ≥ 35 (μg per cubic meter × 10), 0 otherwise
Min S_3 = Min S − 54 (μg per cubic meter × 10) if Min S ≥ 54 (μg per cubic meter × 10), 0 otherwise
Mean P_1 = Mean P − 67 μg per cubic meter if Mean P ≥ 67 μg per cubic meter, 0 otherwise
Mean P_2 = Mean P − 95 μg per cubic meter if Mean P ≥ 95 μg per cubic meter, 0 otherwise
Mean P_3 = Mean P − 123 μg per cubic meter if Mean P ≥ 123 μg per cubic meter, 0 otherwise.

The coefficients and *t* statistics were:

Variable	Regression 7.4-5	7.4-11
Min S_1	1.078 (.23)	1.494 (.36)
Min S_2	-1.203 (-.50)	-2.456 (-1.18)
Min S_3	1.353 (.65)	2.382 (1.32)

Variable	Regression 7.4-5	7.4-11
Mean P_1	-1.381 (-.56)	-1.128 (-.53)
Mean P_2	-1.055 (-.66)	-.438 (-.32)
Mean P_3	-.269 (-.21)	-.428 (-.38)

[c] Based on 103 SMSAs, see chapter 7, footnote 11.

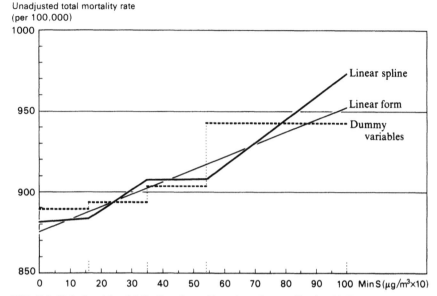

FIG. 7.1. Relationship of Min S and unadjusted total mortality for 1969.

Additional tests of the linear form were also examined. Regression 7.4-4 presents a dummy variable specification for the unadjusted total mortality rate, and regression 7.4-5 presents a linear spline specification. The results from these regressions as well as those of the linear specification are depicted in figure 7.1 for the minimum level of sulfates, and in figure 7.2 for the mean level of suspended particulates. For Min S (figure 7.1), the linear, dummy variable, and linear spline regressions showed similar effects. For Mean P (figure 7.2), the graph corresponding to the linear regression showed a slight rise; the graph corresponding to the dummy variable regression indicated a more uniform rise; and the graph of the linear spline specification was steep initially but eventually became flat. While one might conclude that the linear regression had quite different implications for suspended particulates than did the other specifications, an F test indicated that these differences were not statistically significant.[9] Similar results to those just reported were found when the adjusted total mortality rate was the dependent variable (regressions 7.4-10 and 7.4-11).

In the final test of the linear specification, we used the 1969 data and focused on the sensitivity of the results to outliers, that is, extreme values

[9] The F statistic comparing the dummy variable specification with the linear specification was equal to 0.21, with 4 and 100 degrees of freedom; the F statistic comparing the linear spline form with the linear form was equal to 0.81, with 6 and 98 degrees of freedom. Again, we note that, strictly speaking, the first test is not correct since the linear model is not a subset of the dummy variable specification.

Unadjusted total mortality rate
(per 100,000)

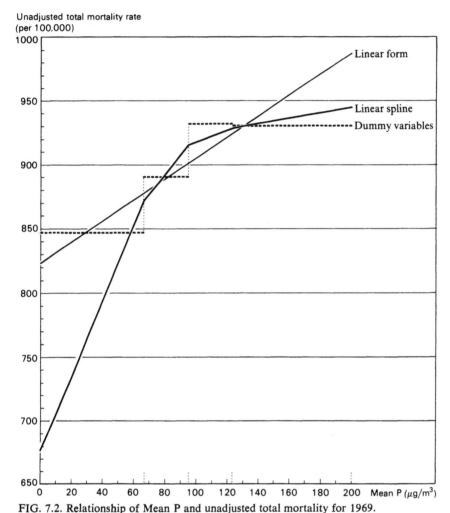

FIG. 7.2. Relationship of Mean P and unadjusted total mortality for 1969.

of one or more variables.[10] Nine SMSAs were dropped from the data set before the regressions were refitted.[11] When these observations were omitted in regression 7.4-6, the explanatory power was slightly higher

[10] While the previous jackknife analysis tested the sensitivity of the regression coefficients to dropping random groups of observations, this analysis was designed to look more directly at the effects of dropping specific observations having variables with extreme values.

[11] The nine SMSAs dropped were Tampa, Honolulu, Jersey City, New York, Davenport, Charleston, West Virginia, Huntington, Chicago, and Wilmington, Delaware. These were chosen since each was an extreme observation on at least one variable and tended to stand apart on that variable. For example, Jersey City's population density was three times higher than that for the next most densely populated SMSA.

than the basic result (R^2 rose from 0.805 to 0.820). The air pollution coefficients became smaller in magnitude and their t statistics were reduced. An F test still indicated that the two air pollution measures made a significant contribution to the regression. Three of the socioeconomic coefficients experienced considerable change in regression 7.4-6. The coefficients for population density and the percentage of poor families in the SMSA dropped considerably and lost statistical significance, while the coefficient for the percentage of nonwhites in the SMSA doubled in magnitude and its t statistic increased substantially. The stability of the air pollution variables relative to the socioeconomic variables instills further confidence in our previously estimated relationship.[12]

Both the jackknife estimates and the estimates derived here indicated that the estimated air pollution coefficients were relatively stable. The jackknife estimates indicated some instability in the socioeconomic coefficients which increased in this analysis when the extreme observations were deleted. We conclude that the two techniques produced consistent results, although systematic deletion of extreme observations resulted in more variation than random exclusion.

Thus, the 1969 analysis of alternatives to the simple linear specification is unequivocal. No formulation significantly dominated the linear specification.[13] In chapter 3, we noted our preference for the linear specification despite mixed statistical results. The results for 1969 tend to support that judgment and, more important, strengthen the conclusions presented throughout the book.

ANALYSIS OF RESIDUALS

The estimated relationships were incomplete in that important explanatory variables were omitted. One way of examining the effects of such omitted factors, as well as testing other hypotheses, is to examine the unexplained portion of the mortality rate—that is, to analyze the residuals.

Table 7.5 presents the residuals corresponding to specific SMSAs from each of four regressions. Reading from top to bottom, the first group of SMSAs are the largest (according to population) in our sample. As can be seen by the relatively small magnitude of their residuals, these SMSAs were well explained by the equation, and there was little evidence of systematic over- or underestimation. The southwestern SMSAs comprise the second group. It was conjectured that these areas would not be well ex-

---

[12] A similar comparison of regressions 7.4-7 and 7.4-12, pertaining to the unadjusted total mortality rate, revealed some reduction in the coefficients and the t statistics corresponding to the pollution variables, although the coefficients for the socioeconomic variables were much less stable.

[13] We replicated the 1960 specifications involving variables for census regions and migration (regressions 3.5-9 and 3.5-10) and found that inclusion of these additional variables had similar effects to those reported in chapter 3; we have not reported these specifications in table 7.4.

TABLE 7.5 Analysis of Residuals

	Unadjusted total mortality rate		Age–sex–race-adjusted total mortality rate	
	1960	1969	1960	1969
Ten largest SMSAs				
New York, N.Y.	−7.06	−26.50	−30.01	−23.29
Chicago, Ill.	35.33	54.76	20.23	45.43
Los Angeles, Calif.	−41.18	−8.16	−55.72	−11.68
Philadelphia, Pa.	11.25	14.29	−12.39	3.96
Boston, Mass.	61.83	15.19	55.07	12.80
Detroit, Mich.	−26.77	9.31	−19.87	9.14
San Francisco, Calif.	31.12	42.74	15.16	32.30
Pittsburgh, Pa.	59.32	—	46.74	—
Saint Louis, Mo.	0.25	−27.50	−13.98	−22.12
Cleveland, Ohio	−29.37	−3.25	−15.72	−17.46
Southwestern SMSAs				
Albuquerque, N.Mex.	−3.30	−52.51	26.15	−49.99
Denver, Colo.	12.95	−82.43	10.29	−76.14
Las Vegas, Nev.	92.12	67.56	54.22	41.00
Los Angeles, Calif.	−41.18	−8.16	−55.72	−11.68
Phoenix, Ariz.	−62.95	−54.38	−70.20	−30.73
Salt Lake City, Utah	−77.14	−90.01	−78.03	−75.52
San Diego, Calif.	−31.20	−69.19	−32.47	−61.65
San Jose, Calif.	−77.74	−53.92	−101.29	−89.74
Ten largest 1960 residuals (unadjusted total mortality rates)				
Tampa, Fla.	−246.09	−202.68	−137.66	−89.13
Wilkes-Barre, Pa.	225.74	175.38	195.06	122.90
Scranton, Pa.	212.09	—	260.72	—
Austin, Tex.	−143.40	—	−159.59	—
Savannah, Ga.	126.41	79.58	112.97	34.40
New Orleans, La.	125.22	78.07	138.52	83.94
Canton, Ohio	−122.63	55.08	−129.57	58.39
Orlando, Fla.	−119.10	—	−107.28	—
Terre Haute, Ind.	113.26	—	79.50	—
Sioux Falls, S.Dak.	−108.00	—	−172.94	—
Ten largest 1960 residuals (age–sex–race-adjusted total mortality rates)				
Scranton, Pa.	212.09	—	260.72	—
Wilkes-Barre, Pa.	225.74	175.38	195.06	122.90
Sioux Falls, S.Dak.	−108.00	—	−172.94	—
Austin, Tex.	−143.40	—	−159.59	—
New Orleans, La.	125.22	78.07	138.52	83.94
Tampa, Fla.	−246.09	−202.68	−137.66	−89.13
Canton, Ohio	−122.63	55.08	−129.57	58.39
Brockton, Mass.	68.87	—	115.18	—
Savannah, Ga.	126.41	79.58	112.97	34.40
Fall River, Mass.	75.84	45.53	108.77	29.77
Ten largest 1969 residuals (unadjusted total mortality rates)				
Duluth, Minn.	62.35	209.72	48.07	161.62
Tampa, Fla.	−246.09	−202.68	−137.66	−89.13
Honolulu, Hawaii	—	−181.21	—	−135.48
Wilkes-Barre, Pa.	225.74	175.38	195.06	−122.90
Fargo, N.Dak.	—	−141.72	—	−152.18
Montgomery, Ala.	7.55	128.70	−10.93	65.64
San Bernardino, Calif.	—	−115.69	—	−106.01
Miami, Fla.	−94.32	−114.94	−105.51	−87.56
Toledo, Ohio	22.09	103.06	11.03	97.89
Albany, N.Y.	—	94.79	—	76.00
Ten largest 1969 residuals (age–sex–race-adjusted total mortality rates)				
Duluth, Minn.	62.35	209.72	48.07	161.62
Fargo, N.Dak.	—	−141.72	—	−152.18
Honolulu, Hawaii	—	−181.21	—	−135.48
Wilkes-Barre, Pa.	225.74	175.38	195.06	−122.90
San Bernardino, Calif.	—	−115.69	—	−106.01
Toledo, Ohio	22.09	103.06	11.03	97.89
Erie, Pa.	—	93.62	—	97.25
Johnstown, Pa.	27.99	91.35	33.99	95.97
Mobile, Ala.	19.05	−81.51	26.73	−94.05
San Jose, Calif.	−77.74	−53.92	−101.29	−89.74

Note: The second column shows residuals from the 1960 unadjusted total mortality rate equation (regression 7.1-1) based on 117 SMSAs; the third column shows residuals from the corresponding 1969 replication (regression 7.1-3) based on 112 SMSAs; the fourth column shows residuals from the 1960 adjusted total mortality rate equation (regression 7.1-6) based on 117 SMSAs; and the fifth column shows residuals from the corresponding 1969 replication (regression 7.1-8) based on 112 SMSAs. The standard deviations for the four sets of residuals were as follows: 63.09 (regression 7.1-1), 65.99 (regression 7.1-3), 63.15 (regression 7.1-6), and 54.43 (regression 7.1-8).

A negative residual indicates that the regression equation overestimated the mortality rate for the particular SMSA.

133

plained by the equation since other air pollutants (for example, photo-chemical oxidants) were likely to be important but could not be included in the regression.[14] In fact, the southwestern SMSAs had residuals that were not particularly large in absolute value, although there was a tendency to overestimate their mortality rates. The third group consists of the ten SMSAs with the largest (in absolute value) residuals from regression 7.1-1 for the 1960 unadjusted total mortality rate. One notes that Tampa, Wilkes-Barre, and Scranton had particularly large residuals.[15] This continued to be the case for Tampa and Wilkes-Barre in the 1969 reestimation (note the residual values in the third column). The remaining three SMSAs, for which there were 1969 data (Savannah, New Orleans, and Canton), were explained satisfactorily in 1969; there apparently was no systematic tendency to under- or overestimate the mortality rates in these areas. The fourth group consists of the ten SMSAs with the largest residuals from regression 7.1-6 for the 1960 adjusted total mortality rate. Noting the values in column four, one sees that the mortality rates for Scranton and Wilkes-Barre were considerably underestimated. Looking across to column five, one notes that this continued to be the case for Wilkes-Barre in 1969. The fifth and sixth groups represent similar analyses for the ten SMSAs with the largest residuals from regression 7.1-3 for the 1969 unadjusted total mortality rate and those from regression 7.1-8 for the 1969 adjusted total mortality rate. As already noted, Tampa and Wilkes-Barre had large residuals in both 1960 and 1969 for the unadjusted total mortality rate (only Wilkes-Barre had large 1960 and 1969 residuals for the adjusted total mortality rate). Only 1969 data were available for Fargo, Honolulu, San Bernardino, Albany, and Erie; hence, comparisons for the two years are not possible. Based on the available comparisons, we conclude that there was limited evidence that an important variable(s) had been omitted, since SMSAs with unexpectedly large (or small) mortality rates in 1960 had large (or small) mortality rates in 1969.

Thus far we have examined only subsets of the residuals. In addition, we performed a more general analysis of the residuals taken from the eighty-one SMSAs common to both the 1960 and 1969 data sets (regressions 7.2-1, 7.2-3, 7.2-6, and 7.2-8). First, we examined the association between the residuals of each regression and the dependent variable, that is, the relationship between the unexplained portion of the mortality rate

[14] Furthermore, measures of sulfates and suspended particulates were not apt to be chemically equivalent to measures of these air pollutants in other regions. For example, suspended particulates are largely due to natural sources rather than to fossil fuel combustion.

[15] The overestimate for Tampa is probably an artifact of its large proportion of older people; the proportion of the population greater than sixty-five was 17.1 percent as opposed to a mean of 8.4 percent for the 117 SMSAs. The underestimates for Wilkes-Barre and Scranton may be due to the amount of coal fuels used in these areas.

and the mortality rate itself. The correlations corresponding to the four regressions were 0.388, 0.358, 0.804, and 0.702, respectively. The magnitudes of these correlations suggests that there are important factors influencing mortality that are absent from the specification. Furthermore, these correlations indicate that the omitted variables are closely correlated with the magnitude of the mortality rates.

In an attempt to identify these omitted factors, we reexamined the residuals from the regressions including the additional independent variables described in chapter 5.[16] The correlations between the residuals and dependent variables were statistically significant for all specifications, even when each set of additional variables from chapter 5 was added. The correlations were much larger for regressions involving the age–sex–race-adjusted than for the unadjusted total mortality rate. Thus, there is additional evidence of important explanatory variables being omitted from the analysis, especially for the adjusted total mortality rate.

Our last examination of the unexplained portions of the mortality rates consisted of correlating the residuals from the 1960 regressions with those from the 1969 regressions for the eighty-one common SMSAs. We hypothesized that some significant variables which were omitted in 1960 would continue to be significant (and omitted) in 1969; and hence, that the correlations would be statistically significant. The results bore this out: the correlation was 0.58 for the unadjusted total mortality rate and 0.52 for the adjusted total mortality rate.

CROSS-LAGGED CROSS-SECTIONAL ANALYSIS

Another test for uncontrolled factors which involves the simultaneous examination of data from two or more time periods, was suggested to us by Donald T. Campbell. Consider the simple case where a single factor A_t is alleged to cause a result B_t (where the subscripts denote time t, and it is assumed that there are no lag effects; that is, A_{t+1} is unrelated to B_t, and B_{t+1} is unrelated to A_t). As stated earlier, a statistically significant correlation between A_t and B_t has four logical possibilities, one being that the association is spurious. It can still be argued that a replication showing a significant correlation between A_{t+1} and B_{t+1} does not rule out the possibility of an uncontrolled factor, since the underlying structure

[16] The correlations between the residuals and dependent variables for the 117 SMSA data set were as follows:

Explanatory variables	Total mortality rate	Age–sex–race-adjusted total mortality rate
6 AP + 5 SE	0.41	0.85
6 AP + 5 SE + home-heating equipment	0.36	0.73
6 AP + 5 SE + home-heating fuels	0.34	0.73
6 AP + 5 SE + water-heating fuels	0.31	0.67
6 AP + 5 SE + occupation	0.28	0.60
6 AP + 5 SE + climate	0.36	0.74

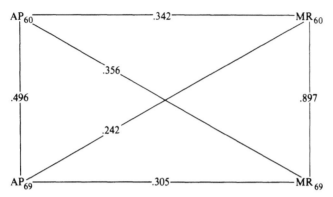

FIG. 7.3. Cross-lagged cross-sectional analysis of the air pollution-mortality relationship in 81 SMSAs.

that produced A_t and B_t is likely to generate data of the same sort in a subsequent period, $t + 1$. If the association between A_t and B_t were due merely to an uncontrolled variable that also operated in period $t + 1$, then A_t could be spuriously associated with B_{t+1}, and A_{t+1} could be spuriously associated with B_t. The "true" factor causing both A and B could result in significant cross-lagged correlations, although one would expect the synchronous correlations between A and B to be greater than correlations of the two variables across time.

In applying Campbell's suggestion to our analysis, we should note that the effect of A on B may continue to hold over time; that is, A_t may cause B_{t+1}. For example, substantial air pollution during one year could be expected to take its toll on mortality both in that year and in future years. In such cases there would be significant correlations between A_t and B_t, A_{t+1} and B_{t+1}, and A_t and B_{t+1}, but not necessarily between A_{t+1} and B_t.

Since our analysis involves more than two independent variables, we followed Tukey's suggestion of defining indexes for the variables in order to perform Campbell's test. For regressions 7.2-5 and 7.2-10, we constructed separate indexes for sulfates, suspended particulates, and the socioeconomic variables. Here we combine the two pollution indexes into a new "air pollution" index. Making use of a single index for air pollution (AP) and a single index for the socioeconomic (SE) factors enables us to compute the necessary statistics. Thus, AP_{60} and SE_{60} were constructed from 1960 data, using weights from regression 7.2-1; AP_{69} and SE_{69} were constructed from 1969 data using the same weights.

Figure 7.3 presents all possible correlations between the 1960 and 1969 air pollution indexes (AP_{60} and AP_{69}) and the 1960 and 1969 unadjusted total mortality rate (MR_{60} and MR_{69}). Figure 7.4 presents analogous correlations for the 1960 and 1969 socioeconomic indexes (SE_{60} and SE_{69}) and the 1960 and 1969 unadjusted total mortality rates. The 1960 air

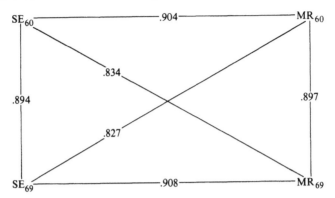

FIG. 7.4. Cross-lagged cross-sectional analysis of the socio-economic-mortality relationship in 81 SMSAs.

pollution index was more highly correlated with the 1960 unadjusted total mortality rate than was the 1969 air pollution index ($\rho = 0.342$ compared with 0.242). Similarly, the 1960 socioeconomic index was more highly correlated with the 1960 mortality rate than was the 1969 socioeconomic index ($\rho = 0.904$ compared with 0.827). These results were in the expected direction.

For the 1969 unadjusted total mortality rate, the results were not all as expected. For example, the 1960 air pollution index was slightly more correlated with the 1969 mortality rate than was the 1969 air pollution index ($\rho = 0.356$ compared with 0.305); this could reflect a lag effect of air pollution on mortality. The two socioeconomic indexes correlated with the 1969 mortality rate in the anticipated way ($\rho = 0.908$ compared with 0.834).

Looking only at the cross correlations, one observes that 1960 air pollution exhibited a stronger association with 1969 mortality than 1969 air pollution exhibited with 1960 mortality ($\rho = 0.356$ compared with 0.242). This provides further evidence of lag effects. The cross correlations associated with the socioeconomic index were almost identical ($\rho = 0.834$ compared with 0.827).

Thus, with one exception—the 1960 air pollution index correlating with the 1969 mortality rate slightly more than did the 1969 air pollution index—the results were in the hypothesized direction. The exception and one cross correlation suggest a possible lag between observed air pollution and observed mortality. We conclude that, in general, the observed association between our measures of air pollution and mortality "passed" the cross-lagged cross-sectional test.

INFANT MORTALITY RATE

In addition to examining replications involving the unadjusted and adjusted total mortality rates, we analyzed 1969 infant mortality data in an effort to replicate our earlier findings pertaining to these death rates. These are shown in table 7.6 (the 1960 results are reported in table 4.1).

Except for the unadjusted infant mortality rate (regressions 7.6-1 and 7.6-2), less than 20 percent of the variation in the infant mortality rates was explained by the independent variables. It is apparent that important causal variables, such as the extent of prenatal care, are omitted in the specification. At the same time, it is apparent that the variables included are not powerful, individually or collectively, in explaining the variation in these infant mortality rates. Regression 7.6-2 was comparable to its counterpart in the 1960 analysis (regression 4.1-2); the mean suspended particulate variable was again the significant pollution variable. In addition, four socioeconomic variables were statistically significant. In general the regressions corresponding to the other 1969 infant mortality rates were also comparable to the 1960 findings, although Mean P was more important in explaining the white infant mortality rate (regression 7.6-6) and less so in explaining the nonwhite infant mortality rate (regression 7.6-8) than it had been in the earlier results.[17] The socioeconomic variables were seldom statistically significant in explaining the race-adjusted or race-specific infant mortality rate.

AGE–SEX–RACE-SPECIFIC MORTALITY

A number of age–sex–race-specific mortality rates were analyzed for 1960 (see table 4.3). This analysis is replicated for 1969 in table 7.7.

The 1969 age–sex–race-adjusted total mortality rate (regression 7.1-9) is reproduced as regression 7.7-1 for comparison. The four sex–race-specific mortality rates for all ages follow (regressions 7.7-2 through 7.7-5). F tests indicated that the two air pollution variables (Min S and Mean P) made a significant contribution to each of these regressions. Compared with the 1960 results, the effect of minimum sulfates on whites decreased, while their effect on nonwhites increased; the reverse was true for the effect of mean suspended particulates. As before, Min S and Mean P tended to be more closely associated with nonwhite than with white mortality. Turning to the socioeconomic variables, P/M^2, Poor, and Log Pop generally had larger coefficients in 1969 than in 1960. The explanatory powers of the 1969 regressions were generally higher than those of the corresponding 1960 regressions. Thus, the replication corroborates the earlier findings and strengthens the hypothesis of causality.

Evaluation of F tests indicated that the two air pollution variables did not make a significant contribution to any of the regressions for the newborn to fourteen-year-old age group (regressions 7.7-6 through 7.7-10). The 1960 results indicated significant contributions of the two air pollution variables for the aggregate rate in this category, as well as for male

---

[17] F tests indicated that the two air pollution variables contributed significantly to the explanatory powers of regressions 7.6-2, 7.6-4, and 7.6-6.

TABLE 7.6. Infant Mortality Rates, 1969

	Unadjusted		Race-adjusted		White		Nonwhite	
	7.6-1	7.6-2	7.6-3	7.6-4	7.6-5	7.6-6	7.6-7	7.6-8
R^2	.407	.396	.187	.160	.191	.165	.146	.077
Constant	184.287	176.840	216.900	196.499	207.712	200.329	264.148	180.077
Air pollution variables								
Min S	.020		−.200		−.096	−.010	−.706	
	(.12)		(−.98)		(−.60)	(−.09)	(−.92)	
Mean S	.095	.133	.236	.034	.044		1.164	.244
	(.87)	(1.18)	(1.72)	(.24)	(.41)		(2.29)	(.46)
Max S	−.007		−.044		.009		−.300	
	(−.29)		(−1.43)		(.38)		(−2.63)	
Sum S elasticities	4.48	2.25	3.39	.58	2.19	−.18	6.77	2.75
Min P	−.196		−.173		−.227		.099	
	(−1.00)		(−.71)		(−1.19)		(.11)	
Mean P	.203	.180	.217	.229	.195	.202	.320	.360
	(1.54)	(2.44)	(1.31)	(2.47)	(1.51)	(2.79)	(.52)	(1.02)
Max P	−.011		−.003		.002		−.025	
	(−.51)		(−.11)		(.09)		(−.25)	
Sum P elasticities	5.18	8.43	7.18	10.76	6.63	10.65	8.95	11.22
Socioeconomic variables								
P/M²	.041	.039	.034	.030	.022	.018	.093	.090
	(2.51)	(2.45)	(1.65)	(1.52)	(1.36)	(1.18)	(1.23)	(1.19)
≥65	.224	.253	.253	.312	.180	.192	.601	.887
	(1.91)	(2.28)	(1.73)	(2.24)	(1.57)	(1.76)	(1.10)	(1.67)
NW	.089	.087	.003	.004	−.009	−.015	.063	.096
	(3.13)	(3.17)	(.09)	(.11)	(−.31)	(−.56)	(.47)	(.73)
Poor	.234	.237	.118	.126	.082	.089	.285	.303
	(3.11)	(3.20)	(1.26)	(1.35)	(1.12)	(1.21)	(.81)	(.85)
Sum SE elasticities	27.28	28.52	17.96	20.83	13.33	13.62	30.97	41.19
Log Pop	−.097	−.092	−.125	−.102	−.115	−.109	−.175	−.074
	(−1.61)	(−1.60)	(−1.66)	(−1.41)	(−1.96)	(−1.92)	(−.62)	(−.27)

Note: All regressions are based on data for 112 SMSAs. The numbers in parentheses below the regression coefficients are *t* statistics.

TABLE 7.7.   Age–Sex–Race-specific Mortality Rates, 1969

	All ages				
	7.7-1 *Total*	7.7-2 *MW*	7.7-3 *FW*	7.7-4 *MNW*	7.7-5 *FNW*
R^2	.348	.308	.218	.350	.376
Constant	918.657	1117.329	725.721	948.761	917.223
Air pollution variables					
Min S	.784 (2.48)	.497 (1.25)	.575 (1.96)	2.702 (2.61)	2.385 (3.44)
Min S elasticities	2.83	1.54	2.42	8.60	10.86
Mean P	.723 (3.48)	.711 (2.73)	.560 (2.91)	1.648 (2.42)	1.054 (2.31)
Mean P elasticities	7.21	6.10	6.50	14.48	13.26
Socioeconomic variables					
P/M²	.092 (2.07)	.070 (1.25)	.103 (2.50)	.191 (1.31)	.076 (.78)
≥65	.315 (1.00)	.391 (.99)	.033 (.11)	1.079 (1.05)	1.016 (1.48)
NW	.109 (1.40)	.155 (1.59)	−.020 (−.28)	.407 (1.60)	.413 (2.42)
Poor	.640 (3.06)	.848 (3.23)	.099 (.51)	2.507 (3.65)	1.275 (2.78)
Sum SE elasticities	11.13	12.21	2.17	35.62	34.66
Log Pop	−.283 (−1.74)	−.389 (−1.92)	.010 (.07)	−.868 (−1.63)	−1.049 (−2.95)

nonwhites. In 1969, air pollution—as measured by the mean level of suspended particulates—was statistically significant for only one specific rate in this category, male whites (regression 7.7-7). (Mean P approached statistical significance for the aggregate rate in regression 7.7-6.) The coefficients for P/M² and Poor were positive and significant for the aggregate category. The coefficient for Poor was also positive and significant in the white regressions. At the same time, the coefficients for nonwhites and Log Pop were generally negative and the former was significant in regressions 7.7-6 and 7.7-7. The only significant coefficient in either of the nonwhite regressions was the proportion of the population aged sixty-five and older (regression 7.7-10); apparently the important causes of death among young nonwhites are omitted from the specification.

F tests indicated that three of the five regressions for the fifteen- to forty-four age group had significantly greater explanatory power when the air pollution variables were added (regressions 7.7-11, 7.7-12, and 7.7-14); the exceptions were for the female white and nonwhite rates (regressions 7.7-13 and 7.7-15). The coefficient of minimum sulfates was

TABLE 7.7.   (*Continued*)

	Newborn to 14 years				
	7.7-6 Total	7.7-7 MW	7.7-8 FW	7.7-9 MNW	7.7-10 FNW
R^2	.252	.215	.147	.045	.120
Constant	192.851	156.095	163.883	408.925	343.060
Air pollution variables					
Min S	−.034 (−.31)	−.067 (−.55)	−.048 (−.48)	−.104 (−.14)	.294 (.55)
Min S elasticities	−.68	−1.33	−1.30	−1.09	3.96
Mean P	.137 (1:88)	.199 (2.45)	.093 (1.42)	.150 (.30)	.010 (.03)
Mean P elasticities	7.48	10.82	6.92	4.37	.38
Socioeconomic variables					
P/M²	.033 (2.12)	.011 (.64)	.021 (1.48)	.151 (1.41)	.100 (1.34)
≥65	.141 (1.29)	.022 (.18)	−.039 (−.40)	.803 (1.06)	1.147 (2.18)
NW	−.054 (−1.98)	−.071 (−2.36)	−.045 (−1.84)	.048 (.26)	−.095 (−.73)
Poor	.271 (3.70)	.306 (3.74)	.172 (2.59)	.349 (.69)	.512 (1.46)
Sum SE elasticities	18.73	11.93	6.01	37.07	56.40
Log Pop	−.109 (−1.93)	−.031 (−.49)	−.087 (−1.70)	−.369 (−.94)	−.421 (−1.55)

(*Continued*)

negative three times and statistically significant twice.[18] The coefficient for mean suspended particulates was always positive and was statistically significant in three regressions. Among the socioeconomic variables, the percentage of poor families had positive and significant coefficients in three regressions; population density and Log Pop each had a single positive and significant coefficient. No coefficient was statistically significant in regression 7.7-15 for female nonwhites; again, this indicated omitted factors. Nevertheless, the results for this age category generally conform to the 1960 results.

For those aged forty-five to sixty-four, one or the other air pollution variable was significant in four of the five categories (regressions 7.7-16, 7.7-17, 7.7-19, and 7.7-20); the exception was for white females (regression 7.7-18). For the aggregate rate, the coefficients of the two air pollution variables were comparable to the 1960 results; the coefficients of the socioeconomic variables displayed less consistency. For the sex–race-

[18] Negative (but statistically nonsignificant) associations had also occurred in the 1960 analysis of these death rates (regressions 4.3-11, 4.3-13, 4.3-14, and 4.3-15).

TABLE 7.7. (Continued)

| | 15 to 44 years | | | | |
	7.7-11 Total	7.7-12 MW	7.7-13 FW	7.7-14 MNW	7.7-15 FNW
R^2	.283	.319	.219	.269	.023
Constant	99.082	131.654	−.728	307.276	355.330
Air pollution variables					
Min S	−.119 (−1.01)	−.342 (−2.23)	−.173 (−1.98)	1.108 (1.65)	.546 (.82)
Min S elasticities	−2.25	−5.64	−5.57	8.07	7.63
Mean P	.269 (3.46)	.343 (3.41)	.094 (1.63)	1.211 (2.74)	.110 (.25)
Mean P elasticities	14.03	15.63	8.35	24.34	4.26
Socioeconomic variables					
P/M^2	.019 (1.15)	.003 (.15)	.001 (.05)	.254 (2.69)	.035 (.38)
≥65	−.002 (−.01)	.063 (.42)	−.103 (−1.19)	−.121 (−.18)	.354 (.54)
NW	.002 (.06)	−.036 (−.95)	.002 (.11)	1.26 (.76)	.125 (.76)
Poor	.303 (3.88)	.459 (4.54)	.087 (1.50)	1.167 (2.62)	−.048 (−.11)
Sum SE elasticities	15.64	20.15	−1.11	27.37	18.72
Log Pop	.059 (.98)	.026 (.33)	.185 (4.13)	−.202 (−.59)	−.318 (−.93)

specific rates, the correspondence between the two years was less similar. Among the socioeconomic coefficients, population density was always positive, but significant only once. The percentage of the population aged sixty-five and older was also always positive and significant twice; the percentage of nonwhites and that of poor families were each always positive and significant in four regressions; Log Pop was generally negative, and in one instance was significant. Taken as a whole, the coefficients for the air pollution variables were more similar to the 1960 coefficients than were the coefficients for the socioeconomic variables.

For those aged sixty-five and older (regressions 7.7-21 through 7.7-25), at least one and, in most cases, both air pollution variables made significant contributions to each regression except that for male nonwhites (regression 7.7-24). In general, the magnitudes and significance of the air pollution coefficients were similar to those displayed in the 1960 analysis; the socioeconomic variables were seldom significant explanatory variables. Therefore, taken as a whole, these results are in accord with the 1960 findings.

TABLE 7.7. (*Continued*)

	45 to 64 years				
	7.7-16 *Total*	7.7-17 *MW*	7.7-18 *FW*	7.7-19 *MNW*	7.7-20 *FNW*
R^2	.458	.444	.169	.344	.371
Constant	934.906	1323.191	529.523	935.745	1371.425
Air pollution variables					
Min S	.967 (1.78)	.348 (.45)	.205 (.59)	8.645 (2.73)	6.036 (3.16)
Min S elasticities	2.90	.80	1.00	13.86	15.68
Mean P	.934 (2.62)	1.322 (2.60)	.379 (1.66)	2.413 (1.16)	1.356 (1.08)
Mean P elasticities	7.72	8.37	5.09	10.68	9.72
Socioeconomic variables					
P/M²	.138 (1.81)	.129 (1.19)	.134 (2.74)	.179 (.40)	.214 (.80)
≥65	1.413 (2.63)	1.810 (2.36)	.410 (1.19)	5.779 (1.84)	3.205 (1.69)
NW	.346 (2.60)	.389 (2.05)	.035 (.40)	1.948 (2.50)	1.332 (2.84)
Poor	1.712 (4.76)	2.616 (5.11)	.117 (.51)	7.063 (3.37)	3.839 (3.03)
Sum SE elasticities	28.96	30.18	8.84	65.28	61.24
Log Pop	−.411 (−1.48)	−.708 (−1.79)	.131 (.74)	−1.244 (−.77)	−2.073 (−2.12)

(*Continued*)

Thus, this 1969 replication of the 1960 age–sex–race-specific mortality rates generally corroborates the 1960 results. It lends further credence to interpreting the association between air pollution (as measured by both sulfates and suspended particulates) and mortality as a causal one.

ADDITIONAL AIR POLLUTANTS

For 69 of the 112 SMSAs in 1969, data were available on three additional air pollutants: nitrates (NO_3), nitrogen dioxide (NO_2), and sulfur dioxide (SO_2). In tables 7.8, 7.9, and 7.10, the unadjusted total mortality rate, the age–sex–race-adjusted total mortality rate, and the race-adjusted infant mortality rate (under one year), respectively, are analyzed, using these additional air pollution variables. Ten regressions are reported for each mortality rate. In each case, the mortality rate was regressed on the five socioeconomic variables together with each of the following:

1. The three sulfate variables
2. The three suspended particulate variables

TABLE 7.7. (Continued)

	65 years and older				
	7.7-21 Total	7.7-22 MW	7.7-23 FW	7.7-24 MNW	7.7-25 FNW
R^2	.199	.147	.193	.102	.203
Constant	6386.452	8426.032	4842.695	8288.991	5797.957
Air pollution variables					
Min S	6.553 (2.82)	6.640 (2.21)	5.212 (2.48)	14.350 (1.27)	14.435 (2.11)
Min S elasticities	3.76	3.06	3.58	7.34	10.49
Mean P	3.853 (2.52)	2.684 (1.36)	3.535 (2.56)	11.262 (1.52)	10.691 (2.38)
Mean P elasticities	6.10	3.41	6.70	15.90	21.44
Socioeconomic variables					
P/M^2	.466 (1.43)	.429 (1.02)	.576 (1.95)	.049 (.03)	−.113 (−.12)
≥65	−.162 (−.07)	−.189 (−.06)	−.013 (−.01)	−1.339 (−.12)	−.661 (−.10)
NW	.526 (.92)	1.240 (1.68)	−.144 (−.28)	.434 (.16)	2.338 (1.39)
Poor	.875 (.57)	.284 (.14)	−.045 (−.03)	12.231 (1.63)	6.701 (1.48)
Sum SE elasticities	2.80	2.69	.50	15.17	17.28
Log Pop	−1.934 (−1.62)	−2.779 (−1.81)	−.595 (−.55)	−7.158 (−1.24)	−5.866 (−1.67)

Note: All regressions are based on data for 112 SMSAs. The numbers in parentheses below the regression coefficients are t statistics.

Abbreviations: FNW, nonwhite females; FW, white females; MNW, nonwhite males; MW, white males; Total, males and females, whites and nonwhites.

3. The three nitrate variables
4. The three nitrogen dioxide variables
5. The three sulfur dioxide variables
6. The three sulfate plus the three suspended particulate variables
7. The three suspended particulate plus the three sulfur dioxide variables
8. The sets of sulfate, suspended particulate, nitrate, and nitrogen dioxide variables
9. The sets of sulfate, suspended particulate, nitrate, and sulfur dioxide variables
10. All fifteen air pollution variables together.[19]

[19] Specification 7 substituted sulfur dioxide for sulfates to provide a direct comparison of the two groups. Specifications 8 and 9 included four of the five air pollution groups.

Unadjusted total mortality

For the unadjusted total mortality rate, regressions 7.8-1, 7.8-2, and 7.8-5 indicate that sulfates, suspended particulates, and sulfur dioxide had net positive effects. (The combined air pollution elasticities were largest for suspended particulates and smallest for sulfur dioxide.) In addition, regression 7.8-3 shows that the sum of elasticities for nitrates was small and negative, while regression 7.8-4 shows that the sum for nitrogen dioxide was comparable to the sum of elasticities for sulfur dioxide. F tests indicated that each set of air pollution variables except the nitrates set made a significant contribution to the regressions.

Regressions 7.8-6 and 7.8-7 indicated that adding sulfate or sulfur dioxide variables to a regression already including suspended particulate variables raised the explanatory power of the regression but did not increase the total estimated effect of air pollution on mortality. The sum of the air pollution elasticities in these two regressions were comparable to the sum of elasticities for suspended particulates alone (regression 7.8-2).

Regressions 7.8-8 and 7.8-9, each excluding one of the five sets of air pollution variables, indicated that the combined effects of sulfates and suspended particulates were comparable but somewhat smaller than their individual effects in regressions 7.8-1 and 7.8-2. Again, nitrates displayed negative summed elasticities. Nitrogen dioxide displayed a large positive summed elasticity in regression 7.8-8, while the summed sulfur dioxide elasticities were slightly smaller than the sum of the sulfate elasticities in regression 7.8-9.

In regression 7.8-10, the sums of elasticities for each of the groups of air pollution variables were as follows: sulfates, 2.45; suspended particulates, 4.71; nitrates, -4.32; nitrogen dioxide, 6.41; and sulfur dioxide, 2.16. The sum of elasticities for all five air pollutants was 11.41. An F test indicated that the fifteen air pollutants together made a significant contribution to the explanatory power of the regression.

Throughout these ten regressions pertaining to the unadjusted total mortality rate, the socioeconomic variables displayed consistent and significant effects. Only the percentage of poor families failed to have a statistically significant coefficient.

Age–sex–race-adjusted total mortality

The results for the adjusted total mortality rate, shown in table 7.9, are quite similar to the results just reported for the unadjusted total mortality rate; hence, we will discuss in detail only the regression containing measures of all five air pollutants (regression 7.9-10). In regression 7.9-10, the sums of the elasticities for each of the groups of air pollution variables were as follows: sulfates, 2.08; suspended particulates, 5.32; nitrates, -3.43; nitrogen dioxide, 3.45; and sulfur dioxide, 0.99. The sum of elasticities for all five air pollutants was 8.41. An F test indicated that the

TABLE 7.8. Unadjusted Total Mortality Rates (the Effects of Additional Air Pollutants), 1969

	7.8-1	7.8-2	7.8-3	7.8-4	7.8-5	7.8-6	7.8-7	7.8-8	7.8-9	7.8-10
R^2	.848	.842	.792	.815	.843	.869	.875	.915	.914	.924
Constant	570.798	567.612	526.489	753.474	702.037	612.791	699.055	743.408	675.191	808.081
Air pollution variables										
Min S	−.821 (−1.44)					−1.201 (−2.08)		−1.761 (−3.26)	−1.834 (−3.40)	−1.949 (−3.61)
Mean S	1.116 (3.48)					1.098 (3.21)		1.142 (3.51)	1.061 (3.28)	1.030 (3.18)
Max S	−.080 (−.91)					−.124 (−1.40)		−.132 (−1.67)	−.092 (−1.15)	−.101 (−1.28)
Sum S elasticities	8.51					5.47		3.61	3.58	2.45
Min P		.230 (.35)				.019 (.03)	.259 (.40)	−.300 (−.51)	.140 (.22)	−.103 (−.16)
Mean P		.656 (1.69)				.044 (.10)	.314 (.79)	.018 (.05)	−.010 (−.02)	−.145 (−.35)
Max P		.136 (2.00)				.153 (2.34)	.139 (2.02)	.223 (3.79)	.181 (2.73)	.226 (3.37)
Sum P elasticities		12.00				5.07	8.47	5.71	5.74	4.71
Min NO_3			2.478 (.63)					2.027 (.66)	−.031 (−.01)	1.245 (.41)
Mean NO_3			−.509 (−.31)					−1.395 (−1.12)	−.203 (−.16)	−.746 (−.59)
Max NO_3			−.290 (−.76)					−.463 (−1.64)	−.507 (−1.77)	−.464 (−1.66)
Sum NO_3 elasticities			−1.98					−5.48	−3.93	−4.32

Variable	(1)	(2)	(3)	(4)	(5)	(6)	(7)	(8)	(9)
Min NO$_2$				−.853 (−1.97)			−.317 (−.91)		−.376 (−1.10)
Mean NO$_2$				.994 (2.60)			.674 (2.13)		.553 (1.76)
Max NO$_2$				−.141 (−.94)			−.008 (−.07)		−.007 (−.06)
Sum NO$_2$ elasticities				6.72			8.45		6.41
Min SO$_2$				5.973 (2.66)		3.703 (1.62)	2.749 (1.31)		1.709 (.80)
Mean SO$_2$				1.134 (1.49)		1.188 (1.66)	1.397 (2.08)		1.158 (1.76)
Max SO$_2$				−1.27 (−.60)		−.156 (−.80)	−.285 (−1.51)		−.227 (−1.23)
Sum SO$_2$ elasticities				5.48		4.17	2.81		2.16
Socioeconomic variables									
P/M^2	.151 (3.28)	.162 (3.42)	.136 (2.55)	.153 (2.82)	.168 (3.56)	.170 (3.73)	.156 (3.67)	.178 (4.34)	.172 (4.03)
≥65	5.616 (14.70)	6.172 (16.34)	5.998 (13.55)	6.167 (14.74)	5.767 (15.44)	5.887 (16.55)	5.845 (16.47)	5.456 (16.21)	5.700 (16.16)
NW	.488 (4.02)	.575 (4.80)	.484 (3.46)	.526 (3.99)	.584 (4.81)	.535 (4.81)	.605 (5.44)	.525 (4.70)	.589 (5.21)
Poor	−.035 (−.11)	−.134 (−.43)	.034 (.09)	.062 (.18)	.199 (.62)	.088 (.30)	−.090 (−.33)	−.057 (−.21)	−.045 (−.17)
Sum SE elasticities	64.33	70.28	68.60	71.34	67.46	69.11	67.82	63.34	66.75
Log Pop	−.552 (−2.30)	−.693 (−2.88)	−.380 (−1.30)	−.945 (−3.06)	−.777 (−3.06)	−.909 (−3.85)	−.960 (−3.66)	−.710 (−2.97)	−1.039 (−3.88)

Note: All regressions are based on data for sixty-nine SMSAs (see table C.1, pp. 317–320). The numbers in parentheses below the regression coefficients are t statistics.

fifteen air pollution variables together contributed significantly to the regression.

Of the socioeconomic variables, population density and the percentage of nonwhites in the population were consistently significant in the regressions for the adjusted total mortality rate. (Log Pop was significant seven times.)

Race-adjusted infant mortality

The results of examining the effects of additional air pollutants on the race-adjusted infant mortality rate, shown in table 7.10, were comparable to those reported earlier for the infant mortality rate (see table 7.6). F tests indicated that the air pollution variables never made a significant contribution to the regressions. The elasticities of the air pollutants were small or negative, with the exception of suspended particulates, and the sum of all the elasticities in the final regression was close to zero. Log Pop was the only socioeconomic variable that exerted a consistently significant effect in the regressions; the larger the SMSA, the smaller was the race-adjusted infant mortality rate.

Thus, when three additional air pollutants were examined (nitrates, nitrogen dioxide, and sulfur dioxide), nitrates were not found to be important in explaining the variation in the three mortality rates across SMSAs. While nitrogen dioxide and sulfur dioxide often had positive net effects, many of their coefficients were negative (some statistically significant). Thus, sulfates and suspended particulates continued to be the most important air pollutants.

INTERACTIONS BETWEEN AIR POLLUTANTS

A natural question concerning the sixty-nine SMSAs having data on five air pollutants is the extent to which there is evidence of an interaction effect between air pollutants. That is, do two air pollutants have a multiplicative effect on the mortality rate in addition to the sum of the two individual effects? To examine this question, we estimated series of regression triplets, in which the first specification had the two air pollutants entered linearly, the second added a term that was the product of the two air pollutants, and the third had only the multiplicative term.[20] The results are shown in table 7.11. Since results for the unadjusted total mortality rate and age–sex–race-adjusted total mortality rate were similar, we report only the latter results. Thirty regressions were necessary in order to show the results for all possible combinations.

Comparing regressions 7.11-1 and 7.11-2, the product of Mean S and Mean P (Mean S × Mean P) added little when both Mean S and Mean P were present individually. However, it is interesting to note that regression

---

[20] Only the mean measure of each air pollutant was used since it was thought to be the most characteristic measure, and we wanted to lessen the number of parameters to be estimated.

7.11-3, with the product variable alone, had a slightly higher R^2 than did regression 7.11-1, with the two variables entered separately. This also took place with the product of NO_3 and SO_2 and the product of NO_2 and SO_2 (comparing regressions 7.11-25 with 7.11-27, and 7.11-28 with 7.11-30, respectively). In addition, there were two occasions when a product term significantly increased the coefficient of determination of a regression including the individual air pollutants: Mean S $\times$ Mean $\overline{NO}_3$ and Mean $\overline{NO}_3$ $\times$ Mean $\overline{SO}_2$ (regressions 7.11-5 and 7.11-26, respectively). Thus, there appeared to be four cases where the product of two air pollution variables was worthy of further consideration: the two just defined and Mean S $\times$ Mean P and Mean NO_2 $\times$ Mean SO_2.

Upon closer inspection, the equations involving sulfates and nitrates (regressions 7.11-4 through 7.11-6) were of little interest. The coefficient of nitrates was uniformly negative, and regression 7.11-6—with only the product term—explained relatively little of the variance in the adjusted total mortality rate. In the equations with nitrates and nitrogen dioxide (regressions 7.11-22 through 7.11-24), the interaction term was negative (and approached statistical significance in one case and was completely nonsignificant in the other). Looking at the separate equations involving each of the two nitrogen oxides in combination with sulfur dioxide (regressions 7.11-25 through 7.11-30), one notes that the four regressions including product terms had elasticities smaller than the two regressions including the respective pollutants alone. Again, there was no evidence of synergism.

The remaining interaction term of interest was the product of Mean S and Mean P. Looking once more at the relevant regressions, one notes that the summed air pollution elasticities for the regressions including the interaction term (regressions 7.11-2 and 7.11-3) were lower than the summed air pollution elasticities for the regression with the two pollutants entered alone (regression 7.11-1).[21] Taken together, the results indicated that adding the interaction term, Mean S $\times$ Mean P, did little to improve the basic specification we have highlighted throughout. Finally, it should be noted that sulfur dioxide did not show as significant effects as sulfates; the regressions involving sulfur dioxide were each inferior to analogous regressions involving sulfates.

SUMMARY OF THE CROSS-SECTIONAL ANALYSES

In this section we have performed a number of cross-sectional analyses on SMSAs in the United States for the years 1960, 1961, and 1969. In

[21] For the 1960 data set of 117 SMSAs, adding the variable Mean S $\times$ Mean P raised the coefficient of determination from 0.245 to 0.285; the coefficient of the new variable was negative and statistically significant. However, the coefficients of both Mean S and Mean P increased substantially, and the joint effect of a 10 percent decrease in Mean P and Mean S was also substantially increased. With the interaction term alone, R^2 was only 0.205. For the 1969 data set of 112 SMSAs, adding Mean P $\times$ Mean S raised the R^2 from 0.360 to 0.369. The interaction term coefficient was negative. When only the interaction term was included, R^2 was 0.335.

TABLE 7.9. Age–Sex–Race-adjusted Total Mortality Rates (the Effects of Additional Air Pollutants), 1969

	7.9-1	7.9-2	7.9-3	7.9-4	7.9-5	7.9-6	7.9-7	7.9-8	7.9-9	7.9-10
R^2	.516	.531	.355	.434	.497	.594	.607	.689	.702	.728
Constant	1067.027	1057.043	1014.537	1205.630	1166.708	1102.833	1154.284	1193.226	1110.729	1205.511
Air pollution variables										
Min S	−.761					−1.062		−1.486	−1.466	−1.501
	(−1.45)					(−2.03)		(−2.80)	(−2.85)	(−2.85)
Mean S	.979					.889		.901	.920	.827
	(3.32)					(2.87)		(2.82)	(2.98)	(2.62)
Max S	−.078					−.118		−.122	−.094	−.082
	(−.96)					(−1.48)		(−1.56)	(−1.23)	(−1.06)
Sum S elasticities	6.71					3.33		1.84	2.98	2.08
Min P		.298				.094	.086	−.201	−.134	−.281
		(.52)				(.16)	(.14)	(−.34)	(−.22)	(−.45)
Mean P		.604				.182	.516	.155	.317	.218
		(1.76)				(.46)	(1.43)	(.41)	(.78)	(.54)
Max P		.126				.142	.099	.187	.120	.143
		(2.09)				(2.40)	(1.58)	(3.24)	(1.90)	(2.19)
Sum P elasticities		10.78				6.19	8.42	6.17	6.20	5.32
Min NO₃			3.156					2.400	1.362	1.865
			(.89)					(.80)	(.47)	(.64)
Mean NO₃			−.998					−1.486	−1.065	−1.134
			(−.68)					(−1.21)	(−.89)	(−.92)
Max NO₃			−.030					−.212	−.263	−.269
			(−.09)					(−.76)	(−.96)	(−.99)
Sum NO₃ elasticities			−1.00					−3.61	−3.47	−3.43

	(1)	(2)	(3)	(4)	(5)	(6)	(7)	(8)	(9)	(10)
Min NO$_2$	−.888 (−2.27)	−.417 (−1.22)	−.522 (−1.57)							
Mean NO$_2$	.923 (2.69)	.658 (2.12)	.544 (1.78)							
Max NO$_2$	−.170 (−1.26)	−.066 (−.58)	−.071 (−.64)							
Sum NO$_2$ elasticities	4.40	5.64	3.45							
Min SO$_2$				6.201 (3.00)	4.329 (2.09)	3.548 (1.77)	3.141 (1.52)			
Mean SO$_2$				.978 (1.39)	.963 (1.48)	1.079 (1.68)	.976 (1.52)			
Max SO$_2$				−.194 (−.99)	−.225 (−1.27)	−.335 (−1.85)	−.319 (−1.77)			
Sum SO$_2$ elasticities				3.95	2.64	1.35	.99			
Socioeconomic variables										
P/M^2	.110 (2.61)	.118 (2.81)	.100 (2.08)	.117 (2.39)	.133 (3.08)	.129 (3.12)	.139 (3.36)	.126 (3.01)	.146 (3.711)	.150 (3.60)
≥65	−.295 (−.84)	.198 (.59)	.087 (.22)	.143 (.38)	−.194 (−.55)	−.119 (−.35)	−.004 (−.01)	−.047 (−.13)	−.354 (−1.10)	−.206 (−.60)
NW	.329 (2.95)	.399 (3.75)	.334 (2.64)	.337 (2.84)	.335 (3.06)	.424 (3.85)	.377 (3.73)	.431 (3.94)	.364 (3.42)	.385 (3.49)
Poor	.167 (.57)	.088 (.31)	.229 (.69)	.260 (.84)	.320 (1.08)	−.007 (−.03)	.195 (.72)	.087 (.33)	.084 (.32)	.095 (.37)
Sum SE elasticities	4.30	9.27	8.46	9.47	6.97	5.84	8.26	7.46	3.81	5.64
Log Pop	−.363 (−1.65)	−.494 (−2.32)	−.215 (−.81)	−.646 (−2.32)	−.532 (−2.27)	−.496 (−2.32)	−.648 (−3.01)	−.685 (−2.65)	−.436 (−1.91)	−.649 (−2.48)

Note: All regressions are based on data for sixty-nine SMSAs. The numbers in parentheses below the regression coefficients are t statistics.

TABLE 7.10. Race-adjusted Infant Mortality Rates (the Effects of Additional Air Pollutants), 1969

	7.10-1	7.10-2	7.10-3	7.10-4	7.10-5	7.10-6	7.10-7	7.10-8	7.10-9	7.10-10
R^2	.291	.303	.278	.283	.348	.312	.376	.376	.397	.455
Constant	319.604	299.271	289.047	308.521	356.443	313.213	345.444	267.303	328.086	288.655
Air pollution variables										
Min S	−.098 (−.47)					−.033 (−.15)		−.219 (−.88)	−.181 (−.75)	−.270 (−1.10)
Mean S	.173 (1.47)					.095 (.71)		.207 (1.38)	.124 (.85)	.178 (1.21)
Max S	−.030 (−.93)					−.027 (−.80)		−.039 (−1.07)	−.016 (−.45)	−.018 (−.51)
Sum S elasticities	3.81					.97		2.47	1.65	2.88
Min P		.171 (.73)				.123 (.50)	.215 (.87)	.143 (.52)	.150 (.51)	.221 (.76)
Mean P		.126 (.91)				.123 (.73)	.066 (.44)	.132 (.75)	.079 (.41)	.082 (.43)
Max P		−.000 (−.02)				−.001 (−.05)	.003 (.10)	−.007 (−.27)	.001 (.03)	−.014 (−.45)
Sum P elasticities		8.63				7.62	6.83	7.59	6.21	5.55
Min NO₃			1.351 (1.09)					.678 (.48)	.611 (.45)	.271 (.20)
Mean NO₃			−.461 (−.90)					−.522 (−.91)	−.465 (−.83)	−.332 (−.58)
Max NO₃			.006 (.05)					−.003 (−.02)	.005 (.04)	−.010 (−.08)
Sum NO₃ elasticities			−1.76					−4.09	−3.39	−3.18

	(1)	(2)	(3)	(4)	(5)	(6)	(7)	(8)	(9)	(10)
Min NO$_2$				−.118 (−.81)				−.007 (−.04)		−.041 (−.26)
Mean NO$_2$				−.084 (−.65)				−.238 (−1.63)		−.284 (−1.98)
Max NO$_2$				.055 (1.11)				.090 (1.66)		.085 (1.62)
Sum NO$_2$ elasticities				−.25				−3.60		−7.89
Min SO$_2$					.553 (.71)		.243 (.28)		.160 (.17)	.702 (.72)
Mean SO$_2$					.602 (2.28)		.621 (2.29)		.614 (2.03)	.650 (2.17)
Max SO$_2$					−.141 (−1.92)		−.151 (−2.04)		−.168 (−1.99)	−.175 (−2.08)
Sum SO$_2$ elasticities					2.89		1.95		.71	2.08
Socioeconomic variables										
P/M^2	.028 (1.65)	.026 (1.54)	.025 (1.49)	.019 (1.05)	.033 (2.05)	.026 (1.47)	.029 (1.71)	.011 (.56)	.030 (1.62)	.020 (1.01)
≥65	.191 (1.36)	.259 (1.92)	.262 (1.87)	.220 (1.57)	.205 (1.55)	.226 (1.55)	.227 (1.68)	.109 (.67)	.183 (1.21)	.046 (.28)
NW	−.017 (−.39)	−.018 (−.43)	−.024 (−.53)	−.016 (−.36)	−.028 (−.68)	−.016 (−.33)	−.032 (−.76)	−.027 (−.52)	−.037 (−.74)	−.050 (−.96)
Poor	.120 (1.02)	.121 (1.08)	.146 (1.26)	.117 (1.02)	.172 (1.55)	.112 (.92)	.162 (1.43)	.099 (.80)	.150 (1.23)	.119 (.99)
Sum SE elasticities	13.63	16.51	17.33	14.44	16.07	14.86	16.14	7.79	13.43	4.87
Log Pop	−.252 (−2.86)	−.245 (−2.85)	−.193 (−2.09)	−.222 (−2.14)	−.320 (−3.64)	−.263 (−2.85)	−.323 (−3.60)	−.137 (−1.13)	−.271 (−2.53)	−.153 (−1.25)

Note: All regressions are based on data for sixty-nine SMSAs. The numbers in parentheses below the regression coefficients are *t* statistics.

TABLE 7.11. Age–Sex–Race-adjusted Total Mortality Rates (Interactions Between Air Pollutants), 1969

	7.11-1	7.11-2	7.11-3	7.11-4	7.11-5	7.11-6	7.11-7	7.11-8	7.11-9	7.11-10
R^2	.524	.527	.525	.515	.551	.381	.500	.505	.488	.501
Constant	1039.843	1079.640	1111.582	1008.475	1060.075	1105.057	1087.340	1129.172	1219.935	1074.915
Air pollution variables										
Mean S	.369 (2.00)	.148 (.34)		.657 (4.63)	.087 (.29)		.578 (3.98)	.316 (.82)		.544 (3.44)
Mean P	.600 (1.92)	.304 (.50)								
Mean NO_3				−.940 (−1.59)	−4.630 (−2.59)					
Mean NO_2							1.31 (.78)	−.064 (−.20)		
Mean SO_2										.247 (.?6)
Product		.202 (.57)	.361 (4.87)		2.881 (2.18)	.731 (1.95)		.172 (.73)	.282 (4.19)	
Sum AP elasticities	10.66	7.53	4.64	5.80	−1.58	1.98	8.82	5.83	4.80	7.40
Socioeconomic variables										
P/M^2	.108 (2.65)	.109 (2.65)	.109 (2.71)	.091 (2.19)	.097 (2.40)	.117 (2.53)	.099 (2.39)	.101 (2.41)	.102 (2.44)	.098 (2.36)
≥65	−.058 (−.17)	−.034 (−.10)	−.028 (−.09)	−.287 (−.83)	−.449 (−1.30)	.056 (.15)	−.106 (−.30)	−.144 (−.40)	−.024 (−.07)	−.215 (−.62)
NW	.325 (3.01)	.343 (3.04)	.352 (3.39)	.238 (2.15)	.201 (1.86)	.367 (3.10)	.302 (2.72)	.305 (2.74)	.347 (3.22)	.218 (2.60)
Poor	.205 (.73)	.150 (.50)	.116 (.42)	.374 (1.30)	.468 (1.66)	.164 (.52)	.305 (1.06)	.294 (1.02)	.289 (1.01)	.343 (1.17)
Sum SE elasticities	6.82	6.79	6.65	4.84	3.74	8.18	6.87	6.47	8.14	5.90
Log Pop	−.423 (−2.00)	−.439 (−2.04)	−.444 (−.213)	−.257 (−1.17)	−.206 (−.96)	−.414 (−1.71)	−.475 (−1.83)	−.490 (−1.88)	−.656 (−2.85)	−.414 (−1.86)

	7.11-11	7.11-12	7.11-13	7.11-14	7.11-15	7.11-16	7.11-17	7.11-18	7.11-19	7.11-20
R^2	.505	.428	.513	.522	.349	.500	.501	.463	.509	.509
Constant	1034.844	1182.427	1004.866	937.688	1086.527	1093.516	1083.035	1244.175	1087.648	1082.211
Air pollution variables										
Mean S	.646 (2.95)									
Mean P			1.104 (4.59)	1.584 (3.13)		.967 (3.98)	1.053 (1.37)		.899 (3.60)	.920 (2.77)
Mean NO_3			−.945 (−1.60)	1.741 (.68)						
Mean NO_2						.160 (.97)	.218 (.42)			
Mean SO_2	.813 (.92)				.404 (.79)				.380 (1.42)	.451 (.58)
Product	−.367 (−.68)	.436 (3.04)		−2.496 (−1.08)			−.056 (−.12)	.373 (3.72)		−.057 (−.10)
Sum AP elasticities	8.87	2.02	9.32	14.53	.94	12.29	13.20	5.40	10.63	10.88
Socioeconomic variables										
P/M^2	.095 (2.27)	.103 (2.34)	.108 (2.62)	.108 (2.61)	.113 (2.39)	.115 (2.75)	.114 (2.72)	.110 (2.58)	.111 (2.69)	.111 (2.66)
≥65	−.252 (−.711)	−.113 (−.31)	.018 (.05)	.090 (.26)	.098 (.25)	.176 (.51)	.187 (.52)	.194 (.55)	.003 (.01)	−.001 (−.00)
NW	.273 (2.50)	.325 (2.85)	.341 (3.14)	.342 (3.16)	.374 (3.02)	.396 (3.64)	.396 (3.61)	.412 (3.70)	.361 (3.38)	.361 (3.35)
Poor	.394 (1.30)	.319 (1.04)	.180 (.63)	.179 (.63)	.150 (.46)	.138 (.48)	.142 (.49)	.177 (.60)	.217 (.74)	.223 (.74)
Sum SE elasticities	5.89	7.29	7.53	8.21	8.51	9.44	9.58	10.15	8.03	8.04
Log Pop	−.370 (−1.58)	−.532 (−2.23)	−.353 (−1.59)	−.335 (−1.51)	−.371 (−1.45)	−.584 (−2.26)	−.583 (−2.24)	−.740 (−2.97)	−.524 (−2.37)	−.519 (−2.27)

(*Continued*)

155

TABLE 7.11. (Continued)

	7.11-21	7.11-22	7.11-23	7.11-24	7.11-25	7.11-26	7.11-27	7.11-28	7.11-29	7.11-30
R^2	.438	.378	.409	.343	.406	.455	.429	.418	.441	.425
Constant	1195.769	1144.675	1103.472	1053.783	1152.465	1172.532	1196.888	1199.868	1334.081	1219.967
Air pollution variables										
Mean S										
Mean P										
Mean NO_3		−.552 (−.83)	3.315 (1.48)		.207 (.31)	−1.534 (−1.56)			−.008 (−.04)	
Mean NO_2		.328 (1.78)	.876 (2.47)					.210 (1.17)		
Mean SO_2					.730 (2.49)	−.388 (−.70)		.628 (2.22)	−1.521 (−1.10)	
Product	.579 (3.24)		−2.379 (−1.80)	−.047 (−.14)		5.984 (2.34)	3.814 (3.06)		1.184 (1.58)	.418 (2.98)
Sum AP elasticities	2.13	3.41	12.13	−.15	2.98	−.79	2.55	5.14	1.01	2.24
Socioeconomic variables										
P/M^2	.105 (2.40)	.101 (2.15)	.100 (2.18)	.108 (2.28)	.103 (2.25)	.099 (2.25)	.109 (2.47)	.100 (2.22)	.108 (2.41)	.102 (2.31)
≥65	−.068 (−.19)	.159 (.41)	.252 (.65)	.054 (.14)	−.103 (−.27)	−.118 (−.32)	−.021 (−.06)	−.002 (−.01)	.027 (.07)	−.086 (−.24)
NW	.334 (2.96)	.369 (2.98)	.391 (3.20)	.350 (2.80)	.336 (2.80)	.270 (2.27)	.332 (2.92)	.355 (3.00)	.354 (3.03)	.335 (2.93)
Poor	.297 (.99)	.281 (.87)	.282 (.89)	.195 (.60)	.358 (1.12)	.443 (1.42)	.336 (1.10)	.379 (1.20)	.251 (.78)	.348 (1.13)
Sum SE elasticities	7.65	10.09	11.28	8.13	7.88	7.59	8.47	9.26	8.44	7.94
Log Pop	−.563 (−2.36)	−.536 (−1.84)	−.628 (−2.16)	−.291 (−1.08)	−.506 (−1.93)	−.474 (−1.87)	−.585 (−2.39)	−.645 (−2.30)	−.793 (−2.71)	−.610 (−2.45)

Note: All regressions are based on data for sixty-nine SMSAs. The numbers in parentheses below the regression coefficients are t statistics. The thirty regressions above represent ten sets of triplets. The first regression in each set includes two air pollutants entered linearly. The second regression in each set includes the two air pollutants entered linearly as well as a product term of the two air pollutants. The third regression in each set includes only the product term.

chapter 3 an ad hoc relationship was estimated between the unadjusted total mortality rate and both air pollution and socioeconomic variables for 1960, and corroborated by both a principal component analysis and a partial replication for 1961. A number of different functional forms (log-log, quadratic, dummy variable, and linear spline) were examined, as well as splitting the sample into two parts on the basis of suspended particulate pollution.[22] The addition of dummy variables representing census regions of the country increased the explanatory power over the original regression but did not appreciably affect the estimated coefficients of the air pollution variables. The effects of migration were explored by examining the change in SMSA population between 1950 and 1960; there was little effect on the air pollution coefficients. Jackknife estimates indicated that the estimated co-efficients were not sensitive to "extreme" observations. To test whether multicollinearity among the explanatory variables could be responsible for the observed effect of air pollution, a two-stage procedure was undertaken in which the air pollution variables were initially excluded from the regres-sion and then the unexplained portion of the mortality rate was regressed on only the air pollution variables. The air pollution measures continued to be significant.

In chapter 4, a number of additional death rates were investigated: the mortality rates for infants under one year of age (total, race-adjusted, and race-specific); age–sex–race-adjusted total mortality rates; twenty-four age–sex–race-specific mortality rates; and fifteen disease-specific mortality rates. The infant mortality rate was more closely associated with suspended particulates than sulfates. The results were satisfactorily replicated for 1961. Air pollution (as measured by sulfates and suspended particulates) was also a significant factor in explaining the variation in the adjusted total mor-tality rate across SMSAs. For the age–sex–race-specific rates, air pollu-tion was more closely associated with mortality among nonwhites than among whites. In addition, the mortality rates for the older age groups were most closely associated. Using these results, it was estimated that if the relationships were causal, a 50 percent abatement of suspended par-ticulates and sulfates would be estimated to increase life expectancy by slightly less than one year. For the disease-specific death rates, total can-cers and cancer of the digestive system were closely related to sulfate pollution in 1960, although the results did not replicate well for 1961. Total cardiovascular mortality, as well as four subclassifications, were closely associated with sulfate pollution in both 1960 and 1961. The re-sults for the total and five respiratory disease rates often included nonsignifi-cant air pollution effects. We attributed the lack of association largely to

[22] While there was some indication that the linear specification could be improved upon, we decided to emphasize the simple form and reexamine alternative forms using the 1969 data.

difficulties due to sampling variation in examining these extremely small mortality rates.

Sets of additional explanatory variables were added to the regressions in chapter 5. Occupation mix, home-heating equipment, home-heating fuels, water-heating fuels, prevalence of air conditioning, and climate variables were conjectured as possible "true" causes of the association between the measures of air pollution and the mortality rates. The addition of occupation variables had a greater effect on the socioeconomic variables than on the air pollution variables. The addition of the group of home-heating fuels had the most pronounced effect on the estimated air pollution coefficients. We conjecture that this was due to a combination of multicollinearity problems and the possibility that the type of home-heating fuel was a better indication of air pollution exposure than the rather poor data on ambient air quality which were available.

In chapter 6 we analyzed several social ills assumed to be related to urbanization but not to air pollution. Suicides were not associated with air pollution in 1960 or in 1961. For the three venereal disease rates examined, no air pollution variable was statistically significant in both 1960 and 1961. For total crimes, as well as seven subclassifications of crime, no consistent association with air pollution was evident in 1960 (a 1961 replication was not undertaken).

Finally, in this chapter we presented a 1969 replication of the 1960 analysis. The results for the 1969 unadjusted and adjusted total mortality rates were generally similar to the earlier results, although some dissimilarities were noted with respect to the adjusted rate. The jackknife technique and the deletion of outliers was applied to the 1969 data, and it was found that the estimated air pollution effects were not very sensitive to particular data points or "extreme" observations, while the estimated socioeconomic effects exhibited less stability. Alternative specifications to the simple linear form were also reexamined, using the 1969 data. None was found to be superior to the simple linear specification. The residuals from several of the basic 1960 and 1969 regressions were examined in search of systematic relationships. The most highly populated SMSAs were explained well by the regressions. To a lesser extent this was also true for the southwestern SMSAs, although there was a slight tendency to overestimate their mortality rates. There was some evidence that an important variable (or variables) had been omitted, since SMSAs with unexpectedly large (or small) mortality rates in 1960 had large (or small) mortality rates in 1969. Thus, some other factors in addition to those variables used in the analysis were significant in raising or lowering the mortality rate. Cross-lagged cross-sectional correlations indicated a possible lag effect of our measures of air pollution on mortality but did not provide evidence contrary to the hypothesis of causality. The findings in chapter 4 pertaining to infant mortality and age–sex–race-specific mortality were replicated using 1969 data; the results were comparable. Finally, additional air pollutants (nitrates, nitrogen dioxide, and sulfur dioxide) were analyzed. Nitrates were not found to be important in explaining the variation in mortality rates across SMSAs. To a lesser extent this was true for nitrogen dioxide and sulfur dioxide. Both sulfates and suspended particulates continued to be the most significant air pollution measures. Furthermore, interaction variables consisting of the product of pairs of air pollution measures were found to add little to the analysis.

We have performed a number of analyses to test the validity of the original 1960 results. In general, we found that those mortality rates we expected to be closely associated with air pollution were so, whereas rates that we did not expect to be closely associated with air pollution were not. Not all the factors hypothesized to affect mortality have been controlled in the analysis. However, considerable evidence has been presented concerning the relationship between air pollution and various mortality rates. Although it is impossible to prove causality in this case, we believe that the evidence is sufficient to convince an impartial observer that the estimated association between air pollution and mortality is probably a causal one. Further demonstration of this relationship will be presented in section III.

Annual and daily time-series analyses

CHAPTER 8

Cross-sectional
time-series analysis,
1960–69

In section II we presented an extensive analysis of cross-sectional data for more than one hundred SMSAs in order to explore the association between measurements of air pollution and mortality rates. Implicit in the cross-sectional analysis is the assumption that factors causing increases in mortality, which are not constant across observations, are either accounted for explicitly in the analysis or are uncorrelated with the measured air pollutants. Consequently, to control for factors that cause increases in mortality, we added a host of explanatory variables characterizing demography, home-heating characteristics, climate, and occupation mix, and we found that the results were not inconsistent with the hypothesis that air pollution increases the mortality rate.

Since one can never hope to measure all the factors that vary across areas, the possibility remains that one or more of the factors shown in table 1.1, but not included in the analysis, might be correlated with air pollution and thus might be the "true" cause of the relationship we have observed. Another approach to controlling for unmeasured factors is by analyzing an area over a period of time. Whatever the factors are (for example, genetic factors, smoking habits, or medical care) that cause the mortality rate to be lower in Dallas than in New York City, they should be relatively constant over time within each city. This is particularly true when the number of deaths are compared from one day to the next, but to a lesser extent it should also apply to comparisons of mortality rates within a city from one year to the next. Thus, a time-series analysis presents a different method for investigating the association between air pollution and mortality rates while controlling for unmeasured factors.

The relationship between air pollution and mortality is likely to differ between time-series and cross-sectional studies. For example, an analysis of daily deaths and air pollution levels is designed to discover how day-to-day changes in mortality are related to day-to-day changes in air quality. An analysis of annual mortality rates and air pollution levels across cities is designed to discover the long-term effects of air pollution, since cities with relatively good air quality are likely to have had it for many years. An analysis of year-to-year changes in air quality and mortality rates is a hybrid between the pure time-series and cross-sectional analyses. In exploring these time-series relationships here, we provide a different way to control for unmeasured factors affecting mortality and offer new insights into the air pollution–mortality relationship.

We begin this section with an analysis of annual time-series data (1960–69) for twenty-six SMSAs.[1] (Chapter 9 consists of an analysis of daily data for five cities.) The goal of the present chapter is to examine that component of the annual death rate which is associated with annual changes in air quality. The factors that were hypothesized to affect a cross-sectional analysis of mortality rates (discussed in chapter 1) are also assumed to apply to time-series analysis. However, the focus shifts when one moves from cross-sectional to time-series analysis, since variables such as occupation mix and home-heating fuels vary little over time, while variables such as climate and air pollution can vary a great deal. In a cross-sectional time-series analysis of the air pollution–mortality relationship the variation in the mortality rate can be thought of as being comprised of two types of elements. The first type is cross-sectional elements relating to differences in air quality and mortality *across* areas. The second type is time-series elements relating to changing air quality and mortality over time *within* an area. For the annual data analyzed here, the year-to-year variations in the mortality rate and air quality might give rise to a relationship quite different from that of our previous cross-sectional analysis.

The cross-sectional time-series relationship is estimated with the same variables used in chapter 3, supplemented by factors hypothesized to control for changes in the mortality rate over time. The primary air pollution data measures—suspended particulates and sulfates—were available as annual measures for the period 1960–69. In addition, nitrates, nitrogen dioxide, and sulfur dioxide were studied for a subsample of fifteen SMSAs during the years 1962–68. Again, the socioeconomic characteristics were population density, the percentage of population aged sixty-five and older, the percentage of the population that was nonwhite, the percentage of families in the SMSA with incomes below the poverty level, and a population variable. Since these data were taken from the census and were available only every ten years, we used the 1960 and 1970 figures in order to calculate values for the intervening years by linear

---

[1] See table C.1 (pp. 317–320) for a list of the twenty-six SMSAs. The data set was not complete, since missing air pollution data required deleting 19 of the 260 possible observations.

interpolation. The mortality rates we examined were for unadjusted total deaths, age–sex–race-adjusted total deaths, and race-adjusted deaths for infants under one year of age. Because yearly population figures were not reported, the interpolated population figures were used in computing both the unadjusted and adjusted total mortality rates. Consequently, they were both subject to error.[2] The infant mortality rate, calculated from the ratio of deaths to live births should be accurate since statistics for both deaths and live births were published annually.

THE EFFECT OF TIME

Mortality rates change over time for reasons other than the possible effects of air pollution. These include changes in income and in medical care, occurrences of natural disasters, outbreaks of epidemics, and so on. There are several methods of controlling for such factors. One common way is to add a linear time variable, that is, a variable representing the year in which a specific mortality rate was observed. The time variable then acts as a proxy for omitted factors associated with the time of observation. Another procedure used in controlling for time-related factors is to add a vector of time dummy variables. For example, in our analysis, ten variables were defined, one for each year. The first variable assumed a value of one for the 1960 observations and zero for observations in other years; the second assumed a value of one for the 1961 observations and zero for observations in other years; and so on. Statistically, the vector of time dummy variables is more general than the linear time variable discussed above (estimating nine parameters instead of one parameter). The time dummy variables can characterize effects common to most of the areas in any given year, while the linear time variable can characterize only a trend common to most areas over the period of analysis.

Changes in an area's mortality rate can be thought of as being influenced by factors that are uniform across all areas, for example, rising income, better medical knowledge, and national programs such as Medicare, as well as by factors that are peculiar to each area, such as climate and air pollution. Two ways to account for factors that are uniform across areas have been described above; a third way involves using the national mortality rate as an explanatory variable. The mortality rate for the entire United States reflects the influences of some of the factors that are uniform across the nation.

Similarly, there may be characteristics in each SMSA that are important causes of mortality but are either unmeasured or measured inadequately in our data. If so, one might insert a dummy variable for each SMSA.[3]

---

[2] See the discussion in chapter 3 (pp. 40–43) regarding the 1961 reestimation.

[3] This approach is similar to the variance component approach in cross-sectional time-series analysis; see Wallace and Hussain (1969).

We have examined this procedure in a preliminary analysis. The results indicated that the SMSA dummy variables alone explained more than 78.6 percent of the variation in the age–sex–race-adjusted total mortality rate, and that the SMSA and time dummy variables together explained almost 91.1 percent of the variation in the mortality rate (results were somewhat higher for the unadjusted total mortality and the race-adjusted infant mortality rates). Since little variation was left to be explained by the other independent variables, and since all the independent variables were closely associated with the SMSA and time dummy variables, one would not expect the air pollution and socioeconomic variables to contribute significantly to the explanatory power of the regressions. Indeed, when the SMSA and time dummy variables were included, the estimated coefficients of the air pollution variables were statistically nonsignificant in explaining the three mortality rates (the coefficients were generally negative as well). As a consequence of these preliminary findings, we chose to exclude the SMSA dummy variables in the subsequent investigation.

Insertion of the time variable(s) should still be viewed with caution. Its use is testimony to our ignorance and the lack of relevant data. Time is not hypothesized to be a causal factor; rather, it is a surrogate for possible causal factors omitted from the analysis. Specifically, the time variable(s) will represent characteristics common to most SMSAs in a given year. When such characteristics are controlled, they may bias the estimated coefficients of the air pollution variables toward showing no effects. For example, if air pollution is higher (across SMSAs) in some years than in others, increased mortality from increased air pollution might be ascribed to the time variables rather than to the air pollution variables.[4] The same comments apply, although less decidedly, to the U.S. mortality-rate variable.

In cross-sectional time-series analyses, coefficients of determination (R^2) and t statistics are often high. This stems in part from the fact that year-to-year variations within an SMSA are small compared with the variation across SMSAs during any one period. In the limit, if all observations on an SMSA were identical, a cross-sectional time-series regression would overstate the degrees of freedom. Further, the coefficient of determination and the t statistics corresponding to the explanatory variables would be biased upward. The implication on our analysis is that we can expect the following regressions to manifest more favorable significance tests than those of chapters 3 through 7.

---

[4] The data for this period (1960–69) indicate that air pollution rose, then fell or exhibited unsystematic patterns in the SMSAs. In contrast, the adjusted total mortality rate generally fell over the period. Positive and significant coefficients for the air pollution variables will mean that, on the average, increases in these air pollutants were still associated with increases in the mortality rate and that, on the average, decreases in these air pollutants were still associated with decreases in the mortality rate (after controlling for socioeconomic factors and the time trend).

TOTAL DEATHS

In our first analysis of the cross-sectional time-series data pool (table 8.1), we regressed the unadjusted total mortality rate on the factors that were used in our earlier cross-sectional analyses. These included three measures of sulfate air pollution (Min S, Mean S, and Max S), the three measures of suspended particulate air pollution (Min P, Mean P, and Max P), population density (P/M^2), the percentage of the population aged sixty-five and older ($\geqq 65$), the percentage of the population who were nonwhite (NW), the percentage of families with incomes below the poverty level (Poor), and the logarithm of SMSA population (Log Pop).[5] In addition, the U.S. total mortality rate for each year was included. More than 90 percent of the variation in the unadjusted total mortality rate was explained by the variables in regression 8.1-1. An F test indicated that the six air pollution variables contributed significantly to the explanatory power of the regression.

The sum of the elasticities of the three sulfate variables was somewhat smaller than in the 1960 analysis (see regression 3.1-1, page 31), but the sum of elasticities of the three suspended particulate variables was somewhat larger. The sum of the six air pollution elasticities (9.30) was almost identical to the sum of elasticities in 1960 (9.41). Contrary to expectations, the coefficient of population density was negative, while the coefficient of Log Pop was positive and had a numerically larger effect than did population density. All of the other socioeconomic variables had positive and significant coefficients. The coefficient of the U.S. total mortality rate was also positive and significant, indicating that there were national variations in the mortality rate over time that were not controlled in the analysis.

In regression 8.1-2, the regression was rerun with the two air pollution measures included in our earlier analysis, Min S and Mean P. The coefficient of determination fell slightly (from 0.907 to 0.899) and, as expected, the magnitudes and significance of the two air pollution coefficients increased substantially.

Regressions 8.1-3 and 8.1-4 present similar specifications except that a linear time variable was substituted for the U.S. total mortality rate. The results indicated slightly lower elasticities for sulfates in both cases and a slightly higher elasticity for suspended particulates in one case (in the other, it stayed virtually the same). In addition, the coefficient for nonwhites increased, the coefficient for poor became negative (and nonsignificant), and the coefficient for Log Pop became nonsignificant. The coefficients of determination were slightly higher than those for the previous specification.

---

[5] The SMSAs for which cross-sectional time-series data were available were somewhat different from the SMSAs which were used for the purely cross-sectional analysis. Both the twenty-six SMSAs and the subset of fifteen SMSAs tended to be more polluted, more densely populated, and larger in population; they also had higher mortality rates.

TABLE 8.1. Unadjusted Total Mortality Rates (Cross-sectional Time-series), 1960–69

	8.1-1	8.1-2	8.1-3	8.1-4	8.1-5	8.1-6
R^2	.907	.899	.913	.909	.922	.919
Constant	−773.977	−781.716	5.331	16.482	−16.164	−17.467
Air pollution variables						
Min S	.160	.470	.121	.316	.105	.353
	(1.15)	(4.63)	(.90)	(3.20)	(.76)	(3.55)
Mean S	.187		.119		.188	
	(1.75)		(1.16)		(1.81)	
Max S	.004		.008		−.014	
	(.16)		(.34)		(−.54)	
Sum S elasticities	3.50	2.18	2.50	1.47	2.68	1.64
Min P	.517		.415		.347	
	(3.28)		(2.68)		(2.29)	
Mean P	.233	.508	.254	.507	.305	.509
	(1.80)	(6.56)	(2.01)	(6.89)	(2.48)	(7.09)
Max P	−.003		.016		.006	
	(−.11)		(.64)		(.23)	
Sum P elasticities	5.80	6.87	6.14	6.85	6.13	6.89
Socioeconomic variables						
P/M²	−.116	−.087	−.111	−.095	−.116	−.098
	(−3.91)	(−2.93)	(−3.87)	(−3.39)	(−4.20)	(−3.61)
≥65	8.424	8.494	8.958	9.063	8.907	9.050
	(36.56)	(38.14)	(37.41)	(39.73)	(38.57)	(41.29)
NW	.582	.610	.719	.756	.718	.757
	(12.95)	(13.68)	(14.36)	(15.67)	(14.85)	(16.26)
Poor	.243	.247	−.101	−.150	−.108	−.148
	(3.19)	(3.20)	(−1.07)	(−1.60)	(−1.18)	(−1.64)
Sum SE elasticities	88.83	90.30	91.98	93.14	91.34	93.02
Log Pop	.156	.141	.031	.007	.025	.006
	(2.11)	(1.88)	(.41)	(.10)	(.35)	(.08)
U.S. total mortality rate	.727	.733				
	(3.38)	(3.34)				
Linear time			−5.240	−6.033		
			(−5.19)	(−6.13)		
Time dummy variables[a]						
1960					24.129	27.443
1961					9.245	9.852
1962					15.308	17.173
1963					21.755	22.672
1964					−4.715	−1.567
1965					−11.258	−12.865
1966					−2.201	−2.741
1967					−21.881	−23.513
1968					−1.270	−1.136
1969					−31.655	−35.316

Note: All regressions are based on data for twenty-six SMSAs (see table C.1, pp. 317–320). The number of observations was equal to 241. The numbers in parentheses below the regression coefficients are t statistics.

[a] The estimated effects of the time dummy variables were scaled so that they summed to zero.

A set of time dummy variables was substituted for the linear time variable in regressions 8.1-5 and 8.1-6.[6] These two regressions were almost identical to the previous regressions with the linear time variable. The coefficients of the linear time variable, as well as the coefficients of the time dummy variables, reflect the generally decreasing trends in the mortality rate over time after controlling for the other included factors.

These results corroborate those reported in the cross-sectional work of section II. However, it should be noted that, compared to our previous findings, sulfates exerted a slightly smaller estimated effect on the mortality rates, while suspended particulates exerted a slightly larger estimated effect. It is interesting to observe that in some cases the combined estimated elasticities for suspended particulates and sulfates were almost identical to those from the cross-sectional results.

AGE–SEX–RACE-ADJUSTED TOTAL DEATHS

The analysis just reported for the unadjusted total mortality rate was replicated for the age–sex–race-adjusted total mortality rate.[7] The results (shown in table 8.2) were similar to those for the unadjusted total mortality rate. Again, the suspended particulate variables were more closely associated with the adjusted total mortality rate than were the sulfate variables. The socioeconomic variables all tended to be statistically significant (with the exception of Log Pop) and generally had the same signs as in the analysis of the unadjusted total mortality rate. Substituting the linear time variable or the time dummy variables for the U.S. total mortality rate had almost the same effect as that which occurred in the analyses of the unadjusted total mortality rate.

RACE-ADJUSTED INFANT DEATHS

Table 8.3 displays the cross-sectional time-series results for the race-adjusted mortality rate for infants under one year of age. Regressions 8.3-1 and 8.3-2 are analogous to the original 1960 cross-sectional regressions (see regressions 4.1-4 and 4.1-5 on page 54). Comparing the coefficients in the two sets of regressions, one notes that the estimated effect of sulfates was consistently negative in the cross-sectional time-series analysis (though statistically nonsignificant), and the estimated effect of suspended particulates was diminished. The socioeconomic variables displayed mixed results. The U.S. infant mortality rate was highly significant, apparently acting as a surrogate for general factors affecting infant mortality during the 1960s. As expected, the explanatory powers of the

---

[6] These dummy variables are reported so that the sum of the time effects is zero; thus, each coefficient is relative to all others.

[7] Since detailed demographic data are collected only every decade, we calculated the adjusted rates by using linear interpolation of the individual population classes for the period 1960–70 and then applied the direct method of adjustment (see appendix E, pages 346–347).

TABLE 8.2. Age–Sex–Race-adjusted Total Mortality Rates (Cross-sectional Time-series), 1960–69

	8.2-1	8.2-2	8.2-3	8.2-4	8.2-5	8.2-6
R^2	.611	.576	.650	.635	.685	.670
Constant	−32.113	−26.085	766.349	780.734	736.353	736.526
Air pollution variables						
Min S	.159	.521	.104	.328	.081	.372
	(.96)	(4.33)	(.66)	(2.87)	(.51)	(3.20)
Mean S	.223		.148		.232	
	(1.76)		(1.24)		(1.91)	
Max S	−.005		−.003		−.030	
	(−.17)		(−.11)		(−1.00)	
Sum S elasticities	3.46	2.27	2.30	1.43	2.48	1.62
Min P	.618		.472		.403	
	(3.31)		(2.63)		(2.27)	
Mean P	.321	.619	.353	.615	.416	.627
	(2.08)	(6.74)	(2.41)	(7.23)	(2.90)	(7.47)
Max P	−.011		.012		.001	
	(−.35)		(.41)		(.04)	
Sum P elasticities	6.82	7.85	7.18	7.81	7.31	7.95
Socioeconomic variables						
P/M²	−.098	−.062	−.093	−.074	−.099	−.077
	(−2.77)	(−1.78)	(−2.77)	(−2.26)	(−3.06)	(−2.44)
≥65	1.427	1.498	2.105	2.218	2.048	2.205
	(5.22)	(5.67)	(7.57)	(8.40)	(7.59)	(8.61)
NW	.345	.375	.522	.562	.521	.564
	(6.47)	(7.08)	(8.98)	(10.05)	(9.23)	(10.37)
Poor	.204	.217	−.237	−.284	−.249	−.285
	(2.26)	(2.38)	(−2.15)	(−2.61)	(−2.33)	(−2.70)
Sum SE elasticities	17.67	19.24	21.40	22.63	20.67	22.49
Log Pop	.099	.075	−.062	−.094	−.070	−.096
	(1.13)	(.84)	(−.72)	(−1.10)	(−.83)	(−1.17)
U.S. total mortality rate	.721	.715				
	(2.82)	(2.75)				
Linear time			−6.878	−7.772		
			(−5.87)	(−6.82)		
Time dummy variables[a]						
1960					33.128	37.105
1961					11.423	11.617
1962					22.637	24.322
1963					24.365	25.235
1964					−7.484	−3.428
1965					−13.959	−15.121
1966					−3.465	−4.559
1967					−25.467	−26.735
1968					−3.178	−6.087
1969					−38.001	−42.354

Note: All regressions are based on data for twenty-six SMSAs (see table C.1, pp. 317–320). The number of observations was equal to 241. The numbers in parentheses below the regression coefficients are t statistics.

[a] The estimated effects of the time dummy variables were scaled so that they summed to zero.

TABLE 8.3. Race-adjusted Infant Mortality Rates (Cross-sectional Time-series), 1960–69

	8.3-1	8.3-2	8.3-3	8.3-4	8.3-5	8.3-6
R^2	.476	.466	.465	.451	.486	.476
Constant	−32.825	−31.942	142.680	154.974	124.815	133.482
Air pollution variables						
Min S	−.045	−.032	−.030	−.028	−.021	−.023
	(−.53)	(−.52)	(−.35)	(−.46)	(−.24)	(−.36)
Mean S	.020		.002		.001	
	(.31)		(.02)		(.01)	
Max S	−.020		−.019		−.017	
	(−1.28)		(−1.22)		(−1.02)	
Sum S elasticities	−2.40	−.61	−3.07	−.54	−2.69	−.44
Min P	.054		.079		.041	
	(.55)		(.81)		(.41)	
Mean P	.117	.088	.138	.103	.135	.086
	(1.49)	(1.93)	(1.73)	(2.24)	(1.67)	(1.85)
Max P	−.014		−.017		−.017	
	(−.86)		(−1.04)		(−1.03)	
Sum P elasticities	5.92	4.89	7.21	5.74	6.24	4.81
Socioeconomic variables						
P/M²	−.014	−.012	−.015	−.012	−.014	−.012
	(−.79)	(−.67)	(−.82)	(−.70)	(−.76)	(−.67)
≥65	.534	.527	.565	.537	.555	.531
	(3.63)	(3.79)	(3.73)	(3.75)	(3.65)	(3.73)
NW	.086	.086	.088	.084	.089	.086
	(2.80)	(2.92)	(2.76)	(2.78)	(2.81)	(2.86)
Poor	.149	.157	.133	.147	.139	.153
	(−2.64)	(2.83)	(2.23)	(2.49)	(2.32)	(2.61)
Sum SE elasticities	31.32	31.55	31.91	31.34	31.92	31.55
Log Pop	.039	.023	.040	.019	.037	.021
	(.83)	(.51)	(.84)	(.41)	(.77)	(.45)
U.S. infant mortality rate	.656	.684				
	(6.36)	(6.95)				
Linear time			−3.784	−3.927		
			(−5.92)	(−6.37)		
Time dummy variables[a]						
1960					11.831	12.531
1961					10.986	10.109
1962					12.094	11.776
1963					4.812	4.717
1964					9.176	9.978
1965					2.139	3.249
1966					−5.162	−5.272
1967					−10.793	−10.280
1968					−13.399	−14.203
1969					−21.680	−22.606

Note: All regressions are based on data for twenty-six SMSAs (see table C.1, pp. 317–320). The number of observations was equal to 241. The numbers in parentheses below the regression coefficients are *t* statistics.

[a] The estimated effects of the time dummy variables were scaled so that they summed to zero.

cross-sectional time-series regressions were larger than those of the 1960 cross-sectional regressions.

The U.S. infant mortality rate was replaced by a linear time variable in regressions 8.3-3 and 8.3-4 and, later, by time dummy variables in regressions 8.3-5 and 8.3-6. There was little change. Thus, for the race-adjusted infant mortality rate, the cross-sectional time-series results displayed nonsignificant (and even negative) estimated effects for sulfate pollution and nonsignificant estimated effects for suspended particulate pollution compared with the earlier cross-sectional results of chapter 4.

ADDITIONAL AIR POLLUTANTS

Using the subset of SMSAs for which data on three additional air pollutants—nitrates (NO_3), nitrogen dioxide (NO_2), and sulfur dioxide (SO_2)—were available (fifteen SMSAs for 1962–68),[8] we examined the air pollution effects on the unadjusted total, the age–sex–race-adjusted total, and the race-adjusted infant mortality rates. This analysis was similar to that found in chapter 7 (see tables 7.8, 7.9, and 7.10).

Total deaths

The unadjusted total mortality rate is the dependent variable for the regressions shown in table 8.4. Regression 8.4-6 represents a specification similar to the basic one used in the cross-sectional model, with the addition of the total U.S. mortality rate as an explanatory variable.[9] The estimated effects of the air pollution variables were similar to those derived in the earlier cross-sectional time-series and, in turn, in the earlier pure cross-sectional work. The socioeconomic coefficients were positive and significant except for population density and Log Pop. The former was positive and approached statistical significance. The coefficient of determination was slightly higher than that in the previous analysis of twenty-six SMSAs (regression 8.1-1).

Regressions 8.4-1 through 8.4-5 enter three variables for each air pollutant separately. *F* tests indicated that sulfates and suspended particulates, followed by sulfur dioxide, added most to the explanatory powers of the regressions, but that nitrates and nitrogen dioxide made little contribution. Regression 8.4-7 contains both suspended particulates and sulfur dioxide, to provide a comparison with regression 8.4-6 containing suspended particulates and sulfates. The specification containing sulfates and suspended particulates was slightly "superior" to that with sulfur dioxide and sus-

---

[8] See table C.1 (pp. 317–320), for a listing of these.

[9] The specification with the U.S. total mortality rate was chosen because the earlier cross-sectional time-series results (tables 8.1 through 8.3) indicated little difference in the estimated air pollution effects from using any of the three ways to account for changing factors over time; using the U.S. total mortality rate had the clearest interpretation.

pended particulates.[10] Regression 8.4-8 contains three measures each for all five air pollutants. An F test indicated that the group of fifteen air pollution variables together contributed significantly to the explanatory power of the regression. Sulfates, suspended particulates, and sulfur dioxide were most significant; nitrates and nitrogen dioxide were nonsignificant and had a net negative effect on the mortality rate. The sum of elasticities derived from the fifteen air pollution coefficients was 11.74, which is only slightly larger than the sums of elasticities in either regression 8.4-6 or 8.4-7. The coefficients of the socioeconomic variables were of the same sign as in regression 8.4-6 although their statistical significance displayed some variation.

Age–sex–race-adjusted total deaths

A similar analysis was performed for the age–sex–race-adjusted total mortality rate (table 8.5). Regression 8.5-6 again represents a specification similar to the original cross-sectional specification with the addition of the U.S. total mortality rate. The air pollution coefficients were similar to the estimates in table 8.4 for the unadjusted total mortality rate. The socioeconomic variables displayed more variation, although the signs of their coefficients were generally similar to those in table 8.4. The explanatory power of regression 8.5-6 was somewhat higher than in regression 8.2-1, based on data from twenty-six SMSAs ($R^2 = 0.720$ compared with 0.611).

The first five regressions in table 8.5 indicate that sulfates and suspended particulates were again the most important air pollutants, followed by sulfur dioxide. As before, nitrates and nitrogen dioxide contributed little to the regressions. The specification with sulfates and suspended particulates (regression 8.5-6) was again superior to the specification with suspended particulates and sulfur dioxide (regression 8.5-7). When all of the air pollution variables were included (regression 8.5-8), an F test indicated that the fifteen air pollution variables made a significant contribution to the regression. The sum of elasticities of the fifteen air pollution variables was 11.48; this was again similar to the sums of elasticities for regressions 8.5-6 and 8.5-7 with either sulfates or sulfur dioxide, and suspended particulates.

Race-adjusted infant deaths

Similar specifications are presented in table 8.6 for the race-adjusted mortality rate for infants under one year of age. As was true in the previous cross-sectional time-series analyses (see table 8.3), the air pollu-

---

[10] The sum of the air pollution elasticities in regression 8.4-6 was 11.72, and in regression 8.4-7 it was 10.61; however, note that suspended particulates were relatively more important in the presence of sulfur dioxide than in the presence of sulfates.

TABLE 8.4. Unadjusted Total Mortality Rates (the Effects of Additional Air Pollutants), 1962–68

	8.4-1	8.4-2	8.4-3	8.4-4	8.4-5	8.4-6	8.4-7	8.4-8
R^2	.923	.924	.888	.891	.905	.944	.940	.953
Constant	−599.484	−716.352	−694.688	−711.926	−525.602	−668.711	−682.889	−621.914
Air pollution variables								
Min S	.475					.405		.485
	(2.09)					(1.97)		(2.25)
Mean S	.396					.310		.165
	(2.54)					(2.26)		(1.02)
Max S	−.019					−.023		−.032
	(−.50)					(−.73)		(−.92)
Sum S elasticities	6.49					4.96		3.16
Min P		1.161				.758	.887	.512
		(4.73)				(3.32)	(3.87)	(2.18)
Mean P		.090				.202	.341	.579
		(.45)				(1.12)	(1.81)	(2.70)
Max P		.009				.003	−.032	−.037
		(.25)				(.08)	(−.92)	(−1.07)
Sum P elasticities		7.59				6.76	8.23	9.27
Min NO$_3$			1.577					.160
			(.90)					(.12)
Mean NO$_3$			−.056					−.708
			(−.07)					(−1.02)
Max NO$_3$			.051					.012
			(.30)					(.10)
Sum NO$_3$ elasticities			1.09					−1.57

	(1)	(2)	(3)	(4)	(5)	(6)	(7)	(8)
Min NO$_2$				.244 (1.15)				−.154 (−.93)
Mean NO$_2$				−.236 (−1.27)				.168 (1.18)
Max NO$_2$				.001 (.02)				−.092 (−1.91)
Sum NO$_2$ elasticities				−1.78				−1.02
Min SO$_2$					−.103 (−.20)		−.106 (−.25)	−.175 (−.40)
Mean SO$_2$					.561 (2.82)		.482 (2.93)	.355 (1.99)
Max SO$_2$					−.058 (−1.42)		−.035 (−1.05)	−.016 (−.48)
Sum SO$_2$ elasticities					2.41		2.38	1.90
Socioeconomic variables								
P/M^2	.147 (1.81)	.140 (1.72)	.178 (1.84)	.147 (1.53)	.106 (1.17)	.128 (1.75)	.044 (.57)	.066 (.85)
≥65	7.790 (19.75)	8.909 (25.11)	8.661 (19.11)	8.693 (20.16)	7.833 (18.84)	8.273 (23.54)	8.300 (24.17)	7.997 (21.64)
NW	.382 (4.18)	.563 (7.07)	.650 (6.36)	.748 (7.02)	.616 (6.86)	.358 (4.47)	.528 (7.13)	.417 (4.39)
Poor	.470 (3.63)	.173 (1.38)	.181 (1.12)	.036 (.20)	.248 (1.68)	.362 (3.18)	.179 (1.49)	.207 (1.42)
Sum SE elasticities	86.65	96.31	95.38	94.83	86.69	89.76	88.82	85.28
Log Pop	−.203 (−1.36)	−.164 (−1.09)	−.397 (−2.21)	−.414 (−2.45)	−.351 (−2.22)	−.083 (−.61)	−.114 (−.83)	−.073 (−.54)
U.S. total mortality rate	.816 (2.72)	.811 (2.76)	1.003 (2.86)	1.064 (3.05)	.869 (2.70)	.734 (2.78)	.787 (2.96)	.722 (2.67)

Note: All regressions are based on data for fifteen SMSAs (see table C.1, pp. 317–320). The number of observations was equal to 105. The numbers in parentheses below the regression coefficients are t statistics.

175

TABLE 8.5. Age–Sex–Race-adjusted Total Mortality Rates (the Effects of Additional Air Pollutants), 1962–68

	8.5-1	8.5-2	8.5-3	8.5-4	8.5-5	8.5-6	8.5-7	8.5-8
R^2	.604	.658	.488	.516	.531	.720	.700	.755
Constant	21.548	−105.158	−23.873	−95.086	126.150	−87.316	−71.259	−33.935
Air pollution variables								
Min S	.481					.399		.488
	(1.65)					(1.53)		(1.76)
Mean S	.474					.355		.218
	(2.37)					(2.04)		(1.05)
Max S	−.052					−.057		−.069
	(−1.10)					(−1.41)		(−1.53)
Sum S elasticities	6.03					4.13		2.53
Min P		1.382				.977	1.137	.717
		(4.70)				(3.37)	(3.92)	(2.37)
Mean P		.173				.304	.400	.696
		(.73)				(1.33)	(1.68)	(2.51)
Max P		−.001				−.007	−.039	−.048
		(−.02)				(−.16)	(−.88)	(−1.06)
Sum P elasticities		8.89				8.37	9.42	10.78
Min NO₃			1.235					−.640
			(.58)					(−.38)
Mean NO₃			.219					−.741
			(.21)					(−.83)
Max NO₃			.035					.024
			(.17)					(.15)
Sum NO₃ elasticities			1.37					−1.88

	(1)	(2)	(3)	(4)	(5)	(6)	(7)	(8)
Min NO_2				.299 (1.19)				−.110 (−.51)
Mean NO_2				−.331 (−1.50)				.100 (.55)
Max NO_2				−.011 (−.15)				−.098 (−1.57)
Sum NO_2 elasticities				−2.84				−1.70
Min SO_2					−.215 (−.33)		−.228 (−.43)	
Mean SO_2					.560 (2.24)		.462 (2.22)	
Max SO_2					−.061 (−1.19)		−.034 (−.79)	
Sum SO_2 elasticities					2.08		2.03	
Socioeconomic variables								
P/M^2	.123 (1.18)	.082 (.84)	.144 (1.23)	.090 (.78)	.067 (.59)	.092 (.99)	−.010 (−.11)	.023 (.23)
≥ 65	.971 (1.92)	2.333 (5.48)	1.964 (3.57)	2.132 (4.14)	1.196 (2.29)	1.616 (3.62)	1.780 (4.09)	1.345 (2.82)
NW	.163 (1.39)	.353 (3.69)	.450 (3.63)	.614 (4.83)	.434 (3.84)	.132 (1.30)	.326 (3.47)	.233 (1.90)
Poor	.488 (2.94)	.164 (1.09)	.201 (1.03)	−.072 (−.34)	.240 (1.29)	.346 (2.39)	.156 (1.03)	.133 (.70)
Sum SE elasticities	16.55	27.16	25.87	25.71	18.18	20.37	20.68	16.02
Log Pop	−.161 (−.84)	−.041 (−.23)	−.351 (−1.61)	−.351 (−1.74)	−.296 (−1.48)	.004 (.03)	.005 (.03)	−.007 (−.04)
U.S. total mortality rate	.871 (2.26)	.790 (2.24)	.987 (2.32)	1.106 (2.66)	.869 (2.14)	.776 (2.32)	.767 (2.28)	.783 (2.24)

Note: All regressions are based on data for fifteen SMSAs. The number of observations was equal to 105. The numbers in parentheses below the regression coefficients are *t* statistics.

177

TABLE 8.6. Race-adjusted Infant Mortality Rates (the Effects of Additional Air Pollutants), 1962–68

	8.6-1	8.6-2	8.6-3	8.6-4	8.6-5	8.6-6	8.6-7	8.6-8
R^2	.447	.461	.450	.436	.457	.470	.479	.524
Constant	−160.763	−190.649	−170.781	−172.935	−143.781	−179.572	−169.402	−74.151
Air pollution variables								
Min S	.163					.104		.229
	(1.05)					(.64)		(1.30)
Mean S	−.030					−.030		−.190
	(−.27)					(−.27)		(−1.46)
Max S	−.016					−.018		−.014
	(−.62)					(−.71)		(−.50)
Sum S elasticities	−.69					−1.97		−7.57
Min P		.337				.310	.308	.250
		(1.98)				(1.70)	(1.77)	(1.29)
Mean P		−.095				−.058	−.064	−.038
		(−.69)				(−.40)	(−.43)	(−.21)
Max P		.016				.014	.008	−.011
		(.65)				(.54)	(.29)	(−.38)
Sum P elasticities		4.08				5.19	4.03	1.91
Min NO₃			.729					.372
			(.73)					(.35)
Mean NO₃			−.120					.302
			(−.25)					(.54)
Max NO₃			.093					.088
			(.95)					(.84)
Sum NO₃ elasticities			3.00					6.26

	(1)	(2)	(3)	(4)	(5)	(6)	(7)	(8)
Min NO₂	.027 (.20)				.025 (.19)			
Mean NO₂	−.102 (−.73)				.001 (.01)			
Max NO₂	.008 (.21)				.000 (.01)			
Sum NO₂ elasticities	−3.89				.63			
Min SO₂	−.302 (−.85)	−.081 (−.25)	−.065 (−.20)					
Mean SO₂	.376 (2.44)	.194 (1.52)	.205 (1.64)					
Max SO₂	−.041 (−1.50)	−.039 (−1.53)	−.041 (−1.63)					
Sum SO₂ elasticities	5.56	1.49	1.68					
Socioeconomic variables								
P/M²	−.008 (−.12)	−.014 (−.24)	−.016 (−.28)	.015 (.25)	−.009 (−.15)	−.005 (−.09)	−.001 (−.01)	.009 (.16)
≥65	.914 (2.82)	.920 (3.31)	.867 (3.13)	1.061 (3.62)	1.032 (4.04)	1.139 (4.29)	1.071 (4.29)	.988 (3.39)
NW	−.003 (−.04)	−.022 (−.32)	−.007 (.10)	−.016 (−.20)	.024 (.38)	.024 (.37)	−.007 (−.10)	.002 (.03)
Poor	.341 (2.64)	.377 (3.25)	.349 (3.03)	.340 (2.85)	.318 (2.87)	.311 (2.79)	.350 (3.25)	.332 (2.77)
Sum SE elasticities	49.44	50.04	47.90	55.86	54.24	58.34	56.21	53.10
Log Pop	.229 (2.03)	.271 (2.59)	.214 (2.17)	.238 (2.19)	.200 (2.00)	.194 (1.88)	.257 (2.47)	.199 (1.93)
U.S. infant mortality rate	.201 (.55)	.457 (2.15)	.549 (2.79)	.548 (2.64)	.654 (2.42)	.598 (3.18)	.535 (2.74)	.628 (3.14)

Note: All regressions are based on data for fifteen SMSAs. The number of observations was equal to 105. The numbers in parentheses below the regression coefficients are t statistics.

179

tion measures were not strongly related to the infant mortality rates. The coefficients of the socioeconomic variables indicated positive and statistically significant associations with three variables (≥ 65, Poor, and Log Pop). In addition, the U.S. mortality rate for infants was positive and statistically significant (except in regression 8.6-8).

INTERACTIONS BETWEEN POLLUTANTS

Chapter 7 presented an analysis of the contribution of multiplicative terms involving two air pollutants at a time (see table 7.11, page 154). A cross-sectional time-series replication of that analysis is presented in table 8.7. As in chapter 7, we have chosen to concentrate on the age–sex–race-adjusted total mortality rate for this investigation.

Unlike the cross-sectional results, there were no cases in which the product terms alone were associated with higher coefficients of determination than regressions involving single air pollutant variables. The age–sex–race-adjusted total mortality rate was best explained by the combination of the variables Mean S and Mean P, although the variable representing the interaction of these air pollutants did not add significantly to regression 8.7-2.

The product terms significantly increased the explanatory powers of regressions in only two cases: Mean S $\times$ Mean SO_2 and Mean NO_2 $\times$ Mean SO_2. However, in both cases the interaction term was negative. Whether because of poor air pollution data or because of other difficulties, we conclude that there is no evidence from either the 1969 cross-sectional analysis or this cross-sectional time-series analysis to show that interactions between air pollutants are more important in explaining variations in mortality rates than individual air pollutants, that is, we find no evidence of synergism.

THE PROBLEM OF AUTOCORRELATION

One of the crucial assumptions of linear multivariable regression analysis is the serial independence of the error terms; that is, that successive residuals are independent of previous values. If this assumption is not valid (that is, if autocorrelation exists), least-squares estimates are still unbiased, but formulas for the sampling variances of the regression coefficients are no longer appropriate. Hence, significance tests will be subject to error.[11]

Unfortunately, autocorrelation in the variables generally results in a lack of independence in the error terms, and autocorrelation is common in time-series data.[12] The conventional measure of autocorrelation in the residuals is the Durbin–Watson statistic. Although it is not appropriate to

---

[11] See Johnston (1972), pp. 246–254.

[12] The problem is aggravated in our analysis because many of the variables are based on linear interpolations from 1960 to 1970.

apply it to cross-sectional time-series data, it can be used to provide a crude indication of autocorrelation.[13]

For regressions in table 8.1 pertaining to the unadjusted total mortality rate, the Durbin–Watson statistic attained values around 1.0, indicating possible autocorrelation. The Durbin–Watson values for the age–sex–race-adjusted total mortality-rate regressions (table 8.2) also indicated possible autocorrelation. For the race-adjusted infant mortality-rate regressions (table 8.3), the Durbin–Watson statistic attained values around 1.4. In table 8.4, the Durbin–Watson statistic had values around 0.8 for the regressions with only one air pollutant, and higher values (up to 1.5) as the number of air pollutants in the regression increased. Thus, there seemed to be less indication of autocorrelation in the regression for the unadjusted total mortality rate when additional air pollutants were included. Similar results pertained to the analysis of the age–sex–race-adjusted total mortality rate in table 8.5. For the race-adjusted infant mortality rates (table 8.6) there was no evidence of autocorrelation; the Durbin–Watson statistic ranged from 1.8 to 2.0. Finally, in table 8.7, the analysis of interactions between air pollutants produced Durbin–Watson statistics ranging from 0.7 to 1.0, indicating possible autocorrelation. Thus, this is some indication that our cross-sectional time-series specification is inadequate, either because of missing factors or an inadequate functional form.

CONCLUSION

Ten annual observations from twenty-six SMSAs for 1960–69 were investigated in an attempt to verify further some of the relationships found in our earlier cross-sectional analysis. When the cross-sectional time-series model was estimated (adding either the U.S. total mortality rate, a linear time variable, or time dummy variables), almost all variables were statistically significant in explaining the unadjusted total mortality rate; the estimated effects of sulfates and suspended particulates were similar to those from the earlier cross-sectional analysis, although sulfates were somewhat less significant and suspended particulates were somewhat more significant. The estimated air pollution coefficients in the cross-sectional time-series analysis of the age–sex–race-adjusted total mortality rate were statistically significant and similar in magnitude to the results for the unadjusted total mortality rate. For the race-adjusted mortality rate for infants under one year of age, the sulfate measures were usually statistically nonsignificant (and sometimes negative), while the suspended particulate measures were

---

[13] Illustrative calculations by Durbin and Watson (1950, 1951) for regressions involving up to one hundred observations and including as many as five explanatory variables show that the statistic ranges around 2.0 when there is not significant autocorrelation.

TABLE 8.7. Age–Sex–Race-adjusted Total Mortality Rates (Interactions Between Air Pollutants), 1962–68

	8.7-1	8.7-2	8.7-3	8.7-4	8.7-5	8.7-6	8.7-7	8.7-8	8.7-9	8.7-10
R^2	.642	.645	.641	.583	.584	.539	.609	.609	.487	.582
Constant	33.307	63.051	75.506	26.164	36.803	76.478	−86.563	−73.438	75.130	28.534
Air pollution variables										
Mean S	.461 (4.51)	.124 (.33)		.519 (4.71)	.405 (1.56)		.532 (5.05)	.462 (1.89)		.492 (3.67)
Mean P	.581 (4.03)	.276 (.77)								
Mean NO_3				.251 (.52)	−.398 (−.28)					
Mean NO_2							−.266 (−2.59)	−.344 (−1.29)		
Mean SO_2										.057 (.46)
Product		.278 (.93)	.421 (6.62)		.523 (.49)	1.019 (3.54)		.063 (.32)	.083 (1.24)	
Sum AP elasticities	12.69	9.01	6.21	6.74	5.34	2.80	3.14	2.27	1.22	6.21
Socioeconomic variables										
P/M^2	.078 (.81)	.077 (.80)	.072 (.76)	.084 (.80)	.084 (.80)	.144 (1.34)	.042 (.42)	.043 (.42)	.148 (1.30)	.070 (.67)
≥65	1.550 (3.41)	1.671 (3.54)	1.606 (3.79)	1.182 (2.45)	1.208 (2.47)	1.702 (3.54)	1.439 (3.02)	1.432 (2.99)	1.555 (2.87)	1.095 (2.23)
NW	.206 (1.96)	.213 (2.01)	.209 (2.03)	.236 (2.06)	.239 (2.08)	.318 (2.74)	.382 (3.14)	.383 (3.13)	.376 (2.76)	.253 (2.21)
Poor	.320 (2.01)	.316 (1.98)	.353 (2.33)	.444 (2.63)	.446 (2.63)	.349 (2.01)	.171 (.88)	.172 (.88)	.378 (1.76)	.433 (2.54)
Sum SE elasticities	20.06	21.18	20.86	18.28	18.57	23.62	18.92	18.87	23.16	17.37
Log Pop	−.170 (−.97)	−.186 (−1.05)	−.179 (−1.03)	−.175 (−.91)	−.187 (−.96)	−.353 (−1.81)	−.147 (−.80)	−.146 (−.79)	−.328 (−1.59)	−.164 (−.86)
U.S. total mortality rate	.760 (2.16)	.765 (2.17)	.780 (2.23)	.850 (2.24)	.858 (2.25)	.893 (2.26)	.980 (2.65)	.975 (2.62)	.899 (2.14)	.855 (2.26)

	8.7-11	8.7-12	8.7-13	8.7-14	8.7-15	8.7-16	8.7-17	8.7-18	8.7-19	8.7-20
R^2	.602	.522	.576	.581	.505	.575	.582	.482	.625	.625
Constant	79.196	52.623	11.634	-95.579	85.897	-27.990	31.543	61.315	101.773	105.739
Air pollution variables										
Mean S	.675 (4.33)									
Mean P			.844 (4.51)	1.223 (3.01)		.634 (3.97)	.176 (.45)			
Mean NO_3			-.873 (-1.50)	1.377 (.62)					.746 (5.10)	.705 (2.83)
Mean NO_2						-.154 (-1.39)	-.624 (-1.63)			
Mean SO_2	1.067 (2.23)								.370 (3.88)	.278 (.60)
Product	-.631 (-2.19)	.175 (2.96)		-1.685 (-1.05)	.632 (2.25)		.397 (1.28)	.069 (.77)		.076 (.21)
Sum AP elasticities	9.24	1.53	8.47	13.39	1.85	6.02	.44	1.00	11.59	11.07
Socioeconomic variables										
P/M^2	.077 (.75)	.079 (.71)	.115 (1.10)	.103 (.98)	.166 (1.49)	.117 (1.12)	.126 (1.21)	.157 (1.37)	.058 (.58)	.059 (.59)
≥65	.830 (1.67)	1.335 (2.61)	2.172 (4.62)	2.176 (4.63)	1.961 (3.90)	2.320 (4.81)	2.331 (4.85)	1.750 (3.42)	1.586 (3.39)	1.605 (3.35)
NW	.271 (2.40)	.409 (3.66)	.414 (3.87)	.407 (3.81)	.412 (3.60)	.475 (3.88)	.478 (3.91)	.416 (3.14)	.338 (3.38)	.339 (3.37)
Poor	.341 (1.98)	.299 (1.71)	.077 (.45)	.066 (.39)	.228 (1.29)	-.030 (-.15)	-.027 (-.14)	.304 (1.49)	.137 (.88)	.137 (.87)
Sum SE elasticities	14.34	19.91	25.87	25.60	26.01	26.80	27.07	24.74	19.69	19.88
Log Pop	-.247 (-1.29)	-.265 (-1.32)	-.297 (-1.57)	-.224 (-1.11)	-.417 (-2.05)	-.333 (-1.77)	-.374 (-1.97)	-.366 (-1.77)	-.270 (-1.53)	-.266 (-1.48)
U.S. total mortality rate	.853 (2.30)	.914 (2.27)	.844 (2.21)	.864 (2.26)	.908 (2.21)	.923 (2.39)	.941 (2.44)	.924 (2.18)	.765 (2.13)	.762 (2.10)

(Continued)

183

TABLE 8.7. (Continued)

	8.7-21	8.7-22	8.7-23	8.7-24	8.7-25	8.7-26	8.7-27	8.7-28	8.7-29	8.7-30
R^2	.563	.510	.511	.480	.540	.541	.526	.562	.596	.482
Constant	115.313	−66.588	−25.177	−15.766	109.372	116.474	76.128	−43.875	46.827	33.230
Air pollution variables										
Mean S										
Mean P										
Mean NO_3		.525 (1.01)	.012 (.01)		.948 (1.84)	1.276 (1.50)				
Mean NO_2		−.250 (−2.17)	−.348 (−1.35)					−.318 (−2.89)	.054 (.32)	
Mean SO_2					.359 (3.35)	.488 (1.72)		.366 (3.53)	1.110 (3.94)	
Product	.347 (4.31)		.392 (.42)	−.132 (−.44)		−.596 (−.49)	1.381 (3.11)		−.602 (−2.83)	.054 (.73)
Sum AP elasticities	2.62	−1.80	−3.08	−.36	4.43	5.17	1.87	−1.52	2.78	.43
Socioeconomic variables										
P/M^2	.058 (.54)	.124 (1.10)	.125 (1.11)	.138 (1.19)	.091 (.83)	.095 (.85)	.092 (.83)	.029 (.26)	.051 (.49)	.135 (1.17)
≥65	1.273 (2.64)	2.132 (4.13)	2.135 (4.12)	1.814 (3.55)	1.290 (2.51)	1.266 (2.44)	1.430 (2.86)	1.537 (3.01)	1.503 (3.05)	1.651 (3.02)
NW	.401 (3.78)	.574 (4.40)	.582 (4.39)	.491 (3.90)	.379 (3.37)	.376 (3.33)	.402 (3.60)	.592 (4.93)	.600 (5.17)	.443 (3.70)
Poor	.232 (1.40)	−.015 (−.07)	−.028 (−.13)	.199 (1.02)	.277 (1.61)	.271 (1.56)	.284 (1.64)	−.067 (−.33)	−.101 (−.52)	−.274 (1.45)
Sum SE elasticities	18.36	26.28	26.29	24.81	19.14	18.88	20.70	19.40	19.13	23.53
Log Pop	−.254 (−1.33)	−.368 (−1.81)	−.378 (−1.84)	−.345 (−1.65)	−.333 (−1.69)	−.346 (−1.73)	−.308 (−1.55)	−.276 (−1.44)	−.284 (−1.54)	−.346 (−1.67)
U.S. total mortality rate	.847 (2.20)	1.071 (2.59)	1.047 (2.50)	1.004 (2.36)	.875 (2.20)	.871 (2.18)	.904 (2.26)	1.058 (2.71)	.927 (2.44)	.959 (2.29)

Note: All regressions are based on data for fifteen SMSAs. The numbers of observations was equal to 105. The numbers in parentheses below the regression coefficients are t statistics. The thirty regressions above represent ten sets of triplets. The first regression in each set includes two air pollutants entered linearly. The second regression in each set includes the two air pollutants entered linearly as well as a product term of the two air pollutants. The third regression in each set includes only the product term.

generally diminished in magnitude and significance compared to the analogous cross-sectional analyses.

Data on five air pollutants were investigated for a subsample of fifteen SMSAs (for 1962–68) in an attempt to isolate the relative cross-sectional time-series effects of the air pollutants on mortality. In addition, interactions between the air pollutants were analyzed. For the total mortality rate (unadjusted and adjusted), the results were similar. Sulfates, suspended particulates, and sulfur dioxide exhibited separate, statistically significant associations with mortality; nitrates and nitrogen dioxide were nonsignificant. The air pollution measures were not strongly associated with the race-adjusted mortality rate for infants under one year of age. Finally, there was no evidence of synergism from the analysis of the adjusted total mortality rate and variables representing interaction between air pollutants.

In general, we conclude that the analysis in this chapter tends to support the association between the specific measures of air pollution and the mortality rates estimated in the previous cross-sectional work. The estimated air pollution elasticities were surprisingly similar.

CHAPTER 9

The relationship
between daily mortality
and daily air pollution

Severe air pollution episodes have had unmistakable effects on health status in general and on mortality in particular. These occurrences suggest the possibility that episodes of lesser severity might also have smaller, but nevertheless, important effects on health (and mortality). While the health effects during major episodes are readily observed, careful statistical analysis is needed to identify and estimate possible effects during less severe conditions.

In earlier chapters we noted a number of factors hypothesized to influence the mortality rate in a geographical area. Further, we discussed and employed methods of controlling for these factors in our attempts to estimate the air pollution–mortality association across a number of areas at a given time. In chapter 8, we then estimated the air pollution–mortality relationship, using annual data for a number of SMSAs over a decade. This chapter is focused on the relationship between daily air pollution levels and the number of daily deaths occurring in five cities (Chicago, Denver, Philadelphia, Saint Louis, and Washington, D.C.).

Many of the problems encountered in the previous cross-sectional analyses disappear in a time-series investigation, while other problems arise. Over the course of a year, there is little variation in the genetic composition of a population, its nutritional history, or similar factors; hence, such factors can be assumed constant in analyzing day-to-day data. Other factors, such as climate, day-of-the-week effects, and seasonal influences are much more important in a daily analysis and must be controlled.

Thus, one problem in analyzing day-to-day effects is not to confound the effects of air pollution with the influences of such factors as weekly cycles. For example, if air pollution tends to be lower on weekends because of less industrial activity, care must be taken not to confuse differences in weekend mortality figures due to changes in activities associated with weekends with those due to changes in air pollution levels.

Other difficulties surround the estimation procedures necessary to analyze daily time-series data. Time-series data often display autocorrelation as well as collinearity between the explanatory variables. As discussed in chapter 8, autocorrelation makes it difficult to obtain efficient estimates. At the same time, collinearity between such factors as air pollution levels, climatological measures, and day-of-the-week factors, makes it difficult to isolate the effect of any single explanatory factor, such as air quality.

In earlier chapters we also discussed the notion that the number of people dying during a period can be modeled as a stochastic process. (In particular, it can be described formally as a Poisson process.) For example, a city with a population of one million would experience approximately twenty-seven deaths per day with a standard deviation of 5.2 deaths per day, while a city of 100,000 would experience approximately 2.7 deaths per day with a standard deviation of 1.6 deaths per day. To illustrate this, assume that the estimated time-series effect of air pollution were similar to the estimated cross-sectional effect that we have previously determined; if this is so, a highly polluted day compared with a "clean" day would lead to three extra deaths in the large city and only 0.3 extra deaths in the small city. The implication is that it will be difficult to disentangle the effects of day-to-day changes in air quality in all but the largest cities.

A related conceptual problem is that of determining whether an air pollution episode merely "harvests" deaths, that is, shifts the time of death of marginally viable people by a few days, or actually lowers the life expectancy of the entire population by some decrement. If the former occurs, one would expect to see the mortality rate fall below average after an air pollution episode. If the latter takes place, the mortality rate should be higher following an episode because permanent damage has been done. The answer to this question can have important policy implications. Since we have little a priori information about the magnitude of these two effects, it is difficult to conjecture as to their joint effect. Whatever the case, the analytical problem remains one of separating the relatively subtle effect of air pollution from the effects of the other factors affecting mortality.

For all the above reasons, it is difficult to be specific regarding the relationship between our previous cross-sectional estimates and the estimates based on these daily time-series data. As we stated before, if the current air quality in a city is indicative of its past air quality, a cross-sectional analysis should uncover primarily the long-term effects of exposure to air pollution; whereas, an analysis of daily data might identify a "harvesting" effect or a more serious phenomenon in which life expectancy is shortened by a few days for large segments of the population.

SOME FAMOUS AIR POLLUTION EPISODES

A number of "killer fogs" and other acute air pollution episodes have occurred in the past fifty years.[1] The highly industrialized Meuse valley of Belgium experienced climatic conditions permitting the buildup of abnormally high levels of air pollutants (particularly sulfur dioxide) during December 1930. Over a five-day period, approximately 6,000 people became ill and perhaps 60 died (most of them elderly or persons with previous heart and lung conditions), more than ten times the number of deaths normally expected (Firket, 1931). In October 1948, a similar episode took place in Donora, Pennsylvania. Within three days, almost 6,000 people (over 40 percent of the population) became ill; about 20 deaths were reported. This again was approximately ten times the expected number of deaths and, again, the aged were most susceptible (the average age of the dead was sixty-five).[2] McCabe and Clayton (1952) reported on a 1950 Mexican incident in which large quantities of hydrogen sulfide emitted from a sulfur-removal plant resulted in 22 deaths and 320 hospitalizations. In December 1952, London was enveloped by a dense fog; in a two-week period 4,000 excess deaths occurred, which were attributed to the abnormally high concentrations of sulfur dioxide and smoke. Unlike the previous episodes, all age groups were affected.[3]

Lesser episodes occurred in London during January 1956 and December 1962. Logan (1956) analyzed the first of these and attributed approximately 1,000 excess deaths to the incident. The greatest *percentage* increase in deaths was among infants; in absolute numbers, the greatest increase was among elderly persons. Bronchitis mortality exhibited the highest increase among specific causes of death.[4]

METHODS USED TO INVESTIGATE DAILY RELATIONSHIPS

Numerous studies have hypothesized that air pollution causes increased numbers of deaths, physician visits, work absences, and hospitalizations.

[1] For a detailed review of the episodes we discuss, as well as several other air pollution incidents, see Ashe (1959) and McCarroll (1967), as well as appendix A.

[2] See Brinton (1949), and Schrenk and co-workers (1949). In a follow-up study, Ciocco and Thompson (1961) found that persons who became ill during the smog episode demonstrated subsequently higher mortality and morbidity than other persons living in the community. There was evidence that this was particularly true for persons with diseases of the cardiorespiratory system.

[3] For a detailed description of the episode, see Wilkins (1954) and the London Ministry of Health (1954). Scott (1953) presented the breakdown of death by certain causes and discussed the abnormally large numbers among respiratory categories. Abercrombie (1953) reported on hospital admissions in London. For the week ending December 13, 1952, 2,019 patients were admitted; the previous weekly high was 1,169 for the week ending January 2, 1951. Fry (1953) commented on the effects of the fog on a general practice of 4,500 patients in the outskirts of London. During the week of the fog, the practice experienced 125 patient visits, compared with a weekly average of 75 for that time of year.

[4] For a description of the 1962 episode, see Prindle (1963). Davies (1963) discussed nine case histories of patients exhibiting respiratory symptoms during this incident.

One of the most common techniques used to relate daily air pollution levels to daily measures of health status has been graphical analysis, that is, the number of deaths and the levels of pollution are graphed for each day, in search of an association.[5]

Unfortunately, graphical techniques are unlikely to reveal the "true" daily effects of air pollution. There are a number of other factors that determine the daily level of mortality, for example, climate variables and life-style patterns relating to the day of the week and to holidays. Several studies can be used to illustrate this. McCarroll and Bradley (1966) examined daily mortality, air pollution (sulfur dioxide and smokeshade), and weather data for New York City during a three-year period (1962–64). The time interval included five air pollution episodes. Using only graphical techniques, McCarroll and Bradley concluded that the periodic peaks in mortality were associated with periods of high air pollution.[6] They further noted that such peaks were not followed by drops sufficiently sharp to compensate for the excess deaths; hence, they inferred that what they were detecting was more than a hastening effect. They also remarked that the influence on death rates occurred among those aged forty-five to sixty-four as well as among the elderly sixty-five and older. Finally, they pointed out the need for studying other relevant factors.

During Thanksgiving of 1966 another episode occurred in New York City. Glasser, Greenburg, and Field (1967) investigated the relationship between morbidity and indexes of sulfur dioxide and smokeshade during this episode. Using a number of different control periods, some of which took into account possible lag effects, they found a total of 168 excess deaths over a seven-day period and an increase in the number of clinic visits for bronchitis and asthma at seven New York hospitals. The rise in temperature at the time of the episode, though possibly a contributing factor, could not account for the observed increase in mortality. Regarding the Thanksgiving study, Eckhardt (1968, page 837) remarked that "lung cancer deaths can hardly be related to air pollution unless the following factors have been investigated: Is the case postoperative? How many days postoperative? How long did the patient have lung cancer?" In addition to these factors, the researchers were aware of the difficulty in assessing the effects of the holiday itself. Eckhardt again commented: "Increased food intake and relaxation of salt restrictions for cardiacs on festive days like Thanksgiving, I am sure exact their toll. . . . Psychiatrists tell us that suicides increase over holidays, and the National Safety Council tells us that highway deaths go up with four-day weekends." Ideally, all these factors should be accounted for, but data are seldom available.

---

[5] A detailed review of mortality (and morbidity) studies using daily, weekly, and monthly observations is found in appendix A, pp. 299–305.

[6] In an attempt to control for variations in climatic and other conditions, they included a fifteen-day moving average as a baseline from which to judge mortality peaks. Graphs of temperature and wind speed were included for comparison.

For this same Thanksgiving episode, Becker, Schilling, and Verma (1968, page 419) used questionnaires in a study of 2,052 executive and clerical personnel and found that "as the air pollution levels increased, a greater response to symptoms of dyspnea, cough, sputum, wheeze, eye irritation, and general discomfort was elicited from study subjects." The direct effects of weather conditions were not accounted for, although the smoking histories of individuals were considered.[7]

The above studies are difficult to evaluate for several reasons. Ad hoc procedures for analyzing small data sets require extreme care in interpretation; often the same authors used different ad hoc assumptions (such as different lag structures) in analyzing other data sets. The use of questionnaires and other voluntary responses to measure the effects of air pollution may also have inherent problems. For example, awareness of high pollution levels is increased by news coverage and other publicity; consequently a major part of the measured response is likely to be due to the type and extent of news coverage. Finally, another problem involves estimating the number of "excess" deaths during a pollution episode. Expected mortality is estimated by computing averages for adjoining periods or for a previous period. Since no adjustments are usually made for population changes or variations in other factors known to affect the mortality rate, the resulting computations may be subject to considerable error. The number of deaths is a stochastic process, so that total deaths over a short period may over- or underestimate the number of excess deaths.

Multivariable statistical analysis offers one way to cope with the possible effects of a number of "relevant" variables on mortality. It has been demonstrated that climate affects mortality (Bonkonjić and Zec, 1968; Boyd, 1960; Rogot and Blackwelder, 1970), that air pollution affects climate (Georgii, 1970), and that air pollutants and climate may have synergistic effects (Lewis, 1965). A multivariable statistical model can consider these interrelationships simultaneously.

Such a model was employed by Hodgson (1970). Using multivariable regression, he analyzed mortality, air pollution (suspended particulates and sulfur dioxide), and certain meteorological factors between 1962–65 in New York City, and found that, for all ages, mortality from respiratory and heart diseases was significantly related to the level of air pollution, whereas mortality from other causes was not. Furthermore, the effects of the environmental factors on mortality occurred on the day of increased pollution and extreme temperature, with lesser effects on the day following. Finally, he concluded that the increase in mortality observed was not merely the bunching together of deaths of persons already ill.

---

[7] After removing time trends, Verma, Schilling, and Becker (1969) could not detect a strong relationship between respiratory absences at an insurance company and daily air pollution (sulfur dioxide, carbon monoxide, and smokeshade) in New York City over the period 1965–66.

Some questions arise with regard to Hodgson's analysis. Although the author professes concern with day-to-day variations in the health effects of pollution, most of his analysis is based on monthly averages. Detailed analysis of the acute reaction is lost in this aggregation. In addition, aggregating the daily data into months enhances the multicollinearity problems among the explanatory variables, especially when lagged periods are included. To counter this difficulty, Hodgson used moving averages of the monthly means. However, as he points out, this sacrifices much in the way of analyzing the short-term effects. In defense, he stated that the index will then reflect the cumulative effect of air pollution. The moving averages will indeed represent the mean pollution levels for the number of months included, but we cannot be sure whether they will reflect long-term or day-to-day effects.

Hodgson did analyze daily observations at the end of his paper, but, again, he used moving averages, and the interesting lag effects were masked. The daily results were not found to be significantly different from the monthly regressions. As we mentioned above, one underlying hypothesis in such a study is that air pollution merely hastens the death of those who would have died shortly. Hodgson (1970, page 593) remarked that "if the sole effect of air pollution [were] to redistribute the deaths within a short time interval, for example, a month or less, then the average daily mortality for a given month would be independent of the concentration of air pollution during the month, and no statistically significant relation would be observed between monthly mortality and air pollution." But monthly averages would only mask such an effect, not eliminate it. At both the beginning and end of the month there would be days where one- or two-day shifts in deaths would still be present. To examine the redistribution question, a more complicated lag structure is needed.

Another related technique that has been used is cross-spectral analysis. Hexter and Goldsmith (1971) used this method to relate daily mortality in Los Angeles County to carbon monoxide and photochemical oxidant concentrations and to maximum temperature for a four-year period (1962–65). A significant association between mortality and carbon monoxide pollution was found, but no association was demonstrated between mortality and photochemical oxidants.[8]

Although Hexter and Goldsmith included maximum temperature as a factor likely to be important in explaining mortality, they failed to account

---

[8] They made no attempt to resolve the conflict with the Hechter and Goldsmith study (1961), which found that daily Los Angeles deaths from 1956–58 were not correlated with either daily oxidant or carbon monoxide concentrations. Many investigators have detected an association with daily data. Mills (1957) found a significant association between Los Angeles smog and day-by-day respiratory and cardiac deaths, as did Brant and Hill (1964) and Brant (1965), when they examined the effects of oxidants on weekly admissions for respiratory and cardiovascular dysfunction in Los Angeles hospitals.

for other possibly relevant factors. This was emphasized in a subsequent exchange published in *Science*. Mosher, Brunelle, and Hamming (1971) found that, for the period corresponding to the Hexter and Goldsmith study, correlations between carbon monoxide and nitric oxide or nitrogen dioxide in Los Angeles were significant at a level of more than 99.9 percent. Thus, none of the three pollutants could be isolated as the true cause of illness. Ellsaesser (1971) questioned Hexter and Goldsmith's procedure, arguing that their ad hoc method and failure to take account of other important factors made their results suspect. For instance, the population (and, therefore, the population at risk) increased over time. Ellsaesser also cited the interrelationships among carbon monoxide, traffic fatalities, and mortality. In a further analysis, Hexter and Goldsmith (1971b) showed that changes in population structure during the time periods studied did not affect their previous results. They also found a negative association between carbon monoxide and traffic fatalities when a death-specific regression was analyzed.

THE MODEL AND DATA

From day to day, within a single city, we hypothesize that many of the factors affecting mortality—genetic characteristics, personal habits, and socioeconomic characteristics—remain essentially constant. Thus, for examining day-to-day changes in mortality, we assume the following function to be applicable:

$$MR = MR(P, W, D, e) \qquad 9.1$$

where MR is the mortality rate; P represents environmental air pollution; W represents climate characteristics; D measures day-of-the-week effects; and e is all other factors. We expect mortality at time t to be associated with current air pollution (at time t) and air pollution levels on immediately preceding days, as well as with a number of meteorological variables. The coefficients of the lagged pollution variables should shed light on the short-term effects of pollution. More precisely, we considered models with finite lags which were linear, multiplicative, or quadratic (including interaction terms). One such model is shown in Equation 9.2:

$$MR_t = 118.875 + 0.882\ SO_{2_t} + 1.375\ SO_{2_{t-1}} + 0.714\ SO_{2_{t-2}}$$
$$\ (0.81)\qquad\ \ (1.30)\qquad\quad\ (0.67)$$
$$-\ 1.260\ SO_{2_{t-3}} + 0.470\ SO_{2_{t-4}} + 3.052\ SO_{2_{t-5}} - 1.535\ Mean\ temp$$
$$(-1.17)\qquad\quad\ (0.44)\qquad\quad\ (3.03)\qquad\quad\ (-2.31)$$
$$+\ 12.316\ Rainfall - 0.374\ Wind + 2.078\ Sun + 2.587\ Mon$$
$$(2.33)\qquad\qquad (-0.16)$$
$$-\ 0.517\ Tues - 2.477\ Wed - 1.760\ Thurs - 0.348\ Fri$$
$$+\ 0.437\ Sat\quad (R^2 = 0.270) \qquad 9.2$$

This model and an explanation of the variables are discussed below.

As with our work in earlier chapters, the research here was limited by the availability of air pollution data and, to a lesser extent, of mortality data. Daily observations on air pollution levels (twenty-four-hour averages) were obtained from the Continuous Air Monitoring Program (CAMP). Data were collected for seven cities and eleven pollutants, but complete data for a single pollutant in a single city were not even available for a full year. Thus, we restricted ourselves to the most complete data series available.[9] The cities remaining under consideration were Chicago, Denver, Philadelphia, Saint Louis, and Washington, D.C. The pollutants remaining were carbon monoxide, nitric oxide, nitrogen dioxide, sulfur dioxide, and hydrocarbons. No single city had data on all five pollutants and no pollutant was available for all five cities.

From a special study by the Environmental Protection Agency, we obtained daily death counts for the five cities, from 1962–66, corresponding to the daily air pollution readings. These deaths were classified into forty-seven causes, ranging from tuberculosis to motor vehicle accidents; however, in this investigation we limited ourselves to analyzing total deaths in order to minimize the problems associated with small samples.

Finally, we secured data on daily climate factors for the cities from the Department of Commerce. Air pollution, mortality, and climate information constituted our data base. (See tables 9.1 and 9.2 and appendix D for information on the individual data sets.)

METHOD AND RESULTS

Having little a priori knowledge of the underlying relationships among daily mortality, air pollution, and climate factors, we initially fit models, like that in Equation 9.2, to Chicago, Denver, Philadelphia, Saint Louis, and Washington, D.C., using ordinary least squares. In each case we regressed the daily deaths on the level of air pollution at time t, at time $t - 1$, and so on, up to time $t - 5$. We included a number of climate factors similar to those included in the Glasser and Greenburg (1971) study: average wind speed (Wind), precipitation (Rainfall), and mean temperature (Mean temp). We also included a set of dummy variables characterizing the days of the week, hypothesizing that both air pollution and mortality are cyclical over the week.[10]

Analysis for Chicago
Results for Chicago are shown in table 9.1.

Four criteria were used to judge whether there was a significant air pollution effect. The first was the statistical significance of an air pollution

---

[9] Missing daily observations were estimated by linear interpolation.

[10] We postulated that air pollution would be lower on weekends due to decreased industrial activity. Silverman (1973a and 1973b) detected a day-of-the-week influence on emergency hospital admissions, which we thought might carry over to daily deaths.

TABLE 9.1. Time-series Analysis Comparing the Effects of Various Air Pollutants on Daily Deaths in Chicago

	9.1-1	9.1-2	9.1-3	9.1-4	9.1-5	9.1-6	9.1-7	9.1-8	9.1-9
R^2	.270	.266	.284	.166	.124	.129	.179	.174	.114
Constant	118.875	95.312	98.831	110.321	129.067	109.431	110.532	128.102	126.729
Air pollution variables									
AP_t	.882	2.574	2.188	14.687	8.228	-3.010	-2.768	1.317	1.269
	(.81)	(2.90)	(2.45)	(2.29)	(.94)	(-1.03)	(-.90)	(1.02)	(.81)
AP_{t-1}	1.375	.382	.505	10.280	-5.639	.327	.866	-1.623	-.492
	(1.30)	(.39)	(.52)	(1.41)	(-.58)	(.12)	(.31)	(-1.09)	(-.28)
AP_{t-2}	.714	2.831	2.780	9.654	10.254	4.087	5.320	1.942	1.762
	(.67)	(2.87)	(2.81)	(1.33)	(1.06)	(1.48)	(1.92)	(1.31)	(1.02)
AP_{t-3}	-1.260	-.701	-.673	-2.814	-18.284	4.344	4.002	-1.111	-2.101
	(-1.17)	(-.71)	(-.69)	(-.39)	(-1.89)	(1.57)	(1.45)	(-.75)	(-1.22)
AP_{t-4}	.470	2.823	2.606	6.101	6.991	1.055	.253	.132	-.015
	(.44)	(2.88)	(2.66)	(.84)	(.73)	(.38)	(.09)	(.09)	(-.01)
AP_{t-5}	3.052	-1.142	-1.132	-3.513	-13.308	4.060	3.943	-2.077	-1.261
	(3.03)	(-1.38)	(-1.37)	(-.59)	(-1.62)	(1.67)	(1.64)	(-1.65)	(-.88)
Sum AP elasticities	7.19	10.72	10.67	13.55	-4.13	8.53	9.92	-3.73	-2.13
Climate variables									
Mean temp	-1.535	1.816	1.161	-2.581	-1.820	-.727	-1.165	-2.393	-1.958
	(-2.31)	(3.38)	(2.06)	(-6.84)	(-4.22)	(-1.37)	(-2.20)	(-6.18)	(-4.73)
Rainfall	12.316	5.383	5.143	-.038	2.083	1.800	3.163	.308	.821
	(2.33)	(1.25)	(1.17)	(-.01)	(.43)	(.51)	(.67)	(.07)	(.17)
Wind	-.374	-.419	-.407	2.439	.137	-.770	-.561	2.087	.698
	(-.16)	(-.22)	(-.21)	(1.21)	(.06)	(-.33)	(-.22)	(1.00)	(.31)
Sum climate elasticities	-5.39	7.30	4.33	-9.80	-6.75	-4.00	-4.87	-7.84	-6.79
Day-of-the-week variables									
Sunday	2.078	.744	.929	-.614	.386	-1.915	-.773	.290	.340
Monday	2.587	2.983	2.923	3.226	2.023	3.206	2.551	2.101	2.278
Tuesday	-.517	2.205	1.437	2.390	1.678	3.072	2.574	1.967	2.145
Wednesday	-2.477	-2.124	-1.875	-1.803	-1.480	-1.107	-.741	-1.084	-1.196
Thursday	-1.760	-1.736	-1.412	-.590	-.798	-.650	-1.077	-.705	-1.055
Friday	-.348	-3.575	-3.420	-3.358	-3.184	-2.840	-2.976	-3.471	-3.456
Saturday	.437	1.504	1.416	.749	1.376	.235	.441	.903	9.44

Note: The above regressions are based on the following data sets:

Regression	Air pollutant	Dates	Number of observations
1	Sulfur dioxide	9/62–6/63	298
2	Sulfur dioxide	9/63–6/64	299
3	Sulfur dioxide	9/63–5/64	269
4	Nitrogen dioxide	8/63–8/64	392
5	Nitrogen dioxide	9/63–5/64	269

Regression	Air pollutant	Dates	Number of observations
6	Nitric oxide	8/63–8/64	392
7	Nitric oxide	9/63–5/64	269
8	Hydrocarbons	8/63–5/64	300
9	Hydrocarbons	9/63–5/64	269

The numbers in parentheses below the regression coefficients are t statistics. The estimated effects of the day-of-the-week variables were scaled so they summed to

coefficient, the second was the sign and magnitude of the sum of the air pollution elasticities,[11] the third was the significance of an F statistic testing the contribution of the air pollution variables, and the fourth was the consistency of a replication for another time period when data were available. In the first regression, which corresponds to Equation 9.2 above, the number of daily deaths in Chicago from September 1962 through June 1963 was regressed on sulfur dioxide, climate variables, and day-of-the-week variables; only 27 percent of the variance was explained, implying that important factors affecting mortality are missing from the regression or that the inherent stochastic element in daily mortality is of considerable importance. The coefficient of the first sulfur dioxide variable suggested a contemporaneous effect of high levels of air pollution on the number of deaths, but the association was not statistically significant. In addition, when high levels of sulfur dioxide occurred, one, two, four, and five days prior to the day of observed deaths, there was a positive correlation with deaths; only the five-day lag was statistically significant. Summing the air pollution elasticities of the sulfur dioxide variables revealed a positive effect of air pollution on mortality (Sum AP elasticities = 7.19). In addition, the F statistic confirmed the significance of the contribution of the air pollution variables ($F = 4.08$). Of the climate variables, mean temperature was statistically significant (indicating that as the daily mean temperature increased, the daily number of deaths decreased). Rainfall was also statistically significant (indicating that days with greater rainfall had greater numbers of deaths). In Chicago during this period, the greatest number of deaths seemed to occur on Mondays, the smallest on Wednesdays.

Regression 9.1-2 reports similar results for the effects of sulfur dioxide in Chicago during the period September 1963 through June 1964. Again, approximately 27 percent of the variation in the number of daily deaths was explained by the right-hand-side variables ($R^2 = 0.266$). In addition, three of the coefficients for sulfur dioxide were positive and statistically significant, indicating a close association between daily deaths and current and lagged sulfur dioxide levels. The sum of the sulfur dioxide elasticities was 10.72, providing further evidence of an important effect from air pollution levels.[12] The F statistic for testing the contribution of the sulfur dioxide variables was again significant ($F = 12.50$). In this regression, the only statistically significant climate variable was mean temperature. Its coefficient now indicated a positive relationship between the daily temperature and the daily number of deaths. This time, the day-of-the-week

[11] In view of the high correlations between day-to-day levels of air pollution, we believe that the sum of elasticities is a better indication of the air pollution effect than the statistical significance of isolated coefficients.

[12] The magnitude of this association for Chicago is revealed by considering a 50 percent reduction in the mean level of sulfur dioxide pollution. A decrease of 0.092 ppm in the mean values of the pollution variables was estimated to lead to a decrease of 6.3 deaths per day (approximately 5.4 percent).

variable suggested that the highest number of daily deaths occurred on Mondays and the fewest on Fridays. (Regression 9.1-3 represents a subset of the data analyzed in regression 9.1-2. It is shown for comparison, since this subset is analyzed in detail below.)

When we applied the four criteria to the other three pollutants in Chicago, the evidence of significant mortality effects was less strong than for sulfur dioxide. For example, regression 9.1-4 reports the effects of nitrogen dioxide on daily deaths in Chicago between August 1963 and August 1964. The concurrent level of nitrogen dioxide (NO_{2_t}) was positive and statistically significant and the sum of the air pollution elasticities (13.55) indicated a substantial effect of nitrogen dioxide levels on daily mortality. Furthermore, an F test confirmed the significance of the six air pollution variables in the regression ($F = 6.82$). Since regression 9.1-5 represented a subset of the data analyzed in regression 9.1-4, we could not adequately test the fourth criterion. Regressions 9.1-6 and 9.1-7 report the results for nitric oxide (NO). In both regressions all of the nitric oxide coefficients were positive, although none was statistically significant. The sums of the air pollution elasticities were relatively large (8.53 and 9.92, respectively), and in both regressions, F tests indicated that the contributions of the air pollution variables were significant ($F = 3.85$ and $F = 4.15$, respectively).[13] The effects of hydrocarbons (HC) on daily mortality are investigated in regressions 9.1-8 and 9.1-9. The air pollution coefficients had mixed signs, although none was statistically significant. The sums of their elasticities were negative (-3.73 and -2.13, respectively), and F tests indicated that the hydrocarbon variables did not make a significant contribution to either regression ($F = 1.20$ and $F = 0.78$, respectively).

Analysis for Denver, Philadelphia, Saint Louis, and Washington, D.C.

When the four criteria described above were applied to the data for the remaining four cities—Denver, Philadelphia, Saint Louis, and Washington, D.C.—there was no consistent evidence of a daily effect of the air pollutants on daily mortality.

Table 9.2 summarizes the results for the other cities. As can be seen from the coefficients of determination (R^2) corresponding to the twelve data sets, in only two cases (Philadelphia/nitric oxide and Washington, D.C./hydrocarbons) was more than 7 percent of the variation in the mortality rates explained. Further, the sums of elasticities of the air pollution variables were generally small and often negative. Finally, F tests indicated that the six air pollution variables did not make a significant contribution to the analyses except in one case (Philadelphia/nitric oxide).

---

[13] This suggested association between nitric oxide and daily deaths will be explored in more detail later.

TABLE 9.2. Summary of Results of Daily Time-series Analysis for Denver, Philadelphia, Saint Louis, and Washington, D.C.

City/pollutant	Dates	Number of observations	Pollution variable (mean)[a]	Daily deaths (mean)	R^2	Sum AP elasticities	F statistic
Denver/sulfur dioxide	3/65–7/66	518	.174	25.168	.056	−2.44	0.73
Denver/nitrogen dioxide	3/65–7/66	518	.336	25.168	.061	−12.04	1.20
Denver/hydrocarbons	4/65–7/66	487	2.379	25.160	.062	−3.82	1.06
Philadelphia/nitrogen dioxide	9/65–9/66	395	.370	25.267	.066	1.24	1.02
Philadelphia/nitric oxide	9/64–4/65	242	.559	24.848	.104	−2.95	2.82
Philadelphia/carbon monoxide	9/65–10/66	426	.726	25.209	.063	−7.37	0.79
Saint Louis/sulfur dioxide	1/65–6/66	546	.475	14.381	.050	0.17	1.21
Saint Louis/nitrogen dioxide	9/64–6/66	668	.278	14.311	.034	−0.34	1.15
Saint Louis/nitric oxide	9/64–4/65	242	.383	14.645	.070	−0.22	1.42
Saint Louis/carbon monoxide	4/64–2/66	699	.650	14.183	.026	1.05	0.28
Washington, D.C./carbon monoxide	4/65–10/66	579	2.354	27.194	.024	−13.79	1.45
Washington, D.C./hydrocarbons	11/64–7/65	273	.340	27.916	.160	−7.01	1.00

Note: Since $F_{0.05} = 2.10$, with 6 and ∞ degrees of freedom, it can be seen that in only one case (Philadelphia/nitric oxide) the contribution of the air pollution variables was statistically significant.

[a] Sulfur dioxide, nitrogen dioxide, and nitric oxide, in parts per million $\times$ 10; hydrocarbons, in parts per million; and carbon monoxide, in parts per million $\times$ 0.1.

Further analysis for Chicago

The question arises as to why the Chicago results differed from the results for the other cities.[14] One possible explanation is the relative size of
the cities. Because of its larger population, the mean number of deaths
per day in Chicago was more than four times as large as that for any other
city in our sample (see table D.13, page 338). Since deaths occur in dis-
crete units (one at a time), effects of air pollution in a smaller city may
be lost when scattered over a five-day period.[15] Another possibility is the
relative level of air pollution in each city. For each air pollutant under
consideration, the mean level in Chicago exceeded that in any other city
(see table D.13, page 338). Chicago's mean levels of sulfur dioxide were
almost ten times as high as those in Denver and almost four times as high
as those in Saint Louis. It may be that at levels of air pollution substantially below those found in Chicago, acute effects are not important. We
shall examine these conjectures in more detail below. [Most of the remaining estimation relates to data from a nine-month period (September
1963 through May 1964) for a Chicago data set containing measures of
four air pollutants (nitric oxide, nitrogen dioxide, sulfur dioxide, and
hydrocarbons).]

Aside from the explanations suggested by Chicago's relatively higher
air pollution levels and larger population, it was possible that we had mis-
specified the relation. We examined this possibility in a number of ways.
First, we included all four air pollutants simultaneously, as is shown in
the first regression of table 9.3. Only sulfur dioxide possessed statistically
significant coefficients (these were positive); nitric oxide possessed positive coefficients approaching statistical significance. (The sum of the air
pollution elasticities was equal to 8.17, indicating that the combined effect
of the four air pollutants was substantial.) As expected from the results
of regression 9.1-3, the mean temperature variable was positive and
statistically significant. Similarly, the day-of-the-week variables indicated that the greatest number of deaths occurred on Mondays, the smallest on Fridays. Approximately 36 percent of the variation in daily deaths
was explained by the variables in regression 9.3-1 ($R^2 = 0.357$).

Second, we explored a number of functional forms: we fit log-log,
quadratic (including interaction terms), dummy variable, and linear spline
specifications. The log-log specifications exhibited results similar to the
linear specifications; the elasticities at the mean were relatively close to the
coefficients of the corresponding untransformed air pollution variables.
The coefficients of the quadratic air pollution variables were generally nonsignificant and added little to the explanatory powers of the regressions.

---

[14] Close associations between daily mortality and air pollution have also been
found for New York City and Los Angeles, both large cities with high levels of air
pollution (see Glasser and Greenburg, 1971; and Hechter and Goldsmith, 1961).

[15] See the previous discussion of difficulties resulting from small samples (p. 25).

TABLE 9.3. Alternative Specifications Analyzing Daily Deaths in Chicago

	All pollutants 9.3-1	Deaths as deviations from a moving average 9.3-2	Episodic pollution 9.3-3
R^2	.357	.165	.301
Constant	98.636	−16.959	101.937
Air pollution variables			
SO_{2t}	2.160 (2.31)	1.867 (2.18)	2.304 (2.50)
SO_{2t-1}	.695 (.66)	−.230 (−.24)	−.306 (−.30)
SO_{2t-2}	2.013 (1.92)	1.877 (1.97)	1.695 (1.61)
SO_{2t-3}	−.640 (−.61)	−1.400 (−1.47)	.085 (.10)
SO_{2t-4}	2.253 (2.16)	2.573 (2.71)	
SO_{2t-5}	−1.354 (−1.52)	−1.754 (−2.17)	
NO_{2t}	5.257 (.58)		
NO_{2t-1}	−12.819 (−1.22)		
NO_{2t-2}	1.035 (.10)		
NO_{2t-3}	−15.503 (−1.49)		
NO_{2t-4}	.872 (.08)		
NO_{2t-5}	−7.917 (−.94)		
NO_t	−2.736 (−.86)	−3.472 (−1.24)	−2.694 (−.88)
NO_{t-1}	.741 (.23)	.504 (.20)	−1.408 (−.50)
NO_{t-2}	2.885 (.90)	2.740 (1.09)	3.180 (1.14)
NO_{t-3}	5.796 (1.82)	2.589 (1.03)	3.373 (1.39)
NO_{t-4}	−.748 (−.23)	−1.588 (−.62)	
NO_{t-5}	4.646 (1.68)	1.471 (.65)	
HC_t	1.240 (.72)		
HC_{t-1}	−.106 (−.05)		
HC_{t-2}	.292 (.14)		
HC_{t-3}	−1.535 (−.74)		
HC_{t-4}	.943 (.45)		
HC_{t-5}	−.586 (−.36)		
$\sum_{k=0}^{3} SO_{2t-k}$			.008 (.98)
$\sum_{k=0}^{3} NO_{2t-k}$			.203 (.29)
Sum AP elasticities	8.17		10.25
Climate variables			
Mean temp	1.710 (2.42)	2.320 (3.85)	.711 (1.07)
Rainfall	6.720 (1.48)	4.984 (1.18)	6.278 (1.40)
Wind	.165 (−.07)	−1.383 (−.58)	−.974 (−.40)
Sum climate elasticities	7.08		2.11
Day-of-the-week variables			
Sunday	.868	−.089	.672
Monday	2.982	2.705	2.481
Tuesday	1.618	1.868	1.954
Wednesday	−2.046	−1.634	−2.081
Thursday	−1.361	−1.485	−1.795
Friday	−3.298	−2.743	−3.103
Saturday	1.237	1.379	1.875

Note: All regressions are based on data for 274 days. The numbers in parentheses below the regression coefficients are *t* statistics. The estimated effects of the day-of-the-week variables were scaled so that they summed to zero.

Of the interaction terms, only sulfur dioxide times hydrocarbons ($SO_2 \times$ HC) was important. Neither the dummy variable nor the linear spline specifications dominated the simple linear form, although there was some evidence that the linear specification was not adequate for describing the effects of nitric oxide. This is examined further in the discussion that follows.

Next, we attempted to see if the structure of the underlying relationship differed between days with high and low levels of air pollution. We divided the Chicago data set on the basis of days with high and low levels of sulfur dioxide and nitric oxide and ran regressions for each of the subsets.[16] The F values indicated no statistically significant difference in the sets of regression coefficients.[17]

Subsequently, we estimated a specification similar to that of Glasser and Greenburg (1971). Specifically, we altered the dependent variable, so that instead of examining deaths at time t we examined deviations of the number of deaths from a fifteen-day moving average centered on the eighth day.[18] Again, we limited the analysis to current and lagged values of the two air pollutants, sulfur dioxide and nitric oxide. Regression 9.3-2 presents the results. The magnitudes and significance of the sulfur dioxide coefficients were not greatly different from those in the previous regression.[19] However, some nitric oxide coefficients diminished substantially in magnitude and remained nonsignificant. The climate and day-of-the-week variables exhibited relatively little change. The explanatory power of the regression (R^2) dropped from 0.357 to 0.165, as might be expected when a dependent variable is transformed into a deviation from a moving average.

It is difficult to compare our results with those of Glasser and Greenburg. They included neither lagged air pollution variables nor day-of-the-week variables.[20] In their study, the coefficients for wind speed displayed mixed signs when they were statistically significant (in our regression, the coefficient was not statistically significant). When rainfall was statistically significant in their study, its coefficient was positive (its coefficient was posi-

---

[16] We limited the analysis to these two air pollutants, since in regression 9.3-1 only they were significant in explaining daily deaths in Chicago.

[17] This result is not inconsistent with the above results which did not uncover a statistically significant association between daily air pollution levels and daily mortality in other cities; even the days with relatively low air pollution levels in Chicago had levels substantially greater than in the other cities.

[18] In notational terms, the left-hand side of Equation 9.2 became

$$MR_t - \sum_{k=-7}^{7} MR_{t+k}/15$$

[19] The coefficient of $SO2_{t-5}$ was negative and statistically significant. This will be discussed below.

[20] They did disaggregate their data by day of the week and run separate regressions.

tive but not statistically significant in our analysis). Because their temperature variable was expressed as a deviation from normal, we cannot compare it with our measure of mean temperature.

Next, we tried other specifications, including moving averages of air pollution levels, as well as variables representing the change in air pollution levels on consecutive days. None proved as satisfactory as the simple linear structure in terms of either explanatory power or the significance of the air pollution coefficients.

Then, we investigated whether a consecutive period of several days of high levels of air pollution was more detrimental than isolated days of high levels. (Many of the episodic studies cited above have found significant effects on mortality during such occurrences.) We defined a new sulfur dioxide variable as the product of the sulfur dioxide levels for the current day and the three preceding days.[21] We also created a similar nitric oxide variable.

The results of adding these new pollution variables are presented as regression 9.3-3. The magnitude and significance of the individual air pollution coefficients exhibited little change. The new air pollution variables were statistically nonsignificant.[22] The climate variables displayed mixed results; mean temperature became nonsignificant, while both precipitation and wind speed remained nonsignificant. The explanatory power of the regression was 0.301.

Finally, having settled on the linear form with lags of up to five days, we attempted to refine the estimates by using the Almon technique, as programmed and discussed by Gaver (1971). This procedure imposes structure on the lag coefficients by constraining them to fit a polynomial curve of a specified degree. The process often results in the reduction of large standard errors in the distributed lag coefficients which may arise from multicollinearity in the lagged values of the independent variables,[23] and allows considerable flexibility. We began by fitting second- and third-degree polynomials, using lags of five to ten days for the two air pollutants, sulfur dioxide and nitric oxide. The third-degree polynomial added little to the analysis, so we confined our interest to the second-degree polynomials. The only other qualification we imposed was that the current (zero lag) air pollution coefficient be positive, inasmuch as a negative coefficient was deemed unreasonable.[24] In this case the effect of

[21] In notational terms, $\quad P_t = \prod_{k=0}^{3} P_{t-k}.$

[22] We experimented with other similarly defined variables but were unable to detect an episodic effect.

[23] For example, the simple correlations between SO_{2t} and SO_{2t-1} and between NO_t and NO_{t-1} were 0.78 and 0.59, respectively.

[24] In practice, this qualification was unnecessary for sulfur dioxide; however, the zero lag of nitric oxide initially had a negative (although statistically nonsignificant) coefficient. Thus, only the latter variable had such a restriction.

TABLE 9.4.   Refined Air Pollution Lag Structures for Analyzing Daily Deaths in Chicago

R^2	.291	Air pollution variables (continued)	
Constant	87.346	NO_{t-4}	1.7
			(3.00)
Air pollution variables		NO_{t-5}	1.5
SO_{2t}	1.7		(2.94)
	(2.94)	NO_{t-6}	1.0
SO_{2t-1}	1.5		(1.98)
	(5.39)	NO_{t-7}	.38
SO_{2t-2}	1.2		(.51)
	(4.33)	NO_{t-8}	−.46
SO_{2t-3}	.88		(−.39)
	(2.72)		
SO_{2t-4}	.51	Climate variables	
	(1.84)	Mean temp	1.539
SO_{2t-5}	.079		(2.66)
	(.32)	Rainfall	5.325
SO_{2t-6}	−.40		(1.22)
	(−.73)	Wind	1.295
NO_t	.74		(.65)
	(2.53)		
NO_{t-1}	1.3	Day-of-the-week variables	
	(2.61)	Sunday	−1.766
		Monday	.643
NO_{t-2}	1.6	Tuesday	2.778
	(2.71)	Wednesday	1.625
		Thursday	−1.589
NO_{t-3}	1.8	Friday	−3.303
	(2.85)	Saturday	1.612

Note: The regression is based on data for 274 days. The numbers opposite each air pollution variable are Almon lag weights not to be confused with regression coefficients. Regression coefficients appear for the climate variables. The estimated effects of the day-of-the-week variables were scaled so that they summed to zero. The numbers in parentheses below the Almon lag weights and the regression coefficients are t statistics.

such a front-end restriction was simply to shift the polynomial so that the $t + 1$ lag (one future day) had a zero weight.

Table 9.4 shows the results for a regression that employed the Almon technique, using second-degree polynomials to estimate the lag structure of the sulfur dioxide and nitric oxide variables.[25] The t statistics indicate that the weights corresponding to the contemporaneous and first three lag variables for sulfur dioxide were statistically significant,[26] while for nitric oxide the contemporaneous and first six lags were statistically significant. In addition, the contribution of the air pollution variables to the explained sum of squares was computed. The resulting F value was 4.30, with 16

[25] This particular regression was chosen because it had the minimum estimated standard error of disturbances adjusted for the degrees of freedom.

[26] The fact that SO_{2t-5} was no longer statistically significant may be an indication that its previous significance was an artifact of multicollinearity between the lagged air pollution variables. See fn. 19.

and 247 degrees of freedom. Since $F_{0.05} = 1.67$, with 15 and ∞ degrees of freedom, it can be seen that the air pollution variables made a significant contribution to the regression. The coefficients of the climate and day-of-the-week variables were similar to those in regression 9.3-1. It is interesting to examine the magnitude of the air pollution weights. The maximum effect of sulfur dioxide on daily deaths took place simultaneously with peaks in sulfur dioxide levels and then dropped off. (This could have possible implications as to the physiological mechanism involved.) The nitric oxide weights imply a different physical response. The maximum effect on daily deaths occurred at a lag of three days. (Figures 9.1 and 9.2 illustrate the two underlying structures.)

THE INFLUENCE OF AIR POLLUTION ON TIME OF DEATH

Whether the estimated effect of air pollution on mortality has significant policy implications is a basic concern of our study. A statistically significant association between measures of daily air pollution and daily mortality may imply that air pollution is doing nothing more than hastening deaths of susceptible individuals by a few days at the most. Abatement in this case would have little policy significance, since it would merely reallocate deaths within a short time interval.

One way to test the so-called hastening hypothesis is to investigate lag structures for a sufficiently long period in order to reveal decreases in mortality that might follow an air pollution episode. A number of models using lags of five to ten days have been estimated above. None of these results indicated a decrease in deaths following a period of high levels of air pollution. Since the lag may not have been long enough, this test is not conclusive, but it does suggest that the reallocation, if it exists, does not take place over a period as short as ten days.[27]

A more interesting test of the hastening hypothesis involves comparing the time-series results with the cross-sectional and cross-sectional time-series findings. Most of this volume has dealt with an extensive analysis of the association between air pollution levels and mortality rates across areas. Since these analyses relate annual mortality rates to annual air pollution measures (holding other factors constant), the estimated effects are hypothesized to be much longer than day-to-day effects.

In this chapter, the results of a daily analysis for Chicago (regression 9.1-2) indicated that a 50 percent reduction in air pollution (as measured by sulfur dioxide) was associated with a 5.4 percent reduction in daily deaths (see footnote 12). Our basic 1960 cross-sectional regression (regression 3.2-1) was interpreted as indicating that a 50 percent reduction in air pollution (as measured by sulfates and suspended particulates) was

---

[27] Another test is to examine longer time intervals, for example, the monthly periods used by Hodgson (1970), in an attempt to average away day-to-day effects in which increased deaths on one day result in decreased deaths on subsequent days.

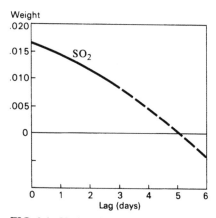

FIG. 9.1. Underlying lag structure for the effects of sulfur dioxide on daily deaths.

associated with a 4.7 percent decrease in the unadjusted total mortality rate.[28] Although these estimated elasticities are similar, a more relevant comparison would be with data sets involving the same air pollutant, sulfur dioxide. The 1969 subset of data having measures of sulfur dioxide was analyzed in chapter 7. For the regression involving sulfur dioxide alone (regression 7.8-5), the effect of a 50 percent reduction in air pollution levels was estimated to be associated with a 2.7 percent decrease in the unadjusted total mortality rate.[29] For the cross-sectional time-series data set having measures of sulfur dioxide, the estimated effect of a 50 percent reduction in sulfur dioxide levels alone was associated with a 1.2 percent reduction in the unadjusted total mortality rate (regression 8.4-5).[30]

As discussed earlier, the daily effect of air pollution on mortality may be composed of two parts: (1) a hastening of deaths of high-risk individuals by a few days; and (2) a reduction in life expectancy of the general population. Presumably, only the latter effect was being estimated in the cross-sectional regressions. A cross-sectional time-series analysis may reveal aspects of both effects. The time-series analysis in this chapter does not clearly indicate whether a harvesting effect was present in the data, although a comparison of the time-series results with our earlier findings suggests the possibility of such an effect on mortality.

[28] The 1969 replication (regression 7.1-3), as well as the 1960–69 cross-sectional time-series finding (regression 8.1-1), suggested similar estimated effects.

[29] It should be noted that when measures of suspended particulates were included, the combined effect of a 50 percent reduction in the levels of both air pollutants was associated with a 6.3 percent decrease in the unadjusted total mortality rate (regression 7.8-7).

[30] Again, when suspended particulates were also included, the combined effect increased substantially. A 50 percent reduction in the levels was associated with a 5.3 percent decrease in the unadjusted total mortality rate (regression 8.4-7).

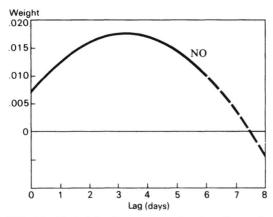

FIG. 9.2. Underlying lag structure for the effects of
nitric oxide on daily deaths.

SUMMARY OF TIME-SERIES ANALYSES

Chapters 8 and 9 investigated annual data on SMSAs over a decade, and day-to-day variations in the level of air pollution and mortality in five cities, respectively. In addition, we have discussed the methods used to analyze the effect of air pollution on health over time. Taken together, the evidence in chapters 8 and 9 supports the conclusion that, in the largest U.S. cities, there are close relationships between the mortality rate and air pollution (as measured by sulfates, sulfur dioxide, suspended particulates, and possibly a nitrogen compound, such as nitric oxide). The air pollutants for which we failed to find consistent, statistically significant time-series relationships with mortality rates were nitrates, nitrogen dioxide, carbon monoxide, and hydrocarbons. These findings were generally consistent with the results in chapter 7.[31]

In addition to the problems of inadequate, badly measured air pollution data, the daily analysis was subject to problems stemming from small samples. Only one of the five cities investigated (Chicago) had a large enough number of daily deaths to allow us to uncover effects of air pollution. While the two most significant air pollutants from our previous investigations—sulfates and suspended particulates—were missing, sulfur dioxide, and to a lesser extent, nitric oxide, were found to be related to daily mortality. Careful investigation of the lag structure revealed that high levels of sulfur dioxide had a relatively large, immediate effect, gradually diminishing over time. For nitric oxide, the effect was delayed by several days, reached its peak, and then diminished. In addition, an examination of the lag structure of the air pollution effects failed to indicate that the number of deaths decreased following a period of high levels of air pollution. How-

[31] In the 1969 analysis, cross-sectional data were not available for nitric oxide, hydrocarbons, and carbon monoxide.

ever, a comparison of these results with our earlier findings suggests the possibility that the mechanism relating air pollution levels to increased mortality might be different in a time-series study than in a cross-sectional or cross-sectional time-series analysis.

Taken as a whole, the time-series results generally support our earlier findings of an important (presumably causal) association between mortality and such air pollutants as sulfates, suspended particulates, sulfur dioxide, and possibly nitric oxide.

Policy implications

CHAPTER 10

The benefits and costs
of air pollution abatement

The costs of abating air pollution are considerable, whether measured in higher prices, lower corporate profits, unemployment, or greater use of scarce resources. These costs are too high for one to conclude casually that an affluent society can afford a clean environment. We can afford much, but not everything we desire. Since economists usually begin with the assumption that the economy is at full employment, diverting resources to air pollution abatement requires that we give up other goods and services we desire. We must establish the priorities for air pollution abatement in relation to other programs that an affluent society would like to undertake. Indeed, the 1970 Amendments to the Clean Air Act and the EPA's administration of them have come under increasing attack as the stringent controls are implemented. These are times for rethinking, reexamination, and perhaps even retreat from current and proposed programs.

The short history of the 1970 amendments is filled with official reexaminations as to their justification (Rall, 1973; NAS, 1974, 1975). High price tags and frequent calls for reexamination should not lead us to the conclusion that expensive programs should be dropped, but rather that we must look carefully at the social benefits and costs of such programs. Oscar Wilde said that a cynic is someone who knows the price of everything and the value of nothing. One might reply that an idealist is someone who knows the value of everything, but the cost of nothing. This is not a time when we can afford to be either cynics or idealists.

We need to know the answers to the following: How much air pollution abatement is justified? What sort of government action is needed? How can such abatement be brought about efficiently? In order to answer these questions, we must decide on a framework for analyzing the problem.

Benefit–cost analysis, and its variations, have been developed and used extensively in the past fifteen years to evaluate proposed public expenditures (Dasgupta and Pearce, 1972; Harberger and coauthors, 1971; Niskanen and coauthors, 1972; Haveman and coauthors, 1974; and Zeckhauser and coauthors, 1975). The basic approach is a systematic search for all effects of a project, which are then classified as either benefits or costs. By hard work, art, and wizardry, the project is judged by some comparison of its associated benefits and costs. The tool is basically a good one, although there are a number of potential dangers. In particular, it is easy to bias the analysis so that a "bad" project can be made to look "good," or vice versa. A good benefit–cost analysis is not easy to do, and even skilled practitioners have difficulty determining and monetizing the more important effects of a proposed project.

It should also be noted that in classic benefit–cost analysis the primary goal is economic or allocative efficiency, where "allocative efficiency as an economic goal [refers] to the fact that it is sometimes possible to reallocate resources—perhaps increasing or decreasing the amount of resources used for [air] pollution control—in ways [that] will bring about an increase in the net value of output produced by those resources" (Haveman and Weisbrod, 1975, page 38).

In practice, it must be recognized that policymakers evaluate alternative programs in terms other than efficiency, for example, equity and political goals. This caveat is especially relevant to air pollution abatement programs. Pollution control is an extremely political issue, and in local areas the distribution of benefits and costs will often be more important (at least for implementation purposes) than aggregate (regional or national) efficiency. This point and previously noted limitations will become more apparent in the context of our analysis of air pollution abatement.

The direct benefits of air pollution abatement include improvements in human health, lessened damage to plants and animals, lower cleaning costs, and longer lives for various materials and structures. In addition, there are other benefits inherently difficult to quantify, such as improved visibility, more frequent clear skies and sunny days, and reduction of noxious odors. These latter benefits are basically ones which enhance the "quality of life."

The direct costs of abatement include the costs of the new capital equipment required, of modifying existing equipment, and of operating the equipment. A more subtle cost relates to the fact that many current or prospective processes and designs can no longer be used since they do not meet the newer regulatory standards. There are also indirect costs associated with air pollution abatement. Abatement regulations will cause plants of limited profitability to shut down if they cannot cover the costs of the new abatement equipment or of modifying existing equipment. These shutdowns impose costs not only on employees who lose their jobs and move away,[1] but also on the cities and other areas whose economic base is dependent on the plants and employees for tax revenues and payrolls. Finally, there are the costs of administering the program itself, although no one has ever attempted to assess them.

MEASUREMENT DIFFICULTIES

It is extremely difficult to quantify the benefits listed above. The underlying relationships are exceedingly complex. We have already shown how difficult it is to prove that air pollution causes ill health, and it is even harder to quantify the nature of the relation. Yet, evaluating the physical effects of air pollution and the associated consequences of abatement are only the preliminary steps in a benefit–cost analysis.

A common metric is needed if we are to make intelligent comparisons of the benefits and costs of air pollution abatement. For example, it is conceivable that the benefit side of an analysis might consist of 10,000 fewer asthma cases per year, 100,000 fewer gallons of paint for repainting, twenty additional clear and sunny days, and so on; the cost side might consist of one million tons of steel, three billion kWh of electricity, and so on. Such a listing of disparate items must be translated to the extent possible into a common unit if one is to make a sensible comparison.

One type of translation could be done by a decision maker applying a set of values he judges to be appropriate. But such a personal assessment would be just that; a statement of what one individual perceives to be the value of the benefits and costs of a given project. A better approach is to use a widely accepted set of values.

Market prices constitute such a set of values. Consumers and producers make decisions every day on the basis of market prices. Prices constitute the major standard used in society for deciding how much of a resource to use in production as well as how much of a final good to produce and consume. In an economist's model world, prices measure the cost to society of producing another unit of a good or service, as well as the extra utility (or satisfaction) a consumer obtains from a unit of the good or service. When markets function well, prices are suitable measures of the benefits and costs of the final goods and services ensuing from a project.

Unfortunately, many goods and services are not valued in the marketplace and consequently cannot be monetized easily. For example, it is difficult to place a value on reduced morbidity and mortality. How much is it worth to experience less sickness each year or even an extra year of

---

[1] The cost of a lost job includes both the forgone wages for the period of unemployment as well as the psychological cost of losing a job (the latter may be greater than the former, but, again, this is difficult to measure).

life expectancy? Individuals rarely make such judgments explicitly; hence, valuation often involves direct query or complicated analyses based on other decisions consumers make, as discussed below. Because of research limitations, in many cases one can list only the nature of the effect without translating it into dollars. For example, valuations of the benefits associated with psychic effects and the general quality of life are often omitted, since guesses as to their values would have no sound foundation. A simple listing of potential effects is often as far as the analyst can go. In the context of air pollution abatement, such intangible benefits may be the most important categories. Thus, any calculation of the benefits from pollution abatement is likely to underestimate substantially the "true" benefits.

Benefit–cost analysis is most useful when there is widespread agreement on the nature and values of the benefits and costs. However, some of the effects of a project may not be estimated with precision (for example, only a range of the quantitative effects may be presented), while others may be very difficult to assess in dollar terms (for example, the dollar value of a clear and sunny day). Consequently, a benefit–cost analysis should differentiate between "hard" estimates of benefits and costs (those for which the relationships and valuations appear to be well established) and "soft" estimates (those for which the relationships are uncertain or valuations differ among individuals). A benefit–cost study is most convincing when the same decision would be made on the basis of either the hard figures alone or on the basis of both hard and soft estimates; that is, when the verdict does not depend on the exact quantification or assessment of the soft benefits and costs. At the other extreme, benefit–cost analysis is of little use when there is no agreement on the quantification or assessment of a project's effects.

Decision makers should recognize that there is an inherent bias in benefit–cost analysis toward underestimating the benefits and overestimating the costs of a project (see Lave, 1972). For example, the most common way of measuring the costs of abatement is to estimate the cost of adding devices that would reduce emissions from existing facilities. But adding an abatement device to an industrial smokestack is often economically inefficient, since it may also decrease the operating efficiency of the firm. In the long-run, it is often more economical to construct a new plant designed to control emissions even if the initial investment is quite high. Furthermore, present cost estimates are usually based on current technology; at best, the analyst can make only educated guesses as to the effects of advancing technology. Because such guesses are subject to considerable uncertainty, they are seldom used in cost estimates. Consequently, cost estimates of pollution abatement are likely to be overestimated, since one expects major technological advances in the efficiency of control systems (for example, improvements in the control of automobile emissions).

Since benefits tend to be underestimated and costs overestimated, a carefully done benefit–cost analysis of air pollution abatement is inherently biased toward rejection. If, despite these biases, the analysis shows that abatement is justified, a strong case can be made for prompt action.

BENEFITS

Although some benefit estimates have received extensive publicity, their quality has not always warranted the attention given them. One of the most widely quoted numbers, $11 billion per year as the value of abatement, originated from a 1913 Mellon Institute study. The figure was arrived at by taking the estimated cost of smoke damage per capita to Pittsburgh residents, updated to 1958 by the consumer price index and then multiplied by the nation's population (see Mellon Institute, 1913, and Gustavson, 1959). Other widely cited figures have no more foundation. Rather than continuing to quote such figures, researchers should undertake more careful analyses.

In order to obtain better estimates of the benefits of pollution abatement, effects must be investigated in detail. In the following sections, we will examine briefly benefit estimation associated with the effects of air pollution on (1) cleaning, maintenance, materials life, and the general value of property; (2) plants and animals; and (3) human health. Our primary interest is focused on the last category; we have not attempted to cover the other classifications in depth.

Effects on cleaning, maintenance, materials life, and value of property

In determining cleaning costs associated with air pollution[2]—for example, frequency of repainting—the essential questions to be answered are, How much more often must surfaces be painted as a result of polluted air, and how much would this additional painting cost? Either experimental or statistical approaches could be used to obtain the answer. Experimentally, one might expose a painted surface to polluted air in a city and compare its lifetime with that of a control surface exposed to relatively unpolluted air. Unfortunately, a number of other factors could be expected to influence the experiment (for example, exposure to sunlight). In addition, it is necessary to determine when repainting is necessary. Is discoloration sufficient to require painting? Whose judgment should determine when the useful life of the painted surface is over?

---

[2] Summaries of some of the literature pertaining to this category can be found in Kneese (1967), Ridker (1967), and Yocum and McCaldin (1968). Ridker (1967) also presented an excellent discussion on the nature of some of the difficulties in quantifying air pollution damage. Studies on specific materials include Robbins (1970) on electrical contacts; ITT (1971) on electrical components; Mueller and Stickney (1970) on rubber products; Fink, Buttner, and Boyd (1971) on metals; Salvin (1970) on textiles; Spence and Haynie (1972) on paints; and Salmon (1970), who conducted a general survey.

Statistically, one might collect data for different areas on the frequency of repainting, the levels of air pollution, and other relevant factors such as meteorology. Multivariable statistical analysis could then be used to infer what component of the repainting frequency could be attributed to air pollution. Although this approach appears feasible, it is not without its difficulties. It requires accurate data on both repainting rates and air pollution levels; data must be extensive enough to average away individual peculiarities. Perhaps, in the past, these data requirements have discouraged investigations of this sort.

The same approaches can be used to ascertain other maintenance and materials-life expenses associated with air pollution. Statistical analyses, as well as individual experiments, should be undertaken to determine these effects. Studies such as the one reported by Yocum and McCaldin (1968), in which unprotected metals and materials stretched on frames were exposed to polluted air, are of limited use in assessing the effects of pollution on materials in current use; conditions were artificial and the experimenter, not the consumer, judged the extent of deterioration.

In another study, Michelson and Tourin (1966) compared cleaning expenditures in two cities and attempted to infer how these costs were related to the different levels of air pollution (primarily suspended particulates) prevailing in the cities. They concluded that $84 per capita more per year was spent on cleaning in the highly polluted city than in the relatively unpolluted one. If this estimate were applicable to 100 million Americans, $8.4 billion per year would be saved in cleaning costs alone as a result of substantial abatement of suspended particulate pollution.

Thus, the lower cleaning costs and increased life for materials associated with air pollution abatement are difficult to quantify, and few estimates are worth quoting. At the same time, the Michelson–Tourin (1966) study suggests that such benefits might be substantial.

Since the effects of air pollution on cleaning, maintenance, and materials life are specific to the place where the materials (and the air pollution) are located, other studies have examined property values in various areas in order to calculate the relationship between property values and environmental amenities.[3] The underlying hypothesis is that, all other things being equal, property in unpolluted areas should be priced higher than property in polluted areas; hence, these studies attempt to estimate consumers' willingness to pay for environmental improvements.

Unfortunately, there are a number of difficulties associated with the property value studies. First, in several studies information could not be obtained on the market value of property. Instead, these studies relied on tax-assessed values. Davis and Wertz (1969), however, found little rela-

---

[3] See, for example, Nourse (1967); Ridker and Henning (1967); Harris, Tolley, and Harrell (1968); Anderson and Crocker (1971); Spore (1972); Wieand (1973); NAS (1974, chap. 4); and Nelson (1975).

tion between assessed value and actual selling price. Second, markets must be functioning well and in equilibrium in order for land values to reflect an air pollution factor properly. But the market is unlikely to function in this way, since property does not change ownership often, and, in any event, its value represents a complex mixture of attributes of which the air pollution component is unlikely to be a systematic part. Third, if purchasers are not aware, explicitly or implicitly, of the effects of air pollution, land prices cannot correctly reflect the differences; most people know little about these effects. Fourth, the effect of pollution on property values must reflect expected future pollution levels at the site and elsewhere; in view of the uncertainty as to future pollution levels, expectations must cover a wide distribution, and, consequently, property values must be subjected to "random shocks." Last, even if the above problems could be overcome, one must be able to isolate that portion of the property value associated with pollution; it is extremely difficult to control for all the many factors that determine the price of land (for example, transportation costs, quality of schools).[4]

Property value studies are of particular interest because benefit estimates based on them can embody, at least conceptually, values attached by consumers to esthetic as well as more tangible benefits associated with locations in better environments. However, as mentioned above, there remains the problem of determining which effects are perceived by consumers and, hence, which are internalized in their locational decisions. Consequently, if the benefit estimates derived from property value studies are simply added to those associated with materials damage, vegetation damage, or even health damage, there is the likelihood that an element of double counting will be introduced into the analysis.

Since the extent of overlap, or double counting, is not known, we have chosen not to emphasize any particular benefit estimate derived by analyzing property values. Instead, we prefer to note that the effects of air pollution in terms of cleaning, maintenance, materials life, and the general value of property (including any esthetic effects) might be quite substantial, although current evidence is not sufficient to disentangle and evaluate these effects.[5]

Effects on plants and animals

A number of cases document the damaging effects of air pollution on plants or animals. For example, Crocker and Rogers (1971) described

---

[4] For an excellent discussion of these, as well as other difficulties associated with using market data in the form of property values or wage differentials to estimate economic benefits from air quality improvement, see NAS (1974, chap. 4). See also Smith (1976) for a review of empirical studies in this area as well as of those investigating the air pollution–mortality association.

[5] More will be said on this issue when the estimates derived by the EPA and those presented in the NAS (1974) study are discussed later.

the effects of fluoride emissions (from heating phosphate rock) on citrus trees and cattle in an area of Florida.[6] Such accounts, though interesting, do little to enable the analyst to assess the quantitative impact of air pollution.

Excellent work was done by O'Gara (1922) in quantifying the relationship between sulfur dioxide concentrations and plant damage. He found that traces of damage appeared in alfalfa when the dose of sulfur dioxide (SO_2) in parts per million satisfied the equation: $SO_2 = 0.92/t + 0.33$, where time (t) was expressed in hours. O'Gara went on to determine similar functions for other plants. In plants whose commercial yield is the leaf, such as tobacco, or for which leaf damage can be related to yield, these formulations might be used to predict yield reduction related to concentrations of sulfur dioxide.

Later experimenters found that the amount of damage was highly dependent on weather factors (for example, heat, sunlight, and humidity), as well as on the growing stage of the plant. They also discovered that many plants can repair air pollution damage caused early in the growing cycle. Thus, the problem has become considerably more complex since O'Gara's original analysis, and major progress has been slow.

Subsequent attempts to assess the economic losses resulting from plant damage by air pollution have relied on two basic approaches. The first involves surveys of actual plant damage in specific areas;[7] the second predicts potential damage using data on air pollution measures, crop statistics, and other relevant factors.[8]

There are several weaknesses associated with areawide surveys. First, by their very nature they are highly subjective, in that field investigators must evaluate both the extent and cause of any observed damage. Second, damage observed in one year may have been caused by environmental factors in a previous year. Consequently, simple analyses of air pollution levels and concurrent damages may be misleading. Third, and perhaps most important, pest damage, drought, and various plant diseases can produce effects quite similar to those caused by certain air pollutants. Thus, it is extremely difficult to isolate the amount of damage caused by air pollution vis-à-vis other factors.

The difficulties with such surveys are exemplified by a comparison of damage assessments for Pennsylvania, which were undertaken by Weid-

[6] Summaries of other literature on damage to plants and animals can be found in the Environmental Health Service study for HEW (1970); in Hershaft, Morton, and Shea (1976); and Heck and Brandt (1976).

[7] See Weidensaul and Lacasse (1970); Lacasse (1971); Feliciano (1972); Pell (1973); Naegele, Feder, and Brandt (1972); and Millecan (1971).

[8] In probably the most comprehensive study to date, Benedict, Miller, and Olson (1971) of the Stanford Research Institute (SRI) used this method to arrive at estimates of air pollution damage to agriculture that were considerably smaller than earlier EPA estimates.

ensaul and Lacasse (1970), and Lacasse (1971). In the first study, direct annual losses attributable to air pollution in Pennsylvania were estimated at $2.5 million for 1969. In the later study, direct losses were valued at a little over $200,000 for 1970–71.[9]

Problems also occur with studies attempting to estimate potential damages to vegetation. For example, the study by Benedict, Miller, and Olson (1971) measured air pollution on the basis of emissions and fuel consumption data rather than on ambient air quality data. This required various questionable assumptions, relating levels of ambient air pollution to either pollution emissions or fuel consumption. Other arbitrary assumptions involved the method of crop valuation, as well as the allocation of specific types of vegetation to certain locations. Finally, the estimates of plant sensitivity to specific air pollutants (which form the basis for the whole analysis) were little more than "best guesses," given the scarcity of information relating measured air pollution to plant damage. In short, one must use extreme care before placing too much emphasis on the Stanford Research Institute's valuations of potential air pollution damage to agriculture.

Thus, taken as a whole, we conclude that although there is evidence that air pollution damages both commercial plants and animals, at present it is difficult to estimate the extent of this damage and to translate it into dollars. In later sections, estimates for this category derived by the EPA, and others found in the NAS (1974) report, will be discussed.

Effects on health from stationary-source pollutants

We have discussed a number of studies documenting an association between ill health and air pollution, as measured by sulfur oxides and suspended particulates, air pollutants primarily attributed to stationary sources.[10] From the literature, as well as our own empirical results, we have concluded that a significant association exists between mortality rates across the United States and air pollution, as measured by suspended particulates and some sulfur compounds (especially suspended sulfates and, to a lesser extent, sulfur dioxide). When possible, we have tried every reasonable test to determine whether the estimated relations between these measures of air pollution and mortality were spurious. In general, the associations appear to be genuine and consistent. We shall now attempt to assess some of the economic implications of our results.

[9] Possible explanations for this divergence included occurrence of air pollution episodes at times when crops were less susceptible, as well as climatic differences between the two years; for example, the latter period was characterized by frequent local rains.

[10] A detailed discussion of additional studies is found in the literature review comprising appendix A (see pp. 273–311). See also Anderson (1967), for extensive summaries in this area.

TABLE 10.1. Estimated Effect on Mortality of a 50 Percent Reduction in Sulfates, Suspended Particulates, and Sulfur Dioxide

Data base	Air pollutants	Total mortality rate (% decrease)	
		Unadjusted	Age–sex–race-adjusted
1960 annual cross section (117 SMSAs)	Sulfates Particulates	4.7 (3.1-1)	4.8 (4.2-5)
1969 annual cross section (112 SMSAs)	Sulfates Particulates	5.8 (7.1-3)	5.0 (7.1-8)
1969 annual cross section (69 SMSAs)	Sulfates Particulates	5.3 (7.8-6)	4.8 (7.9-6)
	Sulfur dioxide Particulates	6.3 (7.8-7)	5.5 (7.9-7)
1960–69 annual cross-sectional time-series (26 SMSAs)	Sulfates Particulates	4.7 (8.1-1)	5.1 (8.2-1)
1962–68 annual cross-sectional time-series (15 SMSAs)	Sulfates Particulates	5.9 (8.4-6)	6.3 (8.5-6)
	Sulfur dioxide Particulates	5.3 (8.4-7)	5.7 (8.5-7)
1963–64 daily time-series (Chicago)	Sulfur dioxide	5.4 (9.1-2)	

Note: Parenthetical figures are the regressions from which the percentages were estimated.

The estimated effect from our basic 1960 annual cross-sectional regression, that included all six measures of sulfates and suspended particulates (regression 3.1-1), was that a 50 percent reduction in air pollution would be associated with a 4.7 percent decrease in the unadjusted total mortality rate. A similar calculation was made for the age–sex–race-adjusted total mortality rate which indicated that such a reduction in air pollution would be associated with a 4.8 percent reduction in this death rate. Table 10.1 summarizes these two results, as well as similar computations based on our other findings. These findings indicate that abatement of air pollution (as measured by sulfates, suspended particulates, and sulfur dioxide) could save lives. Having concluded this, the next step involves quantifying the effects on health of reducing this type of air pollution and valuing the effects in dollars.

The chief difficulty in valuing lives (or health) stems from the fact that neither life nor health is traded directly in the marketplace; that is, consumers cannot directly purchase better health or increased life expectancy. Under nearly all circumstances, no sum of money is sufficient to compensate a person for the loss of life; lives cannot be bartered and are obviously qualitatively different from commodities produced and normally traded. Nonetheless, to improve resource allocation, systematic analyses of public programs require that uniform values be placed on lives and health for the purpose of decision making.

Economists and others have isolated three basic approaches to placing monetary values on life and health: (1) forgone earnings, (2) willingness to pay, and (3) implicit valuations based on private and public decisions. The forgone-earnings or human-capital approach focuses on the proper compensation to be paid in case of illness or premature death of an individual. Treating an individual as a piece of capital equipment, a calculation is made of projected future earnings (discounted back to the present), taking into account the age, sex, and education of the particular individual (plus any medical costs associated with restoring the individual's health or attempting to save the individual's life).[11] Thus, this approach values life and health in terms of what a person is estimated to earn.

Viewing a human being as a machine is but one of many criticisms of this approach. A related issue involves the fact that, in practice, this method values children, women, and retired persons at low or even zero values; whites have greater value than minorities. In a stable, high-income society, such estimates probably understate by a vast amount how much individuals would be willing to pay to improve their health or lengthen their lives.

This observation leads directly to the second approach for valuing lives and health: that of asking people how much they are willing to pay for better health or increased life expectancy.[12] Some thought should indicate to the reader that this question is not a simple one to answer. This is especially true with regard to environmental programs, since decisions generally involve reducing a small probability of illness or death a bit more. For example, the relevant question might be, What would you pay to reduce your chance of dying from cancer this year from one in 20,000 to one in 30,000?[13] Schelling (1968) explored this type of problem and developed a questionnaire designed to elicit such willingness-to-pay amounts. However, few respondents found it possible to give confident answers to these types of questions.[14]

The theoretical deficiencies with the forgone-earnings or human-capital approach and the intractability of the willingness-to-pay approach have led to a third approach: the examination of values implicit in private and public decisions. For example, the Federal Aviation Administration

[11] In civil law suits involving wrongful injury, detailed sets of rules have been established for such calculations. These involve the proper discount rates to be used, assumptions concerning future earnings, and whether the consumption of the worker should be deducted.

[12] See Schelling (1968); Mishan (1971); Usher (1973); and Conley (1976).

[13] An alternative way in which to frame the question would be, How much would you have to be compensated to accept a small increase in the probability of death this year?

[14] Acton (1973) was able to use this approach in evaluating a public program with potential for saving lives.

(FAA) is charged with regulating air traffic to ensure public safety (Fromm, 1968). By tightening controls, the FAA could reduce accidents further, probably with an accompanying increase in the cost of air transportation. Thus, each FAA decision on a safety issue, implicitly contains a judgment concerning the value of life. Unfortunately, analysts have found both very high values of life and very low values of life implicit in governmental decisions.[15]

By their choices of consumption goods, occupations, recreational activities, and so on, individuals also place implicit values on their lives. In most cases, the risks are not quantitatively known and recognized by the consumer. For example, while installing seat belts in automobiles indirectly involves a tradeoff between money and the probability of injury or death, the decision is complicated by other factors such as convenience and comfort (since the belts must be buckled to be effective). In general, it is difficult to isolate private decisions that are not complicated by a host of extraneous factors. Despite this fact, differences in occupational accident rates are quite marked, and some economists have argued that workers are likely to have information on these risks and are likely to think about them in selecting employment. As a consequence, Thaler and Rosen (1976) have attempted to isolate the component in wages relating to differences in accident hazards across occupations, thereby inferring implicit values of life. They estimated that workers, in selecting their employment, behave as if they were implicitly valuing their lives at more than $200,000. Critics of this work point to the fact that many individuals engage freely in recreational activities that increase the probability of death or injury (for example, skydiving and Alpine skiing). Despite such criticisms, it should be noted that this approach results in values of life several times greater than estimates based on forgone earnings.

The implicit-value approach is theoretically more attractive than the forgone-earnings approach. Nevertheless, although we regard the Thaler and Rosen estimates as worthy of consideration, we are somewhat reluctant to use their figures for two reasons. First, the forgone-earnings approach has the virtue of giving numerical estimates that are indisputable measures of what they say they are. Second, there is good reason to expect forgone earnings to underestimate the true value of health and life. Since we have elected to maintain a conservative posture in estimating the air pollution–mortality association by using estimates at the bottom range of those stemming from our work, we shall continue this position by selecting conservative figures for the value of life (and health).

---

[15] Sinclair and coauthors (1972) reviewed the implicit value of life in governmental programs in Great Britain and obtained estimates for the value of life that ranged from £15,000 for requiring cabs on farm tractors to £20 million for existing building codes. Even a casual look at U.S. governmental programs will reveal implicit values of life that differ by a factor of 1,000.

In applying the forgone-earnings approach to our analysis, we have modified the estimates in one way. We have not systematically calculated the loss in income of each person estimated to be killed or made ill by air pollution. Instead, we have chosen to use the average earnings and medical expenses of a U.S. resident as if they applied to any individual, without regard to age, sex, or race. Since our findings indicate that the mortality effects of air pollution (as measured by sulfates and suspended particulates) are more closely associated with the aged than with the general population, making use of the "average" earnings and medical expenses will result in somewhat higher benefit estimates from abatement. However, we believe this upward bias is greatly outweighed by the fact that the implicit values of life (and health) are still low, particularly when compared with more theoretically correct estimates such as those derived from occupational data. Thus, we regard the dollar estimates that we later calculate as highly conservative.

Effects on health from mobile-source pollutants

In the previous chapters our analysis has concentrated primarily on the health effects of air pollution, as measured by sulfate and suspended particulate levels, neither of which is closely related to automobile emissions.[16] Furthermore, the literature on the health effects of air pollutants from mobile sources is much less extensive than that on the effects of such stationary-source air pollutants as the sulfur oxides and suspended particulates.[17] Nevertheless, in this section we will present our findings and conclusions on the complicated issue of mobile-source emissions and their health effects.

In the 1969 cross-sectional analysis involving sixty-nine SMSAs (see chapter 7), we were able to examine additional air pollutants that can be related to mobile sources. Specifically, we analyzed measures of nitrates (NO_3) and nitrogen dioxide (NO_2).[18] The results across SMSAs indicated that nitrates were unimportant in explaining the variation in either the total mortality rates (unadjusted and adjusted) or race-adjusted mortality rates for infants under one year of age. There was, however, some indication of an association between levels of nitrogen dioxide and the variation

[16] In an EPA report, "Estimated Changes in Human Exposure to Suspended Sulfate Attributable to Equipping Light Duty Motor Vehicles with Oxidation Catalysts," there were preliminary indications that automotive catalytic control systems designed to reduce hydrocarbons and carbon monoxide emissions may convert sulfur dioxide to sulfur trioxide and that direct emissions of sulfur trioxide may result in increased local concentrations of sulfuric acid and sulfate salts in the vicinity of roadways. The EPA has since concluded that the contribution to sulfate levels in urban areas by catalytic-equipped automobiles is negligible.

[17] A review of many of these studies is found in appendix A, pp. 305–311.

[18] We recognize that levels of these pollutants can be taken only as crude surrogates for mobile-source emissions since stationary-source emissions of these pollutants are also important.

in total (unadjusted and adjusted) mortality rates. No association was exhibited between nitrogen dioxide levels and infant mortality.

In our cross-sectional time-series analysis, involving fifteen SMSAs over the period 1962–68 (see chapter 8), we failed to isolate a consistent, significant association between either nitrates or nitrogen dioxide and either the total mortality rates (unadjusted and adjusted) or the race-adjusted mortality rate for infants under one year of age.

Regarding analysis of daily mortality (see chapter 9): although we found an association between levels of nitric oxide (NO) and daily mortality in Chicago, the relationship between sulfur dioxide (SO_2) and daily mortality was even more significant. We found no strong relationships between daily mortality and the observed levels of other mobile-source air pollutants [including carbon monoxide (CO), nitrogen dioxide (NO_2), and hydrocarbons (HC)] in any of the cities examined.

While investigators may later find a strong association between ill health and automobile emissions (as represented by ambient levels of carbon monoxide, nitrogen oxides, hydrocarbons, and photochemical oxidants), current evidence is somewhat to the contrary. This is in contrast to the large number of studies, as well as our own analyses, which document significant associations between ill health (or mortality rates) and ambient levels of various sulfur oxides (particularly sulfates and sulfur dioxide) and suspended particulates.

A number of explanations for this contrast can be suggested. High ambient levels of pollution from mobile sources are a relatively recent phenomenon, and it may be that only the acute effects of these air pollutants could have been observed. Furthermore, measurements of the ambient levels of these air pollutants may have been less scientifically accurate than measurements of sulfur oxides and suspended particulates, in which case even the analyses of acute effects would have been obscured. In addition, the analysis of mortality data may be inherently biased against revealing positive findings on mobile-source pollutants if they exert more important effects on morbidity or acute conditions, such as eye irritation.

Previous studies and our own investigation can be used to place these points in perspective. For example, Los Angeles has experienced high levels of photochemical smog for more than two decades; chronic effects, if they exist, should be observable for that city. However, previous studies of daily deaths in Los Angeles failed to detect an unequivocal relationship, despite the fact that analyses in other cities revealed associations between daily mortality and levels of both sulfur dioxide and suspended particulates (see chapter 9 and appendix A). Moreover, our cross-sectional analyses of the total mortality rate (see chapters 3 through 7) indicated that the death rate in Los Angeles was predicted closely by levels of sulfates and suspended particulates (suggesting that knowledge of the levels of other pollutants would have contributed little).

The possibility of inaccurate pollution measurements is more difficult to evaluate. As we discussed in the earlier chapters, there are inherent difficulties associated with the measurement of ambient levels of air pollution and exposure to air pollutants. However, we find little reason to believe that the data on mobile-source pollutants are systematically poorer than those for the other pollutants.

Similarly, it is not easy to determine the likelihood of inherent biases in mortality investigations involving mobile-source pollutants. Current evidence certainly suggests that mobile-source pollution exhibits more acute than chronic health effects.[19] With regard to such acute effects as eye irritation, it should be noted that, even if there is a strong association between the levels of mobile-source pollutants and these types of effects in certain areas of the country, it is questionable whether this implies a *national* health-benefit category of important magnitude. At the same time, if a severe problem exists in a particular area (for example, Los Angeles), and the health-related benefits from abatement of mobile-source pollution are found to be substantial, then a more stringent regional policy may be justified.[20]

Taken as a whole, we feel that at the present time there is little evidence indicating an important association between automobile emissions and ill health on a nationwide basis. We stress, however, the considerable uncertainty surrounding this issue and the need for further comprehensive research in the area. Finally, we wish to point out that the esthetic effects emanating from mobile-source pollution may be relatively more important than those from other kinds of air pollution. Therefore, even if the health effects are not marked, abatement from mobile sources may still be justified on that ground.

Monetary benefits of air pollution abatement

Stationary sources. To determine whether air pollution abatement is called for, we have outlined a benefit–cost analysis. The EPA has provided its own analysis. Unfortunately, instead of providing benefit estimates, the EPA has calculated national air pollution *damage* figures for 1970. We have emphasized the word "damage" to reflect the fact that such estimates generally represent *total* damages ascribed to air pollution in a given category rather than the *incremental* benefits corresponding to a specific amount of air pollution abatement.[21]

---

[19] Headache, cough, and eye and chest discomfort are probably the most common health effects that have been associated with such pollutants. See, for example, Hammer and co-workers (1965, 1974).

[20] In point of fact, the automobile emissions standards for California have been stricter than the national emission standards over the past several years.

[21] This is especially true of the following estimates for materials; the calculation of health "damages" was not based on total abatement but rather on a 26 percent reduction in sulfates and suspended particulates. See Waddell (1974, p. 146, fn. 78).

TABLE 10.2.   Damage from Air Pollution in the United States, by Source and Effect, 1970
(billions of dollars)

Source class	Health	Materials	Vegetation	Esthetics and soiling	Total
Fossil fuel burning	2.2	0.8	Negligible	3.1	6.1
Industrial	2.1	0.3	Negligible	2.3	4.7
Total damages	4.3	1.1	Negligible	5.4	10.8

Note: Waddell assigned an additional $0.2 billion damages from miscellaneous sources
of air pollution to both the health and the esthetics and soiling class.
Source: Waddell (1974, p. 131).

With this in mind, $10.8 billion was the EPA's "best" estimate for air
pollution damages due to stationary sources in 1970.[22] The estimates for the
individual categories were $4.3 billion for health, $1.1 billion for materials,
and a negligible amount for vegetation. In addition, an estimate of $5.4
billion for 1970 was said to represent the value of the negative effects of
air pollution from stationary sources that are capitalized in residential
urban property.[23] Waddell then distributed the total damage figure among
sources on the basis of the relative level of air pollutant emissions (table
10.2).

We can use our empirical results pertaining to mortality effects together
with EPA's projected reduction in air pollutant emissions to arrive at
another measure of health benefits from abatement of stationary-source
pollutants.

The EPA estimated that by 1979, implementation of the technological
standards associated with the 1970 Clean Air Act Amendments would result in an 88 percent decrease in sulfur oxide emissions and a 58 percent
decrease in particulate emissions from the 1971 control levels.[24] Applying
our estimates of the effects of air pollution on mortality to these figures,[25]

[22] In addition, $1.1 billion worth of air pollution damages were attributed to trans-
portation, and $0.4 billion were attributed to miscellaneous sources.

[23] Waddell argues that costs capitalized in this estimate were primarily those associated with esthetics and household soiling. Since there was likely to be some overlap
between this category and the previous three categories, the figures incorporate adjustments that Waddell made in an effort to minimize double counting.

[24] These estimates are presented in more detail in the next section.

[25] There is a host of difficulties in estimating the resulting increase in air quality.
Current models of diffusion and atmospheric chemistry are not sufficient to give confident estimates of the change in air quality caused by a change in air pollutant emissions. Later, we shall assume that these reductions in emissions would result in equal
percentage improvements in ambient air quality. While this assumption is crude, it is
difficult to arrive at a superior one. We note, however, that since natural sources
also produce air pollution, the assumption may overestimate the "final" improvement
in ambient air quality. (Note that decreases in emissions or reductions in discharges
of particulates and sulfur oxides should be contrasted with ambient concentrations
of suspended particulates, sulfates, and sulfur dioxide.)

we obtain a 7.0 percent reduction in the unadjusted total mortality rate.[26] A more detailed method for estimating the reduction would focus individually on each SMSA. Since we have data on 1969 ambient levels of sulfates and suspended particulates, we could estimate an improvement in air quality for each SMSA to some specified level and use these projections together with our elasticities to calculate the estimated reduction in mortality for each SMSA. Such a calculation would be likely to lead to higher estimates than the estimate we present, since the largest areas tend to be the most polluted; hence, they are likely to experience the greatest absolute improvement in air quality. We believe that this level of detail is not warranted in an analysis of this nature. The mortality effects we have estimated are substantial. It seems doubtful that increasing them further would affect our policy conclusions.

If we assume that air pollution in the form of sulfates and suspended particulates has the same effect on morbidity as on mortality (certainly a very conservative assumption),[27] we can calculate the economic costs associated with a 7.0 percent decrease in total mortality and morbidity. Thus, our "best" estimate of the benefits of a 58 percent abatement of particulates and an 88 percent abatement of sulfur oxides, in terms of improvements in health, is $16.1 billion (1973 dollars) for 1979. This estimate represents 7.0 percent of the total 1979 economic costs of morbidity and mortality (assuming a 6 percent discount rate). These total costs are based on 1972 data, analyzed by Cooper and Rice (1976). The two basic components of these costs involve forgone earnings due to sickness and death and direct medical care expenditures. The 1972 indirect cost estimate was adjusted to 1973 dollars by using the consumer price index, and the 1979 indirect costs were then estimated by adjusting this value under the assumption that the average annual increase in real per capita income would be equal to 1.5 percent through 1979 and that the population would continue to grow at an annual rate of 0.8 percent through 1979. The 1973 direct costs were estimated directly using data from the Social Security Administration. The 1979 direct costs were then estimated by calculating the average annual rate of increase in direct costs over the four years 1973–76 (13.5 percent) and adjusting this for the average annual rise in general prices over the same period (8.6 percent); and then by assuming that this adjusted rate would continue through 1979.[28]

---

[26] This figure was obtained by using the most conservative cross-sectional estimate in table 10.1 (4.7 percent) and applying each percentage reduction noted above to the separate elasticities (from regression 3.1-1) of the relevant air pollutant category: (Percentage decrease in sulfur oxide emissions $\times$ Sum S elasticities) + (Percentage decrease in particulate emissions $\times$ Sum P elasticities) = $(0.88 \times 5.04) + (0.58 \times 4.37) = 6.97$.

[27] People may suffer acute illness or irritation from the effects of air pollution without having their time of death affected; however, it is unlikely that someone whose time of death was affected by air pollution had no periods of previous illness aggravated by the air pollution.

[28] The detailed calculation is shown in appendix F, pp. 348–349.

It should be noted that we have applied the estimate to the entire U.S. population, not just to the population living in SMSAs. Thus, our calculation involves an estimated decrease (quite small) in mortality for people living in rural areas as well as for people living in urban areas. Our justification for this is the linear nature of the association that we have estimated.[29] We would not defend our benefit estimate as a good estimate of the value of the associated reduction in morbidity and mortality. Instead, we would argue that this figure is probably a lower bound for the benefits of a reduction in illness and death associated with a 58 percent abatement of particulates and an 88 percent abatement of sulfur oxides.[30]

If one compares our estimated health benefits of $16.1 billion with Waddell's health-benefit estimate of $4.3 billion, one notes a substantial discrepancy. This difference is due largely to the underlying assumptions regarding the percentage of reduction of air pollution levels. In order to make our estimate compatible with EPA control cost estimates, our calculation was based on the EPA projected decrease in emission levels. Waddell assumed much smaller percentage reductions (see footnote 21, page 223. It should also be noted that our benefit estimate does *not* include damage to materials, vegetation, esthetics, or soiling. In addition, neither estimate accounts for the potential benefits of reduced emissions of nitrogen oxides, hydrocarbons, or other pollutants from stationary sources.

Mobile sources. A study sponsored by the National Academy of Sciences (1974) developed benefit estimates of control of air pollution from mobile sources. These were based on calculations embodying two basic valuation techniques. The first involved an analysis of "cost studies" assessing the economic damages to health, vegetation, and materials by mobile-source air pollution. The second examined market valuation studies (for example, property-value and wage-rate studies) in an effort to estimate the benefits of improved air quality.

The estimated range for the direct damages to health in 1970 from mobile-source emissions was reported as ranging from $360 million to $3 billion.[31] Taking the midpoint of this range as the "best" estimate, we obtain a value of $1,680 million. The "best" estimate of the annual vegetation losses due to mobile-source pollutants was $200 million for 1970 (NAS, 1974, page 378). Finally, the "ballpark" estimate of the 1970 annual

---

[29] That is, we found that a linear specification generally fit the data as well as (or better than) other functional forms. Nevertheless, using the estimated function for an 88 percent reduction in sulfur oxides tests the limits of our faith in the estimated relationship.

[30] See the discussion on valuing health effects, especially pp. 217–221.

[31] This estimate includes morbidity effects (for example, eye and chest discomfort, headache, and cough) as well as mortality effects. With regard to the valuation of the latter effects, the estimate embodies a value of human life equal to $200,000. As was the case in EPA estimates, the health "damages" were not based on total abatement but rather on various scenarios. See NAS (1974), pp. 356–360.

losses to materials due to mobile-source pollutants was said to be approximately $1 billion (NAS, 1974, page 397). These three areas together produced a point estimate of $2,880 million per year for the damages associated with 1970 levels of automobile emissions.[32]

In addition to the estimates for direct damage, the NAS report also analyzed market behavior to arrive at benefit estimates. Specifically, a wage-rate model and a property-value model were examined in order to obtain estimates for the potential benefits achievable from the reduction of automobile emissions. On the basis of an empirical analysis of these two models, the NAS report concluded that the benefits of emission control expressed through market prices and wages were in the range of $1.5 to $5 billion per year (NAS, 1974, page 412). Under the assumption that health, vegetation, and materials effects were not fully embodied in the "market valuation" estimates, this range of benefits was combined with the damage estimates discussed above. The final point estimate for the "benefits" from reducing mobile-source emissions was calculated to be $5 billion per year.[33]

COSTS

Stationary sources. The Clean Air Act (as amended) requires the EPA to submit an annual report on the cost of air pollution abatement. The sixth report (April 1974) details the costs of abatement to meet state and national standards through 1979.[34] Fossil fuel-burning sources would cost $6,109 million, and industrial sources would cost $3,410 million; a total of $9,519 million in 1979 (in 1973 dollars).[35] However, since many of the capital costs of abatement would be incurred throughout 1971–79, the total investment expenditures would be greater than this amount.[36] The annualized costs were estimated by discounting the investment over

---

[32] As with EPA estimates discussed in the preceding section, these estimates represent total damage figures. They cannot be construed simply as the value of the incremental benefits associated with abatement of air pollution from mobile sources.

[33] This figure incorporates a slight downward adjustment, since it was recognized that some double counting was probably involved in combining the estimates. More important, the reader should be aware that damage figures were added to benefit figures in order to arrive at the final estimate of "benefits." This presumably results in an overestimate, since only incremental improvements (benefits) should be expected in certain categories unless total abatement is assumed.

[34] The "standards" referred to here are technological emissions rates to be applied to air pollution emitters. They should not be confused with the automobile emissions control standards or ambient air quality standards discussed later in this chapter.

[35] Projected costs are annual initial investment expenditures from 1971–79 for purchasing and installing control equipment (total investment) and the continuing annual costs for interest, property taxes, insurance, depreciation, etc., and for operating and maintaining equipment (ultimate annual cost).

[36] The report estimated that cumulative investment in controlling emissions from these sources throughout 1971–79 would be $24,185 million.

its useful life (then maintenance and operating costs were added). As noted previously, there are several reasons to believe that these costs overestimate the "true" costs of abatement.

As noted above, the EPA also estimated the percentage decrease in emission levels for 1979 that would be expected with the implementation of the 1971 control measures. For fossil fuel-burning sources, it was estimated that sulfur oxide emissions would decrease by 89 percent and particulate emissions would decrease by 60 percent. For industrial sources, it was estimated that sulfur oxide emissions would decrease by 86 percent and particulate emissions by 57 percent. Aggregating these two source categories, the EPA estimates indicated that by 1979 emissions controls would result in an 88 percent decrease in sulfur oxide emissions and a 58 percent decrease in particulate emissions from the 1971 control levels.

Mobile sources. A major cost of abating air pollution under the 1970 Amendments to the Clean Air Act stems from reduction of automobile emissions containing carbon monoxide, hydrocarbons, and oxides of nitrogen; the last two being precursors of photochemical oxidants. In addition to the benefit estimates of mobile-source air pollution control, the 1974 study sponsored by the NAS also developed cost estimates of abating automobile emissions. The NAS analysis was based on the best data available at the time of the study. However, some of the cost data pertain to technology which is not now in major production and may not be for some years. Consequently, the report notes that the specific cost numbers (all costs were in 1974 dollars) are subject to change, although the general conclusions are likely to remain unaltered (NAS, 1974, page 115).

Keeping these caveats in mind, the major findings were:

1. If the current law is followed, ultimately requiring 0.4 gm per mile (gpm) of NO_x, vehicles meeting that standard may cost about $850 more over their lifetimes than vehicles meeting a 1970 standard. Total national expenditures for control of auto emissions would approximate $8 billion per year by 1985 if no catalyst replacements are required, and $10 to $11 billion if all vehicles are required to change catalysts at 50,000 miles.

2. If the most stringent standard requires only 2.0 gpm of NO_x instead of 0.4 gpm, total national expenditures for control of auto emissions would approximate $4.7 billion per year by 1985 without catalyst replacements and $6 to $7 billion per year with catalyst replacements.

3. If the most stringent standard requires only 3.1 gpm of NO_x (the interim 1975 standards), total national expenditures for control of auto emissions would peak in the middle 1970s, and by 1985 it would amount to $3 billion per year without catalyst replacements and $4.5 billion per year with catalyst replacements.

4. Delaying the 0.4 gpm NO_x standard by two years (for example from 1978 to 1980) might save a total of $6.9 billion between 1975–85 for the situation without catalyst replacement at 50,000 miles.[37] This delay would postpone achievement of a given NO_x emission *rate* by about fourteen months in the early 1980s, but NO_x emissions would fall continuously beyond 1985. Further delay of the standard could save still more (depending on the actions of the automobile industry) and might allow continuous NO_x reductions until 1985 or 1990.

5. No single alternative to the conventional gasoline engine with pollution controls appears to be significantly better in all respects for all standards. More radical technologies, like the diesel, can promise greater long-run savings than conventional technologies.[38] However, since they are radical, they can be introduced only at a slower rate.

6. Varying maintenance requirements across the country can substantially affect costs. If catalyst replacement is required for 37 percent of all vehicles (that is, those in the most seriously polluted areas), *total* costs during the eleven-year period 1975–85 would be $15 billion less than with nationwide maintenance requirement under a 0.4 gpm NO_x emission standard.

7. Building vehicles to two standards can achieve substantial cost savings. If 0.4 gpm NO_x is required only for the 37 percent of vehicles in the most seriously polluted areas, and the 1973 or interim 1975 standard is used elsewhere, $23 billion would be saved (over a uniform 0.4 gpm NO_x standard) during 1975–85 exclusive of any catalyst changes anywhere. About $40 billion would be saved if savings are also counted for omitting catalyst changes in the less polluted areas. By 1985, the savings from this two-car strategy over the uniform strategy would run over $3 billion per year without credit for the elimination of catalyst changes.

8. Switching to smaller cars does not significantly affect pollution control costs, although it has a huge impact on total motoring costs. Reducing the average new-car size from an intermediate to a compact by 1985 would save only $0.56 billion in pollution control costs for 1985 in comparing the uniform 0.4 gpm NO_x standard with the interim 1975 standard.

Thus, cleaning up mobile-source emissions is a costly undertaking. The *annual* costs required to meet the strictest standards of the Clean Air Act (especially the 0.4 gpm NO_x standard) could be as high as $11 billion.

[37] This total cost figure covers the period 1975–85 and should not be confused with the annual costs discussed above.

[38] The 1974 NAS report (pp. 116–117) categorized diesel technology as radical, despite its rather widespread use today.

This assumes that (1) the mix of the U.S. automobile fleet does not change greatly; (2) all cars are subject to the standard; (3) the catalytic reactor remains the primary device for reducing emissions; and (4) catalyst replacement is required at 50,000 miles.

COMPARING THE BENEFITS AND COSTS
OF AIR POLLUTION ABATEMENT

Estimates of the dollar benefits and costs of air pollution abatement from stationary and mobile sources have been presented in the preceding pages.[39] The reader who has examined these carefully should be highly skeptical. Before bringing together these benefit and cost figures, we wish to reiterate two important points. The first is that, for reasons mentioned above, the abatement costs are likely to be overestimates and those for the abatement benefits are likely to be underestimates. The second is that one must evaluate how much confidence should be placed in each estimate in order to determine whether the conclusions are sensitive to questionable assumptions or whether they are independent of individual judgments.[40]

Stationary sources

The estimated air pollution damages due to stationary sources in terms of health, materials, and esthetics and soiling effects were almost $11 billion in 1970, according to Waddell (1974). Our estimate of the benefits of an 88 percent abatement of sulfur oxides and a 58 percent abatement of particulates, in terms of improvements in health, was $16.1 billion (1973 dollars) for 1979.

When these benefit figures are compared with the EPA's 1979 annualized cost estimate of $9.5 billion for air pollution control, the total benefits of abatement from stationary sources exceed the total costs of such abatement, and this result is unlikely to change as estimates are improved. However, this comparison of total benefits and total costs is not a sufficient basis for evaluating the current program of air pollution abatement. First, the analysis compares the benefits and costs at equilibrium. It does not examine what the most efficient abatement strategy is or how fast we should achieve certain standards (see Dolde and coauthors, n.d.). Second, from a theoretical standpoint, social welfare is maximized by choosing an abatement strategy so that the extra cost of an additional unit of abatement (marginal cost) is just equal to the extra benefit of achieving that

[39] In some cases the "benefit" figures would be more accurately described as "damage" estimates.

[40] The problem is further complicated by the fact that data on air pollution levels do not distinguish between man-made sources and natural sources. Consequently, unless background air pollution concentrations are known, potential benefits of air pollution abatement from man-made sources alone are difficult to assess.

additional abatement (marginal benefit).[41] Thus, the forgoing benefit–cost calculation indicates that some degree of air pollution abatement is called for, but it does not specify whether the current EPA program with its emissions standards and timing is adequate.

Unfortunately, we do not have cost figures for other strategies (either more stringent or more lenient) to evaluate. Thus, it is possible that the marginal cost of further abatement (associated with the current strategy) is so high that some relaxation of the standards would be called for. At the same time, it is equally possible that the marginal benefit of cleaner air is sufficiently high to warrant even more stringent standards (NAS, 1974, page 16).

We have attempted to present a conservative analysis of the issues. We base our conclusions primarily on our health-benefit estimate, which (for all the reasons outlined above) is likely to represent an underestimate of the "true" health benefits from abatement of sulfur oxides and suspended particulates. Thus, while available data do not permit a definitive conclusion concerning the appropriateness of the degree of abatement of stationary-source air pollutants called for in the legislation, we believe it is not unduly stringent.

Mobile sources

An analysis of air pollution from mobile-source emissions presents a more complicated picture. According to the 1974 NAS study, the benefits of reduced auto emissions (from 1970 levels) were determined to be in the neighborhood of $5 billion per year (at 1973 price levels).[42] In view of our scrutiny of the relevant literature as well as our own (limited) empirical findings in the area, we believe that this figure represents a liberal interpretation of the current evidence.

Turning to the cost side, the NAS findings indicated that the annualized costs required to meet the present mandate of the Clean Air Act (including a 0.4 gpm NO_x standard) were approximately $8.0 billion by 1985 (in 1973 dollars). If, in addition, a change of catalyst is required at 50,000 miles, these costs could escalate to an annual figure of $11 billion (NAS, 1974, page 12). In short, under the present law, the projected costs of control are considerably higher than the probable benefits from such control. This conclusion should not be interpreted as meaning that no abatement of automobile emissions is worthwhile. Instead, one might conclude that the current strategy for control may be too strict in

---

[41] It seems likely that the *marginal* cost of air pollution abatement rises with the degree of control and that the *marginal* benefit of abatement falls with the degree of control. See Ridker (1967).

[42] NAS (1974, p. 15). Note that there was a slight discrepancy in the report as to whether benefit and damage figures were adjusted to 1970 or 1973 price levels and whether costs were adjusted to 1973 or 1974 price levels.

the aggregate and that a slight relaxation of the emission standards may be called for.

As noted earlier, at least two basic approaches exist for reducing the costs of emissions control. The first is what is sometimes referred to as the "two-car strategy." Under this approach, only those new cars principally operated in metropolitan areas with serious levels of air pollution would be required to meet the strictest standards of the 1970 amendments, while interim standards would be applied elsewhere. Given the assumptions in the NAS study, this would mean that only 37 percent of the total fleet would be required to meet the strictest emission standards, and the estimated total annual costs would be reduced to the vicinity of $5 billion (NAS, 1974, page 16).

The second basic method for reducing the costs of emissions control involves relaxation of the NO_x standard. Specifically, if the standard were reduced from 0.4 gpm to 2.0 gpm (the 1976 level), the associated costs would be reduced to an annual level of about $5 billion (without catalyst changes at 50,000 miles) or $6 to $7 billion (with catalyst changes) (NAS, 1974, pages 16–17). It was also pointed out that at a 2.0 gpm NO_x standard, new engine technologies (for example, stratified charge or diesel engines) might make emission control almost costless by the latter part of the century (NAS, 1974, page 17). What is even more interesting from a benefit–cost viewpoint, the study also concluded that

The best guess from currently available data is that the cost savings gained from easing the NO_x emission standard exceed the loss in benefits from the higher concentration of NO_x. Only a few urban areas, principally Chicago and Los Angeles, now have NO_x levels above estimated thresholds where health-related damages are observed. Most of the benefits from moving to the strict automobile NO_x standards might be achieved by adopting these standards for those areas only. In most cities about half of the NO_x emissions originate from non-automotive sources. An attack on these other sources might be more cost-effective than cleaning up automobile NO_x. [NAS (1974, page 17)].

Thus, while there is considerable uncertainty concerning the effects of ambient concentrations of photochemical smog and nitrogen oxides on health, vegetation, and materials, at present there does not appear to be a significant increase in benefits associated with lowering the NO_x standard below 2.0 gpm.

Taking all this into account, it appears that the current ("one-car strategy") regulations surrounding the control of automobile emissions are difficult to justify on benefit–cost grounds. It is hard to arrive at an annual benefit figure in excess of $5 billion, while, as outlined above, the current legislation entails annual costs ranging from 1.5 to 2 times this amount. Only by adopting some alternative policy—for example, the two-car strategy or relaxation of the NO_x standard—can the costs of control

TABLE 10.3.   The Benefits and Costs of Air Pollution Abatement
(billions of dollars)

Source class	Benefits (or damages)	Costs
Stationary sources		
Waddell (1970$)	11	—
EPA (1973$)	—	9.5
Lave and Seskin (1973$)[a]	16.1	—
Mobile sources		
NAS (1973$)	5	8 (11)[b]

[a] Based on health effects alone.
[b] For scenario with catalyst replacement at 50,000 miles.

be brought in line with the potential benefits of control.[43] Of course, further research may reveal that the benefits have been underestimated (for example, by establishing a closer association between automobile-related pollutants and ill health or by estimating high esthetic benefits associated with control of auto emissions) or that the costs have been overestimated (for example, by discovery of new emission control technologies). If these events should take place, the policy conclusions of our analysis would be likely to change.

Our conclusions are based on current technology. It is evident that the 1970 Clean Air Amendments precipitated a level of effort and achievement in discovering new technologies for the control of automobile emissions. In view of the incentive effects of legislative pressure on the development of abatement technology, some analysts conclude that it is prudent to maintain full legislative pressure. While admitting that there are some merits to this argument, we would point to the 1974-model-year automobiles with their emission-control equipment (and interlock devices) as an illustration of the questionable nature of this technological imperative. Mistakes in this area lead to very high costs to society.

CONCLUSION

In this chapter we have outlined a benefit–cost analysis for air pollution abatement from both stationary and mobile sources. A summary of the important benefit and cost estimates is presented in table 10-3. We quote the EPA's 1979 cost figure of approximately $9.5 billion (1973 dollars) for meeting state and national standards for stationary sources (fossil fuel-burning sources and industrial sources). Although we have argued that this amount is likely to be an overestimate of the "true" cost of abatement from these sources, we have not attempted to furnish our own cost

[43] Despite this conclusion, which we believe is substantiated by all the evidence contained in the NAS study, the report itself has been interpreted as advocating no change in the existing legislation.

figure. Similarly, we have quoted figures from an NAS study on the costs of meeting current emission controls for mobile sources as $8 billion (without catalyst changes) and $11 billion (with catalyst changes).

On the benefit side, we have discussed some of the difficulties in determining the effects of air pollution on (1) cleaning, maintenance, materials life, and the general value of property; (2) plants and animals; and (3) human health. Although we would acknowledge that substantial benefits might accrue from categories 1 and 2, in addition to benefits relating to better visibility, an increase in the number of clear and sunny days, a reduction of noxious odors, and a general improvement in the quality of life if air pollution were reduced, we would not defend any particular estimates for these categories.

With regard to stationary sources of air pollution, we have cited the EPA's damage–benefit figure of $11 billion for 1970 as one estimate of the potential benefits from abatement. In addition, our estimate of the potential benefits from an 88 percent reduction in sulfur oxides and a 58 percent reduction in particulates (corresponding to the EPA's projected decrease in emission levels), in terms of improved health alone, was approximately $16.1 billion for 1979 (1973 dollars). With regard to mobile sources of air pollution, we cited the NAS figure of $5 billion (1973 dollars) as a generous estimate of the potential benefits from control of automobile emissions.

From current evidence, we conclude that presently mandated controls of sulfur oxide and particulate emissions from stationary sources are warranted on benefit–cost terms. At the same time, it appears that the costs of implementing the currently mandated emission controls on mobile sources are in excess of the potential benefits from such controls. Furthermore, only by adopting some alternative policy, such as the two-car strategy or a relaxation of the NO_x standard, can the benefits and costs of mobile-source controls be balanced. We recognize that rapid technological progress is being made in the control of automobile emissions. Nevertheless, on the basis of current technology, we believe that suspending (or at least delaying) the most stringent of the current emissions regulations or continuing a two-car strategy is warranted in view of present estimates of benefits and costs.

Finally, with regard to the setting of national ambient air quality standards, we do not believe that an effort to determine a pollutant threshold (or level) that will protect the public health or welfare is a fruitful approach to the problem.[44] Instead, we believe that society must weigh the benefits and costs of achieving various degrees of clean air and in so doing, establish the national priority for air pollution abatement.

[44] In appendix B we use our empirical results to draw some implications as to the specific levels at which the current standards are set for a number of air pollutants.

CHAPTER 11

Summary and conclusion

We have focused our study on one aspect of air pollution abatement: how human health is affected by a reduction in the levels of certain types of air pollutants. We have concentrated on human health because we believe that if specific forms of air pollution have a significant influence at all, health effects will be quantitatively more significant than such other effects as damage to materials or vegetation; hence, the benefits of air pollution abatement would stem predominately from a reduction in human sickness and death. However, to justify the benefit calculations shown in chapter 10, it is necessary that the association between the measures of air pollution and the mortality rates be a causal one. A detailed examination of this issue is the focus of the next section.

THE AIR POLLUTION–MORTALITY ASSOCIATION

We shall review our extensive analysis of the association between air pollution and health by examining the material in light of the nine criteria formulated by the eminent epidemiologist, Sir Austin B. Hill (1965). These standards have been subsequently used by epidemiologists to judge whether causality was a reasonable interpretation of their findings.

Hill's first criterion is the strength of the association. There is considerable evidence of an urban factor in life expectancy that may be due, in part, to air pollution. Furthermore, severe air pollution episodes result in increases in morbidity and mortality rates. Finally, the statistical associations between specific measures of air pollution and mortality rates existing under a wide variety of circumstances demonstrate additional support for the causal hypothesis. (These assertions are documented throughout the text and in appendix A.)

The second criterion is consistency. Has the association between air pollution and health effects been observed by different investigators, in different situations, and at different times? The literature review (see appendix A) indicates that a significant association has been rather consistently recognized.

The third criterion is specificity. If, as Hill (1965, page 297) reports, "the association is limited to specific workers and to particular sites and types of diseases and there is no association between the work and other modes of dying, then clearly that is a strong argument in favor of causation." Both the literature and our statistical analyses indicate that various disease-specific and age–sex–race-specific mortality and morbidity rates are closely associated with certain types of air pollution. In examining the age- and disease-specific rates, as well as suicide, venereal disease, and crime rates, we found that generally the measures of air pollution were closely associated with those rates one would expect them to be associated with and not associated with those rates for which causation was not hypothesized. Furthermore, extensive studies of occupational groups show specificity at high dose rates. Thus, the air pollution–mortality association displays some degree of specificity.

The fourth criterion has to do with temporality, or the direction in which causation occurs. Since few people would argue that increases in mortality (or morbidity) lead to increases in air pollution, we conclude that this criterion is satisfied.

The fifth criterion concerns the existence of a biological gradient. That is, does the mortality (or morbidity) rate increase when air pollution increases? The evidence from much of the literature, as well as from our own statistical work, indicates that there is a marked gradient. Furthermore, we have found that a linear relationship describes the association in the range of air pollution levels we have examined at least as satisfactorily as other alternatives.

The sixth criterion is plausibility—whether general biological knowledge is consistent with the observed association. This is a more complicated question to deal with. Laboratory experiments have revealed physiological mechanisms by which high concentrations of certain air pollutants can cause acute reactions. Hence, we conclude that the sixth criterion is satisfied.

The seventh criterion is coherence. According to Hill (1965, page 298), "the cause-and-effect interpretation of . . . data should not seriously conflict with the generally known facts of the natural history and biology of the disease." Although biological experimentation has not quantified the magnitude of the air pollution–mortality relationship, neither has it provided information that contradicts any observed association. Consequently, this criterion cannot be readily applied. Amdur (1977) surveyed results from analytic chemistry, toxicology, clinical studies, and epidemiology and found many coherent aspects.

The eighth criterion concerns experimentation. Do the results from natural and other experiments support the hypothesized relationship? For example, does the association hold when the level of air pollution falls, as well as when it rises? Both our analysis of the day-to-day variations in air pollution and mortality and our cross-sectional time-series analysis provide an affirmative answer to this question. Further corroboration is given by the studies in appendix A in which certain occupational groups exhibited characteristics that would tend to confirm an association between occupational exposure and ill health.

The last criterion has to do with analogy. For, as Hill (1965, page 299) remarks, "With the effects of thalidomide and rubella before us we would surely be ready to accept slighter but similar evidence with another drug or another viral disease in pregnancy." Extensive literature documents the effect of cigarette smoking on the incidence of lung cancer and the aggravation of cardiovascular disease and the effect of occupational air pollution on mortality. Neither of these constitute a perfect analogy, since they often involve high dose rates for short periods; however, we conclude that this final criterion is generally satisfied. The studies showing that airborne carcinogens cause lung cancer and aggravate cardiovascular disease make it easier to convince scientists that the air pollution–mortality relationship is causal. Furthermore, the literature enables one to test the estimated gradient to determine if it is roughly consistent with the dose-response relationship observed for cigarette smoking and occupational exposure.

Here then are nine different viewpoints from all of which we should study association before we cry causation. What I do not believe—and this has not been suggested—is that we can usefully lay down some hard-and-fast rules of evidence that *must* be obeyed before we accept cause and effect. None of my nine viewpoints can bring indisputable evidence for or against the cause-and-effect hypothesis and none can be required as a *sine qua non*. What they can do, with greater or less strength, is to help us to make up our minds on the fundamental question—is there any other way of explaining the sets of facts before us, is there any other answer equally, or more likely than cause and effect. [Hill (1965), page 299]

Thus, the research relating air pollution to ill health satisfies Hill's criteria reasonably well. It may prove useful for the reader to keep these criteria in mind as we review in detail our own analyses of the association.

SUMMARY OF STATISTICAL ANALYSES

Background and framework

Chapters 1 and 2 provided the framework for an examination of the effects of air pollution on human health and reviewed the methods that have been used, and that we proposed to use, in exploring the association. The health effects of long-term exposure to low concentrations of air pollutants are hypothesized to be subtle (for example, shortening life expectancy by about one year). Thus, laboratory methods are of little help in estimating the dose-response curve, even though they may be powerful in exploring the underlying physiological mechanisms. We concluded that epidemiological methods were the most reasonable ways of exploring the association. The difficulties in being able to estimate the effect of air pollution on mortality are immense, since other factors hypothesized to affect mortality must be controlled, explicitly or implicitly. A host of difficulties associated with exploring causal models, with errors of measurement, and with unobserved variables were discussed. We concluded that simple, robust models were preferred and that extensive sensitivity analyses and replications were needed if one were to have confidence in the results.

Extensive literature reviews are reported in appendix A. Each study was evaluated with respect to its statistical methods and the adequacy with which other factors affecting health status were controlled. Specific diseases provided the principal guide for organization, although other categories included studies relating daily health status measures to daily air pollution levels and studies exploring the health effects of automobile-related pollution. While few studies can pass the stringent test of adequately controlling for confounding factors, the sheer volume of research and the almost uniform findings of significant associations between specific types of air pollution and ill health are impressive.

Cross-sectional analyses

Chapters 3 through 7 utilized data for each of three years to explore the association between specific measures of air pollution and mortality rates across more than one hundred U.S. SMSAs. The basic exploration was done with data for 1960, and much of the work was then replicated, using 1961 and 1969 data.

The unadjusted 1960 total mortality rate across 117 SMSAs was analyzed, and the effect of air pollution (as measured by sulfates and suspended particulates) was estimated using a simple linear model; socioeconomic variables were used to control for population density, racial composition, age distribution, income, and population. We concluded that the measures of air pollution (sulfates and suspended particulates) were significant factors in explaining variation in the total death rate across areas of the United States. Three measures (the minimum, mean, and maximum of biweekly readings) of each of the two air pollutants were available; specifications with all six measures, the two most significant measures (minimum sulfates and mean suspended particulates), and principal components of the six measures revealed similar results. Jackknife and other statistical procedures indicated that the basic relationship was not sensitive to "extreme" observations. A series of alternative functional forms were also examined. While some had greater explanatory power than the linear model, we decided to continue relying on the linear form because of its simplicity and ease of interpretation. Reestimation of the basic relationship, using 1961 data, corroborated our findings; the estimated coefficients of the 1961 air pollution variables were generally similar to their 1960 counterparts.

In chapter 4, we elaborated on the exploration of chapter 3 by analyzing age–sex–race-adjusted total mortality, infant mortality, age–sex–race-specific mortality, and disease-specific mortality. The results for the age–sex–race-adjusted total mortality rate were similar to those for the unadjusted total mortality rate. The measures of air pollution (sulfates and suspended particulates) continued to be significant factors in explaining the variation in these rates across SMSAs. The mortality rates for infants under one year of age (unadjusted, race-adjusted, white, and nonwhite) were more closely associated with suspended particulates than with sulfates; adjusting for race further enhanced the association with the measures of air pollution. A 1961 replication corroborated the 1960 infant mortality findings. Twenty-four age–sex–race-specific mortality rates were investigated using 1960 data. Air pollution (as measured by suspended particulates and sulfates) was generally a significant factor in explaining the variation in the age–sex–race-specific rates. In general, the measures of air pollution were more closely associated with mortality among nonwhites than among whites. In addition, the mortality rates for the older age groups were most closely associated. Using the age–sex–race-specific results, together with our previous results, we were able to estimate the implications on longevity of our findings: a 50 percent reduction in ambient levels of sulfates and suspended particulates was associated with approximately a 0.8 year increase in life expectancy (at birth).

In chapter 4, we also examined fifteen disease-specific mortality rates, using 1960 and 1961 data. For total cancers and for cancer of the digestive system in particular, there was a close association with air pollution (particularly sulfates) in 1960, although the 1961 replication did not indicate the same level of importance. Deaths from cardiovascular diseases and their subcategories also showed a close association with sulfate pollution in 1960; in this case, the 1961 results tended to strengthen the relationship. For diseases of the respiratory system (other than cancer), the results were often nonsignificant. Only tuberculosis was closely associated with air pollution (suspended particulates) in both 1960 and 1961. We believe that the mortality rates for the aggregate category of respiratory disease, influenza, pneumonia, and bronchitis did not display significant relationships because of the small number of deaths and consequent random variation in the mortality rates for each area in each year. We conclude that the results of the disease-specific analysis support our earlier findings for the unadjusted total mortality rate. In general, the measures of air pollution were significantly associated with mortality even after the total death rate was disaggregated, or adjusted, by age, sex, and race as well as when specific causes of death were examined.

It was still conceivable that a number of omitted factors might have been the "true" cause of the relationships we observed. To test this possibility, in chapter 5, additional variables were added to the original socioeconomic variables in order to control for occupation mix, climate, and home-heating characteristics in each area. The new variables generally increased the explanatory power of the previous regressions and their estimated effects had plausible interpretations. Since many of these variables tended to be correlated with the air pollution and socioeconomic variables, their inclusion caused multicollinearity problems. Consequently, some reduction was expected in both the numerical importance and the statistical significance of the regression coefficients pertaining to the air pollution and socioeconomic variables. In general, adding these variables had more effect on the socioeconomic coefficients than on the air pollution coefficients. However, the additional variables did lower the magnitudes of the air pollution coefficients and generally decreased their statistical significance. In particular, the results indicated that variables representing fuels used for home heating had a greater effect on the estimated coefficients for sulfates and suspended particulates than did other home-heating characteristics, occupation mix, or climate factors. Even with sets of these additional variables in the regressions, the estimated pollution coefficients suggested that the measures of sulfates and particulates were significant factors in explaining variations among most of the mortality rates. Thus, incorporating the new variables did not disprove the previously estimated associations between the measures of particulates, sulfates, and the various mortality rates. We view these results as giving qualified endorsement to the hypothesis of causality; but since important causal factors were still missing from the analysis, spurious correlation was still a possibility.

To further test whether omitted factors or other difficulties with the data might have caused the observed association between air pollution and mortality, in chapter 6 we analyzed rates for suicide, venereal disease, and crime—social ills presumed to be associated with many of the urban factors previously examined and expected to be amenable to the type of analysis performed for the mortality rates. We hypothesized that air pollution would *not* be an important explanatory factor. The analysis showed that the sulfate and suspended particulate measures were not consistent, significant explanatory variables, whereas most of the socioeconomic variables were. We concluded that the air pollution measures were not acting as surrogates for other variables in explaining these rates. This finding lent confidence to the previous evidence that the estimated relationship between the air pollution measures and mortality was not a spurious one.

In chapter 7 we performed a replication of much of the 1960 analysis, using 1969 data. The results of analyzing the 1969 total mortality rate (unadjusted and age–sex–race-adjusted) were comparable to the results of our earlier work; the coefficients for 1960 and 1969 were statistically similar (using two different tests). The reexamination of alternative specifications indicated that the simple linear form dominated. Jackknife estimates indicated that the results were not sensitive to extreme data points. Cross-lagged cross-sectional tests supported the hypothesis that the association between air pollution (primarily sulfates and suspended particulates) and mortality is causal. The analysis of the unexplained portions (the residuals) from the basic 1960 and 1969 regressions revealed that mortality rates for the largest SMSAs were predicted well in the regressions; there was a slight tendency to overestimate the mortality rates of the southwestern SMSAs. Unfortunately, there was evidence that factors giving rise to either unexpectedly large or small mortality rates in 1960 were also present in 1969, suggesting the importance of omitted factors and cautioning against overinterpretation of the results. Age–sex–race-adjusted, infant, and age–sex–race-specific mortality rates were reinvestigated and the earlier cross-sectional work was verified further. Finally, for sixty-nine SMSAs, data were also analyzed for nitrates, nitrogen dioxide, and sulfur dioxide in addition to sulfates and suspended particulates; sulfates and suspended particulates were still the most significant air pollutants, sulfur dioxide and nitrogen dioxide were occasionally significant, while measures of nitrates were never significant. Interactions between the five air pollutants were examined, and in spite of our expectations, there was no evidence of synergistic effects. The inadequacy of the aerometric data preclude drawing strong conclusions regarding the importance of interactions between pollutants; we merely remark that we failed to find significant evidence of synergism.

Thus, we conclude from the cross-sectional analysis in section II that, in general, those mortality rates which we expected to be closely associated with the air pollution measures were so, while rates which we did not expect to be closely associated with the air pollution measures were not. Not all the factors hypothesized to affect mortality were controlled in the analysis, but considerable evidence supports the hypothesis that the relationship between the mortality rates and our air pollution measures is causal.

Annual and daily time-series analysis

Further demonstration of this relationship was presented in section III, with analyses of groups of SMSAs and individual cities over time. Observing a given SMSA over time inherently provides control for more factors, since characteristics such as demographic mix, occupation mix, and home-heating characteristics remain relatively constant over time within an area. Thus, time-series analysis presents a purer comparison than does cross-sectional analysis.

However, time-series analysis also provides a different structure than cross-sectional analysis. The air pollution level currently prevailing in a city is a good approximation of the air pollution levels that have prevailed there for some time. Thus, a cross-sectional analysis tends to characterize the result of many years of exposure to that air pollution level. The time-series analysis relates changes in air pollution levels across time periods to changes in mortality across time periods; the analysis focuses on short-term variations in air pollution and mortality. Prolonged exposure to polluted air might result in the loss of one year of life expectancy but this need have no relationship to whether a one-day increase in pollution levels results in a significant increase in the number of deaths; if there is an increase in the number of daily deaths, part might be ascribed to shifting deaths forward by a few days, while part might be due to shortening everyone's life by a few days. Thus, the time-series analysis was not only interesting in itself, but it also provided information on the general relationship between air pollution and mortality measures by contrasting the estimates of day-to-day (or year-to-year) effects with long-term effects.

In chapter 8, annual observations (1960–69) from twenty-six SMSAs were pooled in an attempt to determine whether a component of the yearly death rate was associated with annual changes in the air pollution measures. The basic model was similar to the cross-sectional formulation used in section II. The variables consisted of the same factors that were in the original analysis. When the model was estimated (adding the U.S. total mortality rate, linear time, or time dummy variables to control for unobserved factors influencing mortality each year), both sulfate and suspended particulate pollution, and three of the socioeconomic variables, were significant in explaining the unadjusted total mortality rate. In contrast to the cross-sectional results, suspended particulates displayed relatively stronger associations with the mortality rates than did sulfates. The cross-sectional time-series results for the adjusted total mortality rate were similar to those for the unadjusted total mortality rate. For the race-adjusted infant mortality rate (under one year), suspended particulates were positively associated with mortality while sulfates were negatively associated; neither set of variables was statistically significant.

For a subsample of fifteen SMSAs, data on three additional pollutants (sulfur dioxide, nitrates, and nitrogen dioxide) were investigated in an attempt to isolate the effects of other air pollutants. In addition, first-order interactions between the air pollutants were analyzed. For the unadjusted total mortality rate, sulfates and suspended particulates continued to be significant; sulfur dioxide was also significant, while nitrates and nitrogen dioxide were nonsignificant and often negatively related. The interaction terms did not display evidence of important synergistic effects. The analysis was repeated, using the age–sex–race-adjusted total mortality rate with similar results. For the race-adjusted infant mortality rate, no category of air pollution made a statistically significant contribution. Nevertheless, taken as a whole, the cross-sectional time-series analysis provided additional evidence that measures of air pollution were associated with mortality and confirmed the importance of sulfates and suspended particulates.

In chapter 9 we investigated whether daily mortality was affected by daily pollution levels. Our method of investigation consisted of examining the relevant literature as well as performing our own statistical analysis. Specifically, we examined the effect of five pollutants (carbon monoxide, nitric oxide, nitrogen dioxide, sulfur dioxide, and hydrocarbons) in five cities (there was no city for which data on all five pollutants were available, and there was no pollutant for which data from all five cities were available). In only one of the five cities investigated—Chicago—was there a significant relationship between the air pollutants and daily mortality, controlling for the effects of weather. We conjectured that this was due to the relatively large number of daily deaths and to the relatively high air pollution levels in Chicago. Examination of a number of alternative formulations failed to produce one that dominated the simple linear form. Sulfur dioxide and nitric oxide were the significant air pollutants for Chicago, the former being much more significant. Careful investigation of lag structures revealed that high sulfur dioxide levels had a large immediate effect on mortality that gradually diminished over time. The effect of nitric oxide was delayed by several days, reached a peak, and then diminished. In examining whether deaths associated with the air pollution measures were merely displaced by a few days, we found that comparing our daily estimate for Chicago to estimates obtained from our previous analyses suggested the possibility that the mechanism relating air pollution levels to increased mortality might be different in a time-series study than in a cross-sectional or cross-sectional time-series analysis. We conclude that air pollution does not simply "harvest" deaths of susceptible individuals but seems to reduce life expectancy in general. Both the cross-sectional time-series analysis and the daily study added further evidence of the close association between measures of air pollution and mortality.

Section III's cross-sectional time-series and daily time-series analyses generally support the earlier cross-sectional results. Sulfates and suspended particulates were the most significant air pollutants in analyzing SMSAs over time, and sulfur dioxide (and, to a lesser extent, nitric oxide) were significant air pollutants in examining daily deaths within individual cities.

Thus, an elaborate statistical analysis of the effects of air pollution on mortality rates across the United States was added to reviews of the existing literature on air pollution and health. Our attempt to investigate thoroughly the 1960 ad hoc relationship between air pollution (as measured by sulfates and suspended particulates) and the total mortality rate has led to a long, perhaps tedious, discussion. However, viewing the accumulation of evidence, we find considerable consistency and corroboration among the individual studies. We conclude that the levels of certain pollutants in the air (as they prevailed in U.S. cities during the period 1960–69) caused increases in mortality, and presumably in morbidity as well.

POLICY IMPLICATIONS

In chapter 10, we presented a framework for a benefit–cost analysis of air pollution abatement. Estimates from the U.S. Environmental Protection Agency of the 1979 costs of stationary-source abatement were included, together with a discussion of the estimated benefits. The figure quoted as the 1979 annualized cost of meeting national standards for stationary sources was approximately $9.5 billion (1973 dollars). Although we have argued that this amount probably overestimates the "true" cost of abatement, we have not endeavored to furnish our own cost figures. On the benefits side, we have discussed some of the difficulties associated with determining the effects of air pollution on (1) cleaning, maintenance, and materials life, and the general value of property; (2) plants and animals; and (3) human health. We concluded that defensible figures do not presently exist for categories 1 and 2, or for benefits relating to better visibility, more frequent clear and sunny days, a reduction of noxious odors, and a generally improved quality of life. These benefits presumably would total many billions of dollars per year, although one would be hard pressed to defend particular estimates. Instead, we have based our justification of abatement programs on the benefits to human health alone. Our most conservative estimate of the effect of a 58 percent reduction in particulates and an 88 percent reduction in sulfur oxides (reductions corresponding to proposed control levels) would lead to a 7.0 percent decrease in total mortality (and presumably at least an equal decrease in total morbidity). This would amount to a national annual benefit of $16.1 billion in 1979 (1973 dollars). We have confidence that substantial abatement of air pollution from the major stationary-source categories of solid waste disposal, stationary fuel combustion, and industrial processes is warranted.

The National Academy of Sciences (NAS, 1974) estimated that the costs of controlling mobile-source emissions (to presently mandated standards) would be in the range of $8 to $11 billion (1973 dollars) per year by 1985. In addition, their "best" estimate for the potential benefits from mobile-source pollution was $5 billion per year (in 1973 dollars). Thus, the anticipated costs clearly exceed the expected benefits, at least on a national aggregate basis. In addition to this, we find that the association between emissions from mobile sources and mortality is less strong than the association between air pollution from stationary sources and mortality. This conclusion holds even for areas such as Los Angeles, where high levels of automobile-related air pollution have existed for two decades. Again, we must be cautious in drawing policy inferences, since available data are poor (even poorer than those used in analyzing the relationship between mortality and air pollution attributed primarily to stationary sources).

Our analysis demonstrates that the benefits associated with a rather substantial abatement of air pollution from stationary sources are greater than the costs of abatement. However, current evidence suggests that the costs of implementing the currently mandated emission controls on mobile sources are in excess of the potential benefits from such controls. Only by adopting some alternative policy, such as the two-car strategy or a relaxation of the NO_x standard, will the expected benefits exceed the anticipated costs. Additional information on the health or other effects of automobile emissions, or new information on abatement technology, may alter these conclusions.

With regard to the national ambient air quality standards, we find that for suspended particulates, evidence on the associated benefits and costs supports the presently mandated standard, while for sulfur dioxide, limited evidence suggests the current standard may not be sufficiently stringent.[1] Our mixed and very limited results do not permit policy conclusions concerning the national standards for nitrogen dioxide, carbon monoxide, and hydrocarbons. However, with regard to standard settings in general, we believe that the development of standards to "protect the public health and welfare" is not the correct way of dealing with the air pollution problem. Rather, society must weigh the benefits and costs of achieving improved air quality to determine its importance relative to other national priorities. Once a desired level is selected, the standards corresponding to it should be determined. (See appendix B, pages 312–316, for a detailed discussion.)

FUTURE RESEARCH NEEDS

This investigation has been an extensive one involving many data sets and a large number of analyses. Both the nature of the data available for statistical analyses and a consideration of the benefits and costs of air pollution abatement have suggested to us future research needs.

Perhaps the most serious deficiency we encountered in investigating the air pollution–mortality relationship was that of obtaining adequate air quality data. As noted in chapter 2, air quality measurements from a single sampling station are taken to represent a large geographical area. Very often faulty equipment is used to take infrequent readings of only a few pollutants. If we are to get better answers in the future to the question of which air pollutants should be abated and by how much, better air quality data are essential. Not only should a wider array of air pollutants be monitored but, where possible, the measurements should also be tailored to

---

[1] Although no sulfates standard currently exists, our research and that of others points to the need for a strong policy to control ambient levels of sulfates in the atmosphere.

what is presently known about the physiological effects of each pollutant. For example, measurements of particulates should include particle size as well as total mass. Very large particulates are filtered out in the upper airways and never reach the lungs [Amdur (1977) and Lave and Seskin (1977)].

A minimum set of pollutants to be monitored include those that are known to be associated with mortality or other measures of health status. These include suspended particulates, sulfur dioxide, sulfates, total oxidant, and perhaps nitrogen oxides. There are also a number of pollutants that appear in specific locations and thus should be monitored at those locations, for example, fluorides. For additional pollutants, there is evidence, from toxicological and epidemiological investigations of special occupational groups, indicating that these pollutants are worth monitoring. This group of pollutants includes trace metals, various sulfates and sulfites, and particulates within a particular size range (those small enough to be respirable). While it would be hopelessly expensive to measure all of these pollutants in thousands of stations across the country, it would be straightforward to set up an experimental design so that the additional pollutants are measured in such a way that evidence can be accumulated to test the hypothesis of causation.

After determining which pollutants are to be measured, the next issue concerns the frequency of sampling and the number of monitoring stations. The objective is to characterize the doses experienced by the exposed population in each area. For example, with respect to frequency, if primary interest is focused on the effects of acute air pollution episodes, continuous monitoring would most likely be required. On the other hand, if the focus is on chronic health effects, our comparison between the daily analyses and the annual analyses suggests that continuous monitoring is probably unnecessary. Instead, weekly or biweekly observations should be satisfactory to examine this health category, provided that the observations are sufficiently accurate. With regard to the number of monitoring stations, it seems clear that one sampling station in a large geographical area is not adequate to permit confident inferences as to the doses received by the area's population. Beyond that somewhat obvious conclusion, it is difficult to generalize. The number of stations required for a sound analysis will in most cases depend on such characteristics of the area as its size, its terrain, the meteorological conditions, and the number of significant point sources of pollution.

A different strategy for characterizing the amount of air pollution received by a population is to employ a personal, portable device to measure precisely what the individual breathes (Speizer, Bishop, and Ferris, 1977). Even an elaborate network of monitoring stations can only characterize outside air quality. The individual is generally inside a building or automobile and may be exposed to even higher concentrations through occupational or other activities. The personal dosimeter would provide a more accurate characterization of the total dose for the individuals over the time periods sampled.

Chapter 2 presented a number of factors that affect the mortality rate in an area. Data on many of these factors, such as the personal habits of smoking and medical care, were unavailable for our analyses. It is important that such data be gathered so that they will be available for future studies. In addition, data on other environmental insults, including radiation exposure and drinking water quality, should be collected. If we are to be more successful in isolating the health effects of air pollution exposure from the socioeconomic factors and other environmental insults, additional data on these factors must be made available.

Thus far we have confined the discussion to data on the explanatory factors of health status. The particular measure of health status is itself an extremely important consideration. For example, morbidity data are much more sensitive indicators of air pollution effects than mortality data. However, there is a host of problems associated with gathering morbidity data.[2] One possible approach to these problems would involve selecting a group of people to be monitored closely for changes in their health status. Variations in the morbidity rate over time of each individual (as a function of changes in air pollution exposure) would provide an almost ideal measure of the air pollution–morbidity association (Speizer, Bishop, and Ferris, 1977). While such data are likely to be expensive to gather, they are likely to be extremely useful in sorting out the health effects of various air pollutants.[3]

One potentially rich data source consists of daily observations of air pollution levels and either or both mortality and morbidity rates within a given geographical area. As discussed in chapters 8 and 9, such a data set controls implicitly many of the unmeasured factors that are inherently difficult to control. However, for these data sets to be useful, measure-

---

[2] For example, the number of days a worker is absent and reports being ill is likely to be influenced more by the number of sick days allowed than by what a physician would observe as illness. Most deviations from good health are minor physical problems, for example, headaches and colds. Whether such a problem causes someone to stay in bed or miss work depends on one's philosophy and type of work as much as the particular problem. Indeed, whether an individual characterizes such a problem as an illness is largely idiosyncratic.

[3] One of the problems with trying to determine the health effects of specific air pollutants is that generally they are present in the environment in extremely low concentrations. Therefore, it might be worthwhile to undertake prospective studies of individuals (or populations) exposed to high concentrations of polluted air associated with their occupation or another situation. If such studies were prospective (for example, for those newly hired), a host of biases could be avoided, such as the failure of studies examining current data to capture individuals who previously quit because of occupational exposure.

ment techniques must remain constant throughout the period under consideration, and that period must be long enough (perhaps a decade of consistent data) to permit significant variations (if they exist) to take place in the measured variables.

In chapters 3 and 7, we explored the functional form of the relationship between air pollution (as measured by suspended particulates and sulfates) and mortality. While the statistical results supporting the linear specification were quite strong, there are a number of reasons for not extrapolating the results far beyond the range of observed air quality. For example, the dose-response relationship is not likely to be linear at extremely low (or extremely high) concentrations. If we are to make intelligent judgments about the degree of air pollution abatement necessary for benefits to exceed costs, it is essential that we learn more about the exact nature of the air pollution–health relationship.

A great deal of work remains to be done on establishing the relationship between air pollution and human health. For epidemiological investigations of the sort reported in this book, more and better data are the key to improved knowledge.

IMPROVING THE MEASUREMENT OF BENEFITS AND COSTS

As reported in chapter 10, a great deal of attention has been focused on investigating categories of air pollution effects that represent relatively small losses (for example, the effects of certain air pollutants on plants), while potentially important areas have been completely neglected. Two crucial areas in need of closer examination are the impacts of air pollution on esthetics and its related impact on the quality of life generally. Until at least a rough calculation of the magnitude of these effects can be estimated, one can never be sure that air pollution standards are sufficiently stringent. This is an area in which new ideas on measurement techniques are needed.

Another issue concerns the evaluation of policy decisions involving long-term, low-probability, and possibly catastrophic events. One example of such an event is the claim by some that the buildup of carbon dioxide in the atmosphere may result in an increase or decrease in the earth's temperature, enough to cause another ice age or to melt the polar ice caps and flood much of the earth's land area. Unfortunately, there is little scientific theory or empirical information available to aid policymakers in decisions involving potentially disastrous outcomes (see Krutilla and Fisher, 1975).

Improved techniques for estimating the impacts of air pollution are also needed. For example, consider the impact on cleaning, maintenance, and materials life. One approach might involve the gathering of detailed expenditure data for consumers. An analysis of consumer expenditures on cleaning, painting, repairing, and replacement across different air quality regions could provide a useful way of estimating the relevant air pollution damages.[4] Furthermore, these data could be supplemented by information as to whether certain materials, colors, or product designs are avoided because of possible air pollution effects; such product substitution is a legitimate cost of air pollution that is often neglected. Similar studies could be undertaken for other air pollution effects and in other sectors of the economy (for example, commercial, agricultural, and industrial sectors).

We argued in chapter 10 that there is a systematic tendency in benefit–cost analyses to underestimate the benefits and to overestimate the costs. Obtaining measures of air pollution's effect on esthetics and life-style would do much to resolve the problem of underestimated benefits. One way to handle the problem of overestimated costs would involve an examination of the difference between estimated and actual air pollution control costs on a microeconomic, that is, on a plant-by-plant level. Such a study would enable one to estimate not only the degree (if any) to which costs are overestimated, but it would also shed more light on the relationship between estimated and realized costs.

One reason future costs are overestimated is that additional resources will be put into research and development to seek less costly air pollution control technologies. Questions to be answered include, How rapidly has technological change been made in the past? How rapidly have solutions to specific problems been developed? To resolve these, a general investigation of air pollution control research and development is needed.

We are all environmentalists in the sense that we all believe that some level of control is warranted. Many industrialists look to the emission standards of a few years ago and characterize these as sensible, while calling the more stringent standards which followed nonsensical. We have argued at length that stringent emission standards for particulates and sulfur oxides appear to be justified in the sense that benefits exceed costs. However, in order to set emission standards, we must know how benefits and costs vary with various air quality (or emission) levels. It is unlikely that the exact change in either benefits or costs can be estimated with precision. However, more accurate estimates than are currently available can, and must, be derived if we are to achieve a basis for sound public policy.

One final area of investigation concerns the "best" sequence of moving from the current state of environmental quality to a new level that is selected on the basis of the equilibrium benefits and costs. A slow time path will allow current equipment to depreciate (wear out) rather than to become technologically obsolete; funds can be accumulated for new

---

[4] Freeman (1975) discusses the use of defensive expenditures in measuring the benefits of water pollution control.

equipment with reduced air pollution emissions; time will allow research and development to devise cheaper, better technologies. However, a slow time path will delay the time at which environmental quality reaches the target level. Clearly, the answer is neither to require immediate compliance with all standards, nor to delay implementation indefinitely. There are vast differences in the costs of alternative time paths, and it is essential to determine a reasonable approximation to the "least-cost" path.

References

Abercrombie, G. F. 1953. "December Fog in London and the Emergency Bed Service," *Lancet* vol. 1, p. 234.

Acton, J. 1973. *Evaluating Public Programs to Save Lives: The Case of Heart Attacks* (Santa Monica, Calif., Rand Corporation), R-950-RC.

Amdur, M. O. 1977. "Toxicological Guidelines for Research on Sulfur Oxides and Particulates," in *Proceedings of the Fourth Symposium on Statistics and the Environment* (Washington, American Statistical Association), pp. 48–55.

Anderson, D. O. 1967. "The Effects of Air Contamination on Health," Pts. 1–3, *Canadian Medical Association Journal* vol. 97, pp. 528, 585, and 802.

————, and B. G. Ferris. 1965. "Air Pollution Levels and Chronic Respiratory Disease," *Archives of Environmental Health* vol. 10, p. 307.

Anderson, R. J., and T. Crocker. 1971. "Air Pollution and Residential Property Values," *Urban Studies* vol. 8, pp. 171–180.

Angel, J. H., C. M. Fletcher, I. D. Hill, and C. M. Tinker. 1965. "Respiratory Illness in Factory and Office Workers," *British Journal of Diseases of the Chest* vol. 59, p. 66.

Aronow, W. S., and S. N. Rokaw. 1972. "Effect of Freeway Travel on Angina Pectoris," *Annals of Internal Medicine* vol. 77, p. 669.

Ashe, W. F. 1959. "Exposure to High Concentrations of Air Pollution. Pt. 1: Health Effects of Acute Episodes," in *Proceedings of the National Conference on Pollution, Washington, D.C., Nov. 18–20, 1958* (Washington, U.S. Public Health Service, no. 654, p. 188).

Ashley, D. J. B. 1967. "The Distribution of Lung Cancer and Bronchitis in England and Wales," *British Journal of Cancer* vol. 21, p. 243.

————. 1969a. "Environmental Factors in the Aetiology of Gastric Cancer," *British Journal of Preventive and Social Medicine* vol. 23, p. 187.

————. 1969b. "Environmental Factors in the Aetiology of Lung Cancer and Bronchitis," *British Journal of Preventive and Social Medicine* vol. 23, p. 258.

251

Beard, R. R., and G. A. Wertheim. 1967. "Behavioral Impairment Associated with Small Doses of Carbon Monoxide," *American Journal of Public Health* vol. 57, p. 2012.

Becker, W. H., F. J. Schilling, and M. P. Verma. 1968. "The Effect on Health of the 1966 Eastern Seaboard Air Pollution Episode," *Archives of Environmental Health* vol. 16, p. 414.

Benedict, H. M., and R. E. Olson. 1970. "Economic Impact of Air Pollutants on Plants" (Palo Alto, Calif., Stanford Research Institute). Working paper.

———, C. G. Miller, and R. E. Olson. 1971. *Economic Impact of Air Pollutants on Plants in the U.S.* (Palo Alto, Calif., Stanford Research Institute).

———, ———, and J. S. Smith. 1973. *Assessment of Economic Impact of Air Pollutants on Vegetation in the United States: 1969–1971* (Palo Alto, Calif., Stanford Research Institute).

Berke, J., and V. Wilson. 1951. *Watch Out for the Weather* (New York, Viking).

Biersteker, K. 1969. "Air Pollution and Smoking as Cause of Bronchitis among 1,000 Male Municipal Employees in Rotterdam, Netherlands," *Archives of Environmental Health* vol. 18, p. 531.

Blalock, H. C., Jr. 1964. *Causal Inferences in Nonexperimental Research* (Chapel Hill, University of North Carolina Press).

Bokonjić, R., and N. Zec. 1968. "Strokes and the Weather: A Quantitative Statistical Study," *Journal of Neurological Science* vol. 6, p. 483.

Box, G. E. P., and S. L. Anderson. 1955. "Permutation Theory in the Derivation of Robust Criteria and the Study of Departures from Assumption," *Journal of the Royal Statistical Society* vol. B17, p. 1.

Boyd, J. T. 1960. "Climate, Air Pollution, and Mortality," *British Journal of Preventive and Social Medicine* vol. 14, p. 123.

Brandt, C. S., and W. W. Heck. 1968. "Effects of Air Pollution on Vegetation," in A. C. Stern, ed., *Air Pollution* vol. 1 (2nd ed., New York, Academic Press), p. 401.

Brant, J. W. A. 1965. "Human Cardiovascular Diseases and Atmospheric Air Pollution in Los Angeles, California," *Air and Water Pollution* vol. 8, p. 219.

———, and S. R. G. Hill. 1964. "Human Respiratory Diseases and Atmospheric Air Pollution in Los Angeles, California," *Air and Water Pollution* vol. 8, p. 259.

Brinton, H. P. 1949. "Morbidity and Mortality," in *Air Pollution in Donora, Pennsylvania,* Public Health Bulletin 306.

Brown, E. B., and J. Ipsen. 1968. "Changes in Severity of Symptoms of Asthma and Allergic Rhinitis Due to Air Pollutants," *Journal of Allergy* vol. 41, p. 254.

Buck, S. F., and D. A. Brown. 1964. *Mortality from Lung Cancer and Bronchitis in Relation to Smoke and Sulfur Dioxide Concentration, Population Density, and Social Index* (London, Tobacco Research Council) research paper no. 7.

———, and A. J. Wicken. 1967. "Models for Use in Investigating the Risk of Mortality from Lung Cancer and Bronchitis," *Applied Statistics* vol. 16, p. 185.

Buechley, R. W., F. W. Oechsli, and R. A. Stallones. 1966. "What Meanings Can Be Read into Geographic Variations in Cardiovascular Mortality?" (Durham, N.C., EPA) draft paper.

Buell, P., and J. E. Dunn. 1967. "Relative Impact of Smoking and Air Pollution on Lung Cancer," *Archives of Environmental Health* vol. 15, p. 291.

———, ———, and L. Breslow. 1967. "Cancer of the Lung and Los Angeles-type Air Pollution," *Cancer* vol. 20, p. 2139.

Burgess, S. G., and C. W. Shaddick. 1959. "Bronchitis and Air Pollution," *Royal Society of Health Journal* vol. 79, p. 10.

Burrows, B., A. L. Kellogg, and J. Buskey. 1968. "Relationship of Symptoms of Chronic Bronchitis and Emphysema to Weather and Air Pollution," *Archives of Environmental Health* vol. 16, p. 406.

Carnow, B. W., M. H. Lepper, R. B. Shekelle, and J. Stamler. 1969. "Chicago Air Pollution Study," *Archives of Environmental Health* vol. 18, p. 768.

———, and P. Meier. 1973. "Air Pollution and Pulmonary Cancer," *Archives of Environmental Health* vol. 27, p. 207.

Cassell, E. J., D. W. Wolter, J. D. Mountain, J. R. Diamond, J. M. Mountain, and J. R. McCarroll. 1968. "Pt. II. Reconsiderations of Mortality as a Useful Index of the Relationship of Environmental Factors to Health," *American Journal of Public Health* vol. 58, p. 1653.

Cederlöf, R. 1966. "Urban Factor and Prevalence of Respiratory Symptoms and Angina Pectoris," *Archives of Environmental Health* vol. 13, p. 743.

Chapman, R. S., B. Carpenter, C. M. Shy, R. G. Ireson, L. Heiderscheit, and W. K. Poole. 1973. "Prevalence of Chronic Respiratory Disease in Chattanooga: Effect of Community Exposure to Nitrogen Oxides" (Research Triangle Park, N.C., National Environmental Research Center, EPA) in-house technical report.

Chapman, T. T. 1965. "Air Pollution and the Forced Expiratory Volume in Chronic Bronchitis," *Irish Journal of Medical Science* vol. 472, p. 189.

Chovin, P. 1967. "Carbon Monoxide: Analysis of Exhaust Gas Investigations in Paris," *Environmental Research* vol. 1, p. 198.

Ciocco, A., and D. J. Thompson. 1961. "A Follow-up of Donora Ten Years After: Methodology and Findings," *American Journal of Public Health* vol. 51, p. 155.

Clayton, G. D., W. A. Cook, and W. G. Frederick. 1960. "A Study of the Relationship of Street-level Carbon Monoxide Concentrations to Traffic Accidents," *Industrial Hygiene Journal* vol. 21, p. 46.

Cohen, C. A., A. R. Hudson, J. L. Clausen, and J. H. Knelson. 1972. "Respiratory Symptoms, Spirometry, and Oxidant Air Pollution in Nonsmoking Adults," *American Review of Respiratory Disease* vol. 105, p. 251.

Cohen, S. I., M. Deane, and J. R. Goldsmith. 1969. "Carbon Monoxide and Survival from Myocardial Infarction," *Archives of Environmental Health* vol. 19, p. 510.

Colley, J. R. T. 1971. "Respiratory Disease in Childhood," *British Medical Bulletin* vol. 27, p. 9.

———, and W. W. Holland. 1967. "Social and Environmental Factors in Respiratory Disease: A Preliminary Report," *Archives of Environmental Health* vol. 14, p. 157.

———, and D. D. Reid. 1970. "Urban and Social Origins of Childhood Bronchitis in England and Wales," *British Medical Journal* vol. 2, p. 213.

Collins, J. J., H. S. Kasap, and W. W. Holland. 1971. "Environmental Factors in Child Mortality in England and Wales," *American Journal of Epidemiology* vol. 93, p. 10.

Conley, B. C. 1976. "The Value of Human Life in the Demand for Safety," *American Economic Review* vol. 66, p. 45.

Cooper, B. S. and D. P. Rice. 1976. "The Economic Cost of Illness Revisited," *Social Security Bulletin* vol. 39, p. 21.

———, and N. L. Worthington. 1972. "National Health Expenditures, Fiscal Year 1972," in *Research and Statistics Note,* U.S. Department of Health, Education and Welfare, Social Security Administration Office of Research and Statistics, HEW no. [SSA] 73-11701, note no. 19.

Cornwall, C. J., and P. A. B. Raffle. 1961. "Bronchitis-sickness Absence in London Transport," *British Journal of Industrial Medicine* vol. 18, p. 24.

Crocker, T., and A. Rogers. 1971. *Environmental Economics* (Hinsdale, Ill., Dryden).

Curphey, T. J., L. P. L. Hood, and N. M. Perkins. 1965. "Carboxyhemoglobin in Relation to Air Pollution and Smoking," *Archives of Environmental Health* vol. 10, p. 179.

Curwen, M. P., and E. L. Kennaway. 1954. "The Incidence of Cancer of the Lung and Larynx in Urban and Rural Districts," *British Journal of Cancer* vol. 8, p. 13.

Daly, C. 1959. "Air Pollution and Causes of Death," *British Journal of Preventive and Social Medicine* vol. 13, p. 14.

Dasgupta, A. K. and D. W. Pearce. 1972. *Cost–Benefit Analysis: Theory and Practice* (New York, Barnes & Noble).

Davies, G. M. 1963. "Fog Bronchiolitis," *Lancet* vol. 1, p. 580.

Davis, O., and K. Wertz. 1969. "The Consistency of Assessment of Property: Some Empirical Results and Managerial Suggestions," *Applied Economics* vol. 2, p. 151.

Dean, G. 1959. "Lung Cancer Among White South Africans," *British Medical Journal* vol. 2, p. 852.

———. 1961. "Lung Cancer Among White South Africans: Report on a Further Study," *British Medical Journal* vol. 2, p. 1599.

———. 1962. "Lung Cancer in Australia," *Medical Journal of Australia* vol. 1, p. 1003.

———. 1964. "Lung Cancer in South Africans and British Immigrants," *Proceedings of the Royal Society of Medicine* vol. 57, p. 984.

———. 1966. "Lung Cancer and Bronchitis in Northern Ireland," *British Medical Journal* vol. 1, p. 1506.

Derrick, E. H. 1970. "A Comparison between the Density of Smoke in the Brisbane Air and the Prevalence of Asthma," *Medical Journal of Australia* vol. 2, p. 670.

Dinman, B. D. 1977. "The SO_2 Ambient Air Quality Standard, with Special Reference to the 24-hour Standard—An Inquiry into the Health Bases," in *Proceedings of the Fourth Symposium on Statistics and the Environment* (Washington, American Statistical Association), p. 42.

Dohan, F. C. 1961. "Air Pollutants and Incidence of Respiratory Disease," *Archives of Environmental Health* vol. 3, p. 387.

————, G. S. Everts, and R. Smith. 1962. "Variations in Air Pollution and the Incidence of Respiratory Disease," *Journal of the Air Pollution Control Association* vol. 12, p. 418.

————, and B. S. Taylor. 1960. "Air Pollution and Respiratory Disease: A Preliminary Report," *American Journal of Medical Science* vol. 240, p. 337.

Dolde, W., D. N. Epple, M. Y. Harris, L. B. Lave, and S. Leinhardt. n.d. "Dynamic Aspects of Air Quality Control Costs," *Journal of Environmental Economics and Management*. In press.

Douglas, J. W. B., and R. E. Waller. 1966. "Air Pollution and Respiratory Infection in Children," *British Journal of Preventive and Social Medicine* vol. 20, p. 1.

Duffy, E., and R. Carroll. 1967. *United States Metropolitan Mortality, 1959–1961,* U.S. Public Health Service no. 969-AP-39.

Durbin, J., and D. S. Watson. 1950. "Pt. I: Testing for Serial Correlation in Least Squares Regression," *Biometrika* vol. 37, p. 409.

————, and ————. 1951. "Pt. II. Testing for Serial Correlation in Least Squares Regression," *Biometrika* vol. 38, p. 159.

Durham, W. E. 1974. "Air Pollution and Student Health," *Archives of Environmental Health* vol. 28, p. 241.

Eastcott, D. F. 1956. "The Epidemiology of Lung Cancer in New Zealand," *Lancet* vol. 1, p. 37.

Eckhardt, R. F. 1968. "Variations Affecting Death Rate," *Archives of Environmental Health* vol. 17, p. 837.

Ellsaesser, H. W. 1971. "Air Pollution in Los Angeles," *Science* vol. 173, p. 576.

Enterline, P. E., A. E. Rikli, M. J. Sauer, and M. Hyman. 1960. "Death Rates for Coronary Heart Disease in Metropolitan and Other Areas," *Public Health Reports* vol. 75, p. 759.

Fairbairn, A. S., and D. D. Reid. 1958. "Air Pollution and Other Local Factors in Respiratory Disease," *British Journal of Preventive and Social Medicine* vol. 12, p. 94.

Feliciano, A. 1972. *Survey and Assessment of Air Pollution Damage to Vegetation in New Jersey* (New Brunswick, N.J., College of Agriculture and Environmental Science of Rutgers University).

Ferris, B. G. 1970. "Effects of Air Pollution on School Absences and Differences in Lung Function in First and Second Graders in Berlin, New Hampshire, January 1966 to June 1967," *American Review of Respiratory Diseases* vol. 102, p. 591.

————, and D. O. Anderson. 1962. "The Prevalence of Chronic Respiratory Disease in a New Hampshire Town," *American Review of Respiratory Diseases* vol. 86, p. 165.

————, and ————. 1964. "Epidemiological Studies Related to Air Pollution: A Comparison of Berlin, New Hampshire, and Chilliwack, British Columbia," *Proceedings of the Royal Society of Medicine* vol. 57, p. 979.

————, and J. L. Whittenberger. 1966. "Environmental Hazards: Effects of Community Air Pollution on Prevalence of Respiratory Disease," *New England Journal of Medicine* vol. 275, p. 1413.

Fink, F. W., F. H. Buttner, and W. K. Boyd. 1971. *Final Report on Technical–Economic Evaluation of Air Pollution Corrosion Costs on Metals in the U.S.* (Columbus, Ohio, Battelle Memorial Institute).

Firket, J. 1958. "The Problem of Cancer of the Lung in the Industrial Area of Liège During Recent Years," *Proceedings of the Royal Society of Medicine* vol. 51, p. 347.

Firket, M. 1931. "Sur les Causes des Accidents Servenus dans la Vallée da la Meuse, Lors des Brouillards de Décembre 1930," *Bulletin de l'Academie Royale de Medecine de Belgique* vol. 11, p. 683.

Fletcher, C. M. 1958. "Disability and Mortality from Chronic Bronchitis in Relation to Dust Exposure," *Archives of Industrial Hygiene* vol. 18, p. 368.

Freeman, A. M., III. 1972. "Distribution of Environmental Quality," in A. Kneese and B. Bower, eds., *Environmental Quality Analysis* (Baltimore, Johns Hopkins University Press for Resources for the Future), p. 243.

———. 1975. "A Survey of the Techniques for Measuring the Benefits of Water Quality Improvement," in H. M. Peskin, and E. P. Seskin, eds., *Cost–Benefit Analysis and Water Pollution Policy* (Washington, Urban Institute), p. 67.

———, and R. H. Haveman. 1972. "Residuals Charges for Pollution Control: A Policy Evaluation," *Science* vol. 177, p. 322.

———, and A. V. Kneese. 1973. *The Economics of Environmental Policy* (New York, Wiley).

Friedman, G. D. 1967. "Cigarette Smoking and Geographic Variation in Coronary Heart Disease Mortality in the United States," *Journal of Chronic Diseases* vol. 20, p. 769.

Fromm, G. 1968. "Civil Aviation Expenditures," in R. Dorfman, ed., *Measuring Benefits of Government Investments* (Washington, Brookings Institution), p. 172.

Fry, J. 1953. "Effects of Severe Fog on a General Practice," *Lancet* vol. 1, p. 235.

Gardner, M. J., M. D. Crawford, and J. N. Morris. 1969. "Patterns of Mortality in Middle and Early Old Age in the County Boroughs of England and Wales," *British Journal of Preventive and Social Medicine* vol. 23, p. 133.

———, and R. E. Waller. 1970. "Environmental Factors in the Aetiology of Lung Cancer and Bronchitis," *British Journal of Preventive and Social Medicine* vol. 24, p. 58.

Gaver, K. M. 1971. "A Note on the Polynomial Technique for Estimating Distributed Lags" (Pittsburgh, Pa., Carnegie–Mellon University).

Georgii, H. W. 1968. "The Effects of Air Pollution on Urban Climates," in World Meteorological Organization, *Symposium on Urban Climates and Building Climatology* (Geneva, World Meteorological Organization), p. 624.

Girsh, L. S., E. Shubin, C. Dick, and F. A. Schulaner. 1967. "A Study on the Epidemiology of Asthma in Children in Philadelphia," *Journal of Allergy* vol. 39, p. 347.

Glasser, M., and L. Greenburg. 1971. "Air Pollution, Mortality, and Weather," *Archives of Environmental Health* vol. 22, p. 334.

——, ——, and F. Field. 1967. "Mortality and Morbidity During a Period of High Levels of Air Pollution," *Archives of Environmental Health* vol. 15, p. 684.

Goldsmith, J. R. 1965. "Epidemiology of Bronchitis and Emphysema I: Factors Influencing Prevalence and a Criterion for Testing Their Interaction," *Medicina Thoracalis* vol. 22, p. 1.

——. 1968. "Effects of Air Pollution on Human Health," in A. C. Stern, ed., *Air Pollution* (New York, Academic Press), p. 547.

Golledge, A. H., and A. J. Wicken. 1964. "Local Variation in the Incidence of Lung Cancer and Bronchitis Mortality," *Medical Officer* vol. 112, p. 273.

Gore, A. T., and C. W. Shaddick. 1958. "Atmospheric Pollution and Mortality in the County of London," *British Journal of Preventive and Social Medicine* vol. 12, p. 104.

Gorham, E. 1958. "Bronchitis and the Acidity of Urban Precipitation," *Lancet* vol. 2, p. 691.

——. 1959. "Pneumonia and Atmospheric Sulphate Deposit," *Lancet* vol. 2, p. 287.

Göthe, C. J., B. Fristedt, L. Sundell, B. Kolmodin, H. Ehrner-Samuel, and K. Göthe. 1969. "Carbon Monoxide Hazard in City Traffic," *Archives of Environmental Health* vol. 19, p. 310.

Greenburg, L., M. B. Jacobs, B. M. Drolette, F. Field, and M. M. Braverman. 1962a. "Report of an Air Pollution Incident in New York City, November, 1953," *Conference Report, Public Health Reports* vol. 77, p. 7.

——, F. Field, J. I. Reed, and C. L. Erhardt. 1962b. "Air Pollution and Morbidity in New York City," *Journal of the American Medical Association* vol. 182, p. 161.

——, C. L. Erhardt, F. Field, J. I. Reed, and N. S. Seriff. 1963. "Intermittent Air Pollution Episode in New York City, 1962," *Public Health Reports* vol. 78, p. 1061.

——, ——, ——, and J. I. Reed. 1965. "Air Pollution Incidents and Morbidity Studies," *Archives of Environmental Health* vol. 10, p. 351.

——, F. Field, J. I. Reed, and M. Glasser. 1967a. "Air Pollution and Cancer Mortality Study on Staten Island, New York," *Archives of Environmental Health* vol. 15, p. 356.

——, ——, C. L. Erhardt, M. Glasser, and J. I. Reed. 1967b. "Air Pollution, Influenza, and Mortality in New York City," *Archives of Environmental Health* vol. 15, p. 430.

Gregory, J. 1970. "The Influence of Climate and Atmospheric Pollution on Exacerbations of Chronic Bronchitis," *Atmospheric Environment* vol. 4, p. 453.

Griswold, M. H., C. S. Wilder, S. J. Cutler, and E. S. Pollack. 1955. *Cancer in Connecticut, 1935–1951* (Hartford, Connecticut State Department of Health).

Gustavson, R. 1959. "What Are the Costs to Society?," in *Proceedings of the National Conference on Air Pollution, Nov. 18–20, 1958*, U.S. Public Health Service no. 654.

Haenszel, W. 1961. "Cancer Mortality Among the Foreign Born in the United States," *Journal of the National Cancer Institute* vol. 26, p. 37.

————, D. B. Loveland, and M. G. Sirken. 1962. "Lung Cancer Mortality as Related to Residence and Smoking Histories, Pt. I: White Males," *Journal of the National Cancer Institute* vol. 28, p. 947.

————, and K. E. Taeuber. 1964. "Lung Cancer Mortality as Related to Residence and Smoking Histories, Pt. II: White Females," *Journal of the National Cancer Institute* vol. 32, p. 803.

Hagstrom, R. M., H. A. Sprague, and E. Landau. 1967. "The Nashville Air Pollution Study, Pt. VII: Mortality from Cancer in Relation to Air Pollution," *Archives of Environmental Health* vol. 15, p. 237.

Hammer, D. I., V. Hasselblad, B. Portnoy, and P. F. Wehrle. 1974. "Los Angeles Student Nurse Study," *Archives of Environmental Health* vol. 28, p. 255.

————, B. Portnoy, F. M. Massey, W. S. Wayne, T. Oelsner, and P. F. Wehrle. 1965. "Los Angeles Air Pollution and Respiratory Symptoms," *Archives of Environmental Health* vol. 10, p. 475.

Hammond, E. C. 1958. "Lung Cancer Death Rates in England and Wales Compared with Those in the U.S.A.," *British Medical Journal* vol. 2, p. 649.

————. 1967. "Epidemiological Evidence on the Effects of Air Pollution." Paper presented at the Sixtieth Annual Meeting of the Air Pollution Control Association, Cleveland.

————, and D. Horn. 1958. "Smoking and Death Rates: Report on Forty-four Months of Follow-up of 187,783 Men, Pt. II: Death Rates by Cause," *Journal of the American Medical Association* vol. 166, p. 1294.

Harberger, A. C., R. H. Haveman, J. Margolis, W. A. Niskanen, R. Turvey, and R. Zeckhauser, eds. 1972. *Benefit–Cost Analysis, 1971* (Chicago, Aldine).

Harman, H. H. 1967. *Modern Factor Analysis* (2nd ed., Chicago, University of Chicago Press).

Harris, R., G. Tolley, and C. Harrell. 1968. "The Residence Site Choice," *Review of Economics and Statistics* vol. 50, p. 241.

Haveman, R. H., A. C. Harberger, L. Lynn, Jr., W. A. Niskanen, R. Turvey, and R. Zeckhauser, eds. 1974. *Benefit–Cost and Policy Analysis, 1973* (Chicago, Aldine).

————, and B. A. Weisbrod. 1975. "The Concept of Benefits in Cost–Benefit Analysis: With Emphasis on Water Pollution Control Activities," in H. M. Peskin and E. P. Seskin, eds., *Cost–Benefit Analysis and Water Pollution Policy* (Washington, Urban Institute), p. 37.

Hechter, H. H., and J. R. Goldsmith. 1961. "Air Pollution and Daily Mortality," *American Journal of Medical Science* vol. 241, p. 581.

Heck, W. W. and C. S. Brandt. 1976. "Effect on Vegetation: Native Crops, Forests," in A. C. Stern, ed., *Air Pollution* vol. 2 (3rd ed., New York, Academic Press).

Heimann, H. 1970. "Episodic Air Pollution in Metropolitan Boston: A Trial Epidemiological Study," *Archives of Environmental Health* vol. 20, p. 230.

Hershaft, A., J. Morton, and G. Shea. 1976. *Critical Review of Air Pollution Dose-Effect Functions* (Rockville, Md., Enviro Control, Inc.).

Hewitt, D. 1956. "Mortality in the London Boroughs, 1950–52, with Special Reference to Respiratory Disease," *British Journal of Preventive and Social Medicine* vol. 10, p. 45.

Hexter, A. C., and J. R. Goldsmith. 1971a. "Carbon Monoxide: Association of Community Air Pollution with Mortality," *Science* vol. 172, p. 265.

———, and ———. 1971b. "Air Pollution in Los Angeles," *Science* vol. 173, p. 576.

Higgins, I. T. T. 1966. "Air Pollution and Chronic Respiratory Disease," *ASHRAE Journal* vol. 8, p. 37.

Hill, A. B. 1965. "The Environment and Diseases: Associations and Causation," *Proceedings of the Royal Society of Medicine, Section on Occupational Medicine* vol. 58, p. 272.

Hitosugi, M. 1968. "Epidemiological Study of Lung Cancer with Special Reference to the Effect of Air Pollution and Smoking Habits," *Institutes of Public Health Bulletin* vol. 17, p. 237.

Hodgson, T. A. 1970. "Short-term Effects of Air Pollution on Mortality in New York City," *Environmental Science and Technology* vol. 4, p. 589.

Hoffman, E. F., and A. G. Gilliam. 1954. "Lung Cancer Mortality," *Public Health Reports* vol. 69, p. 1033.

Holland, W. W. 1971. "The Influence of Climate and Atmospheric Pollution on Exacerbations of Chronic Bronchitis," *Atmospheric Environment* vol. 5, p. 435.

———, ed. 1972. *Air Pollution and Respiratory Disease* (Westport, Conn., Technomatic).

———, and D. D. Reid. 1965. "The Urban Factor in Chronic Bronchitis," *Lancet* vol. 1, p. 445.

———, C. C. Spicer, and J. M. G. Wilson. 1961. "Influence of the Weather on Respiratory and Heart Disease," *Lancet* vol. 2, p. 338.

———, ———, R. Seltser, and R. W. Stone. 1965. "Respiratory Disease in England and the United States," *Archives of Environmental Health* vol. 10, p. 338.

———, ———, ———, and ———. 1969a. "Factors Influencing the Onset of Chronic Respiratory Disease," *British Medical Journal* vol. 2, p. 205.

———, ———, ———, and ———. 1969b. "Respiratory Symptoms and Ventilatory Function: A Family Study," *British Journal of Preventive and Social Medicine* vol. 23, p. 77.

———, and R. W. Stone. 1965. "Respiratory Disorders in U.S. East Coast Telephone Men," *American Journal of Epidemiology* vol. 82, p. 92.

Hueper, W. C. 1956. "Environmental Causes of Cancer of the Lung Other Than Tobacco Smoke," *Diseases of the Chest* vol. 30, p. 141.

Ipsen, J., M. Deane, and F. E. Ingenito. 1969. "Relationships of Acute Respiratory Disease to Atmospheric Pollution and Meteorological Conditions," *Archives of Environmental Health* vol. 18, p. 462.

Ishikawa, S., D. H. Bowden, V. Fisher, and J. P. Wyatt. 1969. "The 'Emphysema Profile' in Two Midwestern Cities in North America," *Archives of Environmental Health* vol. 18, p. 660.

ITT Electro-Physics Laboratories, Incorporated. 1971. *A Survey and Economic Assessment of the Effects of Air Pollutants on Electrical Components* (Washington, U.S. Environmental Protection Agency, Air Pollution Control Office) vol. I, sect. 1–9.

Johnston, J. 1972. *Econometric Methods* (2nd ed., New York, McGraw-Hill).

Jorling, T. 1974. "The Federal Law of Air Pollution Control," in E. L. Dolgin and T. G. Guilbert, eds., *Federal Environmental Law* (Washington, West), p. 1058.

Kenline, P. A. 1966. "October 1963 New Orleans Asthma Study," *Archives of Environmental Health* vol. 12, p. 295.

Klarman, H. E. 1965. "Syphilis Control Programs," in R. Dorfman, ed., *Measuring Benefits of Government Investment* (Washington, Brookings Institution), p. 367.

Kneese, A. V. 1967. "Economics and the Quality of the Environment: Some Empirical Experiences," in M. Garnsey and J. Hibbs, eds., *Costs of Air Pollution* (New York, Praeger).

———, R. U. Ayres, and R. C. d'Arge. 1970. *Economics and the Environment: A Materials Balance Approach* (Baltimore, Johns Hopkins University Press for Resources for the Future).

———, and C. Schultze. 1975. *Pollution, Prices and Public Policy* (Washington, Brookings Institution).

Kreyberg, L. 1956. "Occurrence and Aetiology of Lung Cancer in Norway in the Light of Pathological Anatomy," *British Journal of Preventive and Social Medicine* vol. 10, p. 145.

Krutilla, J. V., and A. C. Fisher. 1975. *The Economics of Natural Environments* (Baltimore, Johns Hopkins University Press for Resources for the Future).

Kuller, L. H., E. P. Radford, D. Swift, J. A. Perper, and R. Fisher. 1975. "Carbon Monoxide and Heart Attacks," *Archives of Environmental Health* vol. 30, p. 477.

Lacasse, N. L. 1971. *Assessment of Air Pollution Damage to Vegetation in Pennsylvania, June 1970–June 1971* (University Park, Pa., Center for Air Environment Studies, Pennsylvania State University).

Ladd, B., and H. W. Phelps. 1963. "Incidence of Air Pollution Bronchitis in Military Personnel in Japan," *Diseases of the Chest* vol. 43, p. 151.

Lambert, P. M., and D. D. Reid. 1970. "Smoking, Air Pollution, and Bronchitis in Britain," *Lancet* vol. 1, p. 853.

Lammers, B., R. F. Schilling, and J. Walford. 1964. "A Study of Byssinosis, Chronic Respiratory Symptoms, and Ventilatory Capacity in English and Dutch Cotton Workers, with Special Reference to Atmospheric Pollution," *British Journal of Industrial Medicine* vol. 21, p. 124.

Lave, L. B. 1968. "Safety in Transportation: The Role of Government," *Law and Contemporary Problems* vol. 33, p. 512.

———. 1971. "A Benefit–Cost Analysis of Air Pollution Abatement," in *1971 Intersociety Energy Conversion Engineering Conference* (Warrendale, Pa., Society of Automotive Engineers, Inc.), p. 337.

———. 1972. "Air Pollution Damage," in A. Kneese and B. Bower, eds., *Environmental Quality Analysis* (Baltimore, Johns Hopkins University Press for Resources for the Future), p. 213.

———, and L. C. Freeburg. 1973. "Health Effects of Electricity Generation from Coal, Oil, and Nuclear Fuel," *Nuclear Safety* vol. 14, p. 409.

———, and E. P. Seskin. 1970. "Air Pollution and Human Health," *Science* vol. 169, p. 723.

————, and ————. 1971a. "Does Air Pollution Shorten Lives?" in *Proceedings of the Second Research Conference of the Inter-University Committee on Urban Economics* (Chicago, University of Chicago), p. 293.

————, and ————. 1971b. "Health and Air Pollution: The Effect of Occupation Mix," *Swedish Journal of Economics* vol. 73, p. 76.

————, and ————. 1972. "Air Pollution, Climate, and Home Heating: Their Effects on U.S. Mortality Rates," *American Journal of Public Health* vol. 62, p. 909.

————, and ————. 1973. "An Analysis of the Association Between U.S. Mortality and Air Pollution," *Journal of the American Statistical Association* vol. 68, p. 284.

————, and ————. 1974. "Does Air Pollution Shorten Lives?," in J. W. Pratt, ed., *Statistical and Mathematical Aspects of Pollution Problems* (New York, Marcel Dekker), pp. 223–244.

————, and ————. 1975. "Acute Relationships Among Daily Mortality, Air Pollution, and Climate," in E. Mills, ed., *Economic Analysis of Environmental Problems* (New York, National Bureau of Economic Research), p. 325.

————, and ————. 1977. "Does Air Pollution Cause Mortality?" in *Proceedings of the Fourth Symposium on Statistics and the Environment* (Washington, American Statistical Association), p. 25.

————, and Silverman, L. P. 1976. "Economic Costs of Energy-related Environmental Pollution," *Annual Review of Energy* vol. 1, p. 106.

Lawther, P. J. 1958. "Climate, Air Pollution, and Chronic Bronchitis," *Proceedings of the Royal Society of Medicine* vol. 51, p. 262.

————, R. E. Waller, and M. Henderson. 1970. "Air Pollution and Exacerbations of Bronchitis," *Thorax* vol. 25, p. 525.

Lepper, M. H., N. Shioura, B. Carnow, S. Andelman, and L. Lehrer. 1969. "Respiratory Disease in an Urban Environment," *Industrial Medicine* vol. 38, p. 36.

Levin, M. L., W. Haenszel, B. E. Carroll, P. R. Gerhardt, V. H. Handy, and S. C. Ingraham II. 1960. "Cancer Incidence in Urban and Rural Areas of New York State," *Journal of the National Cancer Institute* vol. 24, p. 1243.

Lewis, H. R. 1965. *With Every Breath You Take* (New York, Crown).

Lewis, L., M. M. Gilkeson, and R. O. McCaldin. 1962. "Air Pollution and New Orleans Asthma," *Public Health Reports* vol. 77, p. 947.

Logan, W. P. D. 1956. "Mortality from Fog in London, January 1956," *British Medical Journal* vol. 1, p. 722.

Lombard, H. L., and C. R. Doering. 1927. "Cancer Studies in Massachusetts: The Relationship Between Cancer and Density of Population in Massachusetts," *Proceedings of the National Academy of Sciences* vol. 13, p. 728.

London Ministry of Health. 1954. "Mortality and Morbidity During the London Fog of December 1952," in *Reports on Public Health and Related Subjects* No. 95 (London, Her Majesty's Stationery Office).

Loudon, R. G., and J. F. Kilpatrick. 1969. "Air Pollution, Weather, and Cough," *Archives of Environmental Health* vol. 18, p. 641.

Lunn, J. E., J. Knowelden, and A. J. Handyside. 1967. "Patterns of Respiratory Illness in Sheffield Infant School Children," *British Journal of Preventive and Social Medicine* vol. 21, p. 7.

———, ———, and J. W. Roe. 1970. "Patterns of Respiratory Illness in Sheffield Junior School Children: A Follow-up Study," *British Journal of Preventive and Social Medicine* vol. 24, p. 223.

McCabe, L. C., and G. D. Clayton. 1952. "Air Pollution by Hydrogen Sulfide in Poza Rica, Mexico," *Archives of Industrial Hygiene and Occupational Medicine* vol. 6, p. 199.

McCarroll, J. 1967. "Measurements of Morbidity and Mortality Related to Air Pollution," *Journal of the Air Pollution Control Association* vol. 17, p. 203.

———, and W. Bradley. 1966. "Excess Mortality as an Indicator of Health Effects of Air Pollution," *American Journal of Public Health* vol. 56, p. 1933.

———, E. J. Cassell, W. T. Ingram, and D. W. Wolter. 1966. "Health and the Urban Environment: Health Profiles Versus Environmental Pollutants," *American Journal of Public Health* vol. 56, p. 267.

———, D. W. Wolter, J. D. Mountain, and J. R. Diamond. 1967. "Health and the Urban Environment V. Air Pollution and Illness in a Normal Population," *Archives of Environmental Health* vol. 14, p. 178.

McDonald, G. C., and R. C. Schwing. 1973. "Instabilities of Regression Estimates Relating Air Pollution to Mortality." *Technometrics* vol. 15, p. 463.

MacMahon, B., T. Puch, and J. Ipsen. 1960. *Epidemiologic Methods* (Boston, Little, Brown).

McMillan, R. S., D. H. Wiseman, B. Hanes, and P. F. Wehrle. 1969. "Effects of Oxidant Air Pollution on Peak Expiratory Flow Rates in Los Angeles School Children," *Archives of Environmental Health* vol. 18, p. 941.

Mancuso, T. F., and E. J. Coulter. 1958. "Cancer Mortality Among Native White, Foreign-born White, and Nonwhite Male Residents of Ohio: Cancer of the Lung, Larynx, Bladder, and Central Nervous System," *Journal of the National Cancer Institute* vol. 20, p. 79.

———, E. M. MacFarlane, and J. D. Porterfield. 1955. "The Distribution of Cancer Mortality in Ohio," *American Journal of Public Health* vol. 45, p. 58.

Manos, N. E., and G. F. Fisher. 1959. "An Index of Air Pollution and Its Relation to Health," *Journal of the Air Pollution Control Association* vol. 9, p. 5.

Manzhenko, E. G. 1966. "The Effect of Atmospheric Pollution on the Health of Children," *Hygiene and Sanitation* vol. 31, p. 126.

Martin, A. E. 1961. "Epidemiological Studies of Atmospheric Pollution," *Monthly Bulletin of the Ministry of Health* (Great Britain) vol. 20, p. 42.

———. 1964. "Mortality and Morbidity Statistics and Air Pollution," *Proceedings of the Royal Society of Medicine* vol. 57, p. 969.

———, and W. H. Bradley. 1960. "Mortality, Fog and Atmospheric Pollution," *Monthly Bulletin of the Ministry of Health (Great Britain)* vol. 19, p. 56.

Mellon Institute. 1913. *The Smoke Investigation* (Pittsburgh, Pa., Mellon Institute).

Michelson, I., and B. Tourin. 1966. "Comparative Methods for Studying the Costs of Controlling Air Pollution," *Public Health Reports* vol. 81, p. 505.

Millecan, A. A. 1971. *A Survey and Assessment of Air Pollution Damage to California Vegetation in 1970.* (Sacramento, Bureau of Plant Pathology, California Department of Agriculture).

Mills, C. A. 1943. "Urban Air Pollution and Respiratory Diseases," *American Journal of Hygiene* vol. 37, p. 131.

――――. 1952. "Air Pollution and Community Health," *American Journal of Medical Sciences* vol. 224, p. 403.

――――. 1957. "Respiratory and Cardiac Deaths in Los Angeles Smogs," *American Journal of Medical Sciences* vol. 233, p. 379.

――――. 1960. "Motor Exhaust Gases and Lung Cancer in Cincinnati," *American Journal of Medical Sciences* vol. 239, p. 316.

Mishan, E. J. 1971. Cost–Benefit Analysis: An Informal Introduction (New York, Praeger).

Mosher, J. C., M. F. Brunelle, and W. J. Hamming. 1971. "Air Pollution in Los Angeles," *Science* vol. 173, p. 576.

Mosteller, F., and J. W. Tukey. 1968. "Data Analysis Including Statistics," in *The Handbook of Social Psychology*, vol. 2, *Research and Methods* (2nd ed., Reading, Mass., Addison-Wesley), p. 80.

Motley, H. L., and H. W. Phelps. 1964. "Pulmonary Function Impairment Produced by Atmospheric Pollution," *Diseases of the Chest* vol. 45, p. 154.

――――, R. H. Smart, and C. I. Leftwich. 1959. "Effect of Polluted Los Angeles Air (Smog) on Lung Volume Measurements," *Journal of the American Medical Association* vol. 171, p. 1469.

Mueller, W. J., and P. B. Stickney. 1970. *A Survey and Economic Assessment of the Effects of Air Pollution on Elastomers* (Raleigh, N.C., The National Air Pollution Control Administration, U.S. Department of Health, Education and Welfare).

Naegele, J. A., W. A. Feder, and C. J. Brandt. 1972. *Assessment of Air Pollution Damage to Vegetation in New England, July 1971–July 1972*, EPA-R5-72-009 (Washington, Office of Research and Monitoring, U.S. Environmental Protection Agency).

National Academy of Sciences. 1974. *Air Quality and Automobile Emission Control*, vol. 4, *The Costs and Benefits of Automobile Emission Control*. Report by the Coordinating Committee on Air Quality Studies, National Academy of Sciences, National Academy of Engineering, serial no. 93-24 (Washington, GPO).

――――. 1975. *Air Quality and Stationary Source Emissions Control*. Report by the Coordinating Committee on Air Quality Studies, National Academy of Sciences, National Academy of Engineering, serial no. 94-4 (Washington, GPO).

Nelson, J. P. 1975. *The Effects of Mobile-Source Air and Noise Pollution on Residential Property Value* (Washington, U.S. Department of Transportation).

Niskanen, W. A., A. C. Harberger, R. H. Haverman, R. Turvey, and R. Zeckhauser, eds. 1973. *Benefit–Cost and Policy Analysis 1972* (Chicago, Aldine).

Nourse, H. 1967. "The Effect of Air Pollution on House Values," *Land Economics* vol. 43, p. 181.

O'Gara, P. 1922. "Sulfur Dioxide and Fume Problems," *Industrial and Engineering Chemistry* vol. 14, p. 744.

Oshima, Y., T. Ishizaki, T. Miyamoto, T. Shimizu, T. Shida, and J. Kabe. 1964. "Air Pollution and Respiratory Diseases in the Tokyo–Yokohama Area," *American Review of Respiratory Diseases* vol. 90, p. 572.

Paulus, H. J., and T. J. Smith. 1967. "Association of Allergic Bronchial Asthma with Certain Pollutants and Weather Parameters," *International Journal of Biometeorology*. vol. 11, p. 119.

Pearlman, M. E., J. F. Finklea, J. P. Creason, C. M. Shy, M. M. Young, and R. J. M. Horton. 1971. "Nitrogen Dioxide and Lower Respiratory Illness," *Pediatrics* vol. 47, p. 391.

Pell, E. J. 1973. *Survey and Assessment of Air Pollution Damage to Vegetation in New Jersey*, EPA-R5-73-022 (Washington, Office of Research and Monitoring, U.S. Environmental Protection Agency).

Pemberton, J. 1961. "Air Pollution as a Possible Cause of Bronchitis and Lung Cancer," *Journal of Hygiene Epidemiology, Microbiology, and Immunology* vol. 5, p. 189.

————, and C. Goldberg. 1954. "Air Pollution and Bronchitis," *British Medical Journal* vol. 2, p. 567.

Peskin, H. M., and E. P. Seskin, eds. 1975. *Cost–Benefit Analysis and Water Pollution Policy* (Washington, Urban Institute).

Petrilli, F. L., G. Agnese, and S. Kanitz. 1966. "Epidemiologic Studies of Air Pollution Effects in Genoa, Italy," *Archives of Environmental Health* vol. 12, p. 733.

Phelps, H. W. 1961. "Pulmonary Function Studies Used to Evaluate Air Pollution Asthma Disability," *Military Medicine* vol. 126, p. 282.

————. 1965. "Follow-up Studies in Tokyo–Yokohama Respiratory Disease," *Archives of Environmental Health* vol. 10, p. 143.

————, and S. Koike. 1962. "Tokyo–Yokohama Asthma," *American Review of Respiratory Disease*, vol. 86, p. 55.

————, G. W. Sobel, and N. E. Fisher. 1961. "Air Pollution Asthma Among Military Personnel in Japan," *Journal of the American Medical Association* vol. 175, p. 990.

Prest, A., and R. Turvey. 1965. "Cost–Benefit Analysis: A Survey," *Economic Journal* vol. 75, p. 683.

Preston, S. H., Keyfitz, N., and R. Schoen. 1972. *Causes of Death—Life Tables for National Populations* (New York, Seminar Press).

Prindle, R. A. 1963. "Notes Made During the London Smoke in December 1962," *Archives of Environmental Health* vol. 7, p. 493.

Prindle, R. A., G. W. Wright, R. O. McCaldin, S. C. Marcus, T. C. Lloyd, and W. E. Bye. 1963. "Comparison of Pulmonary Functions and Other Parameters in Two Communities with Widely Different Air Pollution Levels." *American Journal of Public Health* vol. 53, p. 200.

Rall, D. P. 1973. *A Review of the Health Effects of Sulfur Oxides* (Research Triangle Park, N.C., National Institute of Environmental Health Sciences).

Reid, D. D. 1956. "Symposium: Chronic Bronchitis," *Proceedings of the Royal Society of Medicine* vol. 49, p. 767.

————. 1958. "Environmental Factors in Respiratory Disease," *Lancet* vol. 1, p. 1289.

————, D. O. Anderson, B. G. Ferris, and C. M. Fletcher. 1964. "An Anglo-American Comparison of the Prevalence of Bronchitis," *British Medical Journal* vol. 2, p. 1487.

————, ————, ————, and ————. 1966. "Studies of Disease Among

Migrants and Native Populations in Great Britain, Norway, and the United States, Pt. 3." *National Cancer Institute Monographs* vol. 19, p. 321.

————, and A. S. Fairbairn. 1958. "The Natural History of Chronic Bronchitis," *Lancet* vol. 1, p. 1147.

Rice, D. 1966. *Estimating the Cost of Illness* (Washington, U.S. Public Health Service) no. 945-6.

Ridker, R. 1967. *Economic Costs of Air Pollution* (New York, Praeger).

————, and J. Henning. 1967. "The Determinants of Residential Property Values with Special Reference to Air Pollution," *Review of Economics and Statistics* vol. 49, p. 246.

Robbins, R. C. 1970. *Inquiry Into the Economic Effects of Air Pollution on Electrical Contacts* (Palo Alto, Calif., Stanford Research Institute).

Rogot, E., and W. C. Blackwelder. 1970. "Associations of Cardiovascular Mortality with Weather in Memphis, Tennessee," *Public Health Reports* vol. 85, p. 25.

Rokaw, S. N., and F. Massey. 1962. "Air Pollution and Chronic Respiratory Disease," *American Review of Respiratory Disease* vol. 86, p. 703.

Rosenbaum, S. 1961. "Home Localities of National Servicemen with Respiratory Disease," *British Journal of Preventive and Social Medicine* vol. 15, p. 61.

Saffiotti, U., F. Cefis, L. H. Kolb, and P. Shubik. 1965. "Experimental Studies of the Conditions of Exposure to Carcinogens for Lung Cancer Induction," *Journal of the Air Pollution Control Association* vol. 15, p. 23.

Salmon, R. L. 1970. *Systems Analysis of the Effects of Air Pollution on Materials* (Kansas City, Mo., Midwest Research Institute).

Salvin, V. S. 1970. *Survey and Economic Assessment of the Effects of Air Pollution on Textile Fibers and Dyes* (Raleigh, N.C., U.S. Department of Health, Education and Welfare, Public Health Service, National Air Pollution Control Administration), contract no. PH-22-68-2.

Sauer, H. T., G. H. Payne, C. R. Council, and J. C. Terrell. 1966. "Cardiovascular Disease Mortality Patterns in Georgia and North Carolina," *Public Health Reports* vol. 81, p. 455.

Schelling, T. 1968. "The Life You Save May Be Your Own," in S. Chase, ed., *Problems in Public Expenditure Analysis* (Baltimore, Johns Hopkins University Press), p. 127.

Schimmel, H., and L. Greenburg. 1972. "A Study of the Relation of Pollution to Mortality," *Journal of the Air Pollution Control Association* vol. 22, p. 607.

Schoettlin, C. E. 1962. "The Health Effect of Air Pollution on Elderly Males," *American Review of Respiratory Disease* vol. 86, p. 878.

————, and E. Landau. 1961. "Air Pollution and Asthmatic Attacks in the Los Angeles Area," *Public Health Reports* vol. 76, p. 545.

Schrenk, H. H., H. Heimann, G. D. Clayton, W. M. Gafafer, and H. Wexler. 1949. "Air Pollution in Donora, Pennsylvania: Epidemiology of Unusual Smog Episode of October 1948," *Public Health Bulletin* no. 306.

Schulte, J. H. 1963. "Effects of Mild Carbon Monoxide Intoxication," *Archives of Environmental Health* vol. 7, p. 524.

Schwing, R. C. 1976. *Risks in Perspective—Longevity as an Alternative to "Lives Saved"* (Warren, Mich., Research Laboratories, General Motors Corp.).

Scott, J. A. 1953. "Fog and Deaths in London, December 1952," *Public Health Reports* vol. 68, p. 474.

Seskin, E. P. 1973. "Residential Choice and Air Pollution: A General Equilibrium Model," *American Economic Review* vol. 63, p. 960.

———. 1976. *Air Pollution and Health in Washington, D.C.: An Analysis of Some Acute Health Effects of Air Pollution in the Washington Metropolitan Area*. (Washington, U.S. Environmental Protection Agency, Office of Research and Development) contract no. 68-01-3144.

———. n.d. "An Analysis of Some Short-term Health Effects of Air Pollution in the Washington, D.C., Metropolitan Area," *Journal of Urban Economics*. In press.

Shy, C. M., J. P. Creason, M. E. Pearlman, K. E. McClain, F. B. Benson, and M.M. Young. 1970a. "The Chattanooga School Children Study. Pt. I: Effects of Community Exposure to Nitrogen Dioxide," *Journal of the Air Pollution Control Association* vol. 20, p. 539.

———. 1970b. "The Chattanooga School Children Study. Pt. 2: Effects of Community Exposure to Nitrogen Dioxide," *Journal of the Air Pollution Control Association* vol. 20, p. 582.

———, L. Niemeyer, L. Truppi, and T. English. 1973. "Reevaluation of the Chattanooga School Children Studies and the Health Criteria for NO_2 Exposure" (Research Triangle Park, N.C., National Environmental Research Center, U.S. Environmental Protection Agency) in-house technical report.

Silverman, L. P. 1973a. "Structural and Naive Models for Forecasting Emergency Admissions" (Ph.D. dissertation, Carnegie–Mellon University, Pittsburgh, Pa.).

———. 1973b. "The Determinants of Daily Emergency Admissions to Hospitals" (Washington, D.C., Public Research Institute of the Center for Naval Analyses) working paper.

Simon, H. 1954. "Spurious Correlations: A Causal Interpretation," *Journal of the American Statistical Association* vol. 49, p. 467.

Sinclair, C., P. Marstrand, and P. Newick. 1972. "Innovation and Human Risk" (London, Centre for the Study of Industrial Innovation).

Skalpe, I. O. 1964. "Long-term Effects of Sulphur Dioxide Exposure in Pulp Mills," *British Journal of Industrial Medicine* vol. 21, p. 69.

Smith, R. B. W., E. J. Kolb, H. W. Phelps, H. A. Weiss, and A. B. Hollinden. 1964. "Tokyo–Yokohama Asthma." *Archives of Environmental Health* vol. 8, p. 805.

Smith, T. J., and H. J. Paulus. 1971. "An Epidemiological Study of Atmospheric Pollution and Bronchial Asthma Attacks." Paper presented at the Sixty-Fourth Annual Meeting of the Air Pollution Control Association, Atlantic City.

Smith, V. K. 1976. *The Economic Consequences of Air Pollution* (Cambridge, Mass., Ballinger).

Speizer, F. E., Y. Bishop, and B. G. Ferris. 1977. "An Epidemiologic Approach to the Study of the Health Effects of Air Pollution," in *Proceedings of the Fourth Symposium on Statistics and the Environment* (Washington, American Statistical Association), p. 56.

———, and B. G. Ferris, Jr. 1963. "The Prevalence of Chronic Non-specific Respiratory Disease in Road Tunnel Employees," *American Review of Respiratory Diseases* vol. 88, p. 204.

Spence, J. W., and F. H. Haynie. 1972. *Paint Technology and Air Pollution: A Survey and Economic Assessment* (Washington, U.S. Environmental Protection Agency, National Environmental Research Center).

Spicer, W. S., Jr. 1967. "Air Pollution and Meteorologic Factors," *Archives of Environmental Health* vol. 17, p. 185.

Spicer, W. S., Jr., and D. H. Kerr. 1966. "Variation of Respiratory Function in Patients and Normal Subjects," *Archives of Environmental Health* vol. 12, p. 217.

————, and ————. 1970. "Effects of Environment on Respiratory Function, Pt. III," *Archives of Environmental Health* vol. 21, p. 635.

————, W. A. Reinke, and D. H. Kerr. 1966. "Effects of Environment upon Respiratory Function, Pt. II: Daily Studies in Patients with Chronic Obstructive Lung Disease," *Archives of Environmental Health* vol. 13, p. 753.

————, P. B. Storey, W. K. C. Morgan, D. H. Kerr, and N. E. Standiford. 1962. "Variation in Respiratory Function in Selected Patients and Its Relation to Air Pollution," *American Review of Respiratory Diseases* vol. 86, p. 705.

Spodnik, M. J., Jr., G. D. Cushman, D. H. Kerr, R. W. Blide, and W. S. Spicer, Jr. 1966. "Effects of Environment on Respiratory Function: Weekly Studies on Young Male Adults," *Archives of Environmental Health* vol. 13, p. 243.

Spore, R. 1972. *Property Value Differentials as a Measure of the Economic Costs of Air Pollution* (University Park, Pennsylvania State University, Center for Air Environment Studies), no. 254-72.

Spotnitz, M. 1965. "The Significance of Yokohama Asthma," *American Review of Respiratory Diseases* vol. 92, p. 371.

Sprague, H. A., and R. Hagstrom. 1969. "The Nashville Air Pollution Study: Mortality Multiple Regression," *Archives of Environmental Health* vol. 18, p. 503.

Sterling, T. D., J. J. Phair, S. V. Pollack, D. A. Schumsky, and I. DeGroot. 1966. "Urban Morbidity and Air Pollution," *Archives of Environmental Health* vol. 13, p. 158.

————, S. V. Pollack, and J. J. Phair. 1967. "Urban Hospital Morbidity and Air Pollution: A Second Report," *Archives of Environmental Health* vol. 15, p. 362.

————, ————, and J. Weinkam. 1969. "Measuring the Effect of Air Pollution on Urban Morbidity," *Archives of Environmental Health* vol. 18, p. 485.

Stewart, R. D., J. E. Peterson, E. D. Baretta, R. T. Bachand, M. J. Hosko, and A. A. Herrmann. 1970. "Experimental Human Exposure to Carbon Monoxide," *Archives of Environmental Health* vol. 21, p. 154.

Stocks, P. 1947. "Regional and Local Differences in Cancer Death Rates," in *Studies on Medical and Population Subjects No. 1* (London, His Majesty's Stationery Office).

————. 1957. "Cancer Incidence in North Wales and Liverpool Region in Relation to Habits and Environment," suppl. to Pt. 2, *Thirty-Fifth Annual Report of the British Empire Cancer Campaign* (London, British Empire Cancer Campaign).

————. 1959. "Cancer and Bronchitis Mortality in Relation to Atmospheric Deposit and Smoke," *British Medical Journal* vol. 1, p. 74.

————. 1960. "On the Relations Between Atmospheric Pollution in Urban and Rural Localities and Mortality from Cancer, Bronchitis and Pneumonia, with Particular Reference to 3:4 Benzopyrene, Beryllium, Molybdenum, Vanadium, and Arsenic," *British Journal of Cancer* vol. 14, p. 397.

————. 1966. "Recent Epidemiological Studies of Lung Cancer Mortality, Cigarette Smoking, and Air Pollution, with Discussion of a New Hypothesis of Causation," *British Journal of Cancer* vol. 20, p. 595.

————. 1967. "Lung Cancer and Bronchitis in Relation to Cigarette Smoking and Fuel Consumption in Twenty Countries," *British Journal of Preventive and Social Medicine* vol. 21, p. 181.

———— and J. M. Campbell. 1955. "Lung Cancer Death Rates Among Nonsmokers and Pipe and Cigarette Smokers: An Evaluation in Relation to Air Pollution by Benzopyrene and Other Substances," *British Medical Journal* vol. 2, p. 923.

Sultz, H. A., J. G. Feldman, E. R. Schlesinger, and W. E. Mosher. 1970. "An Effect of Continued Exposure to Air Pollution on the Incidence of Chronic Childhood Allergic Disease," *American Journal of Public Health* vol. 60, p. 891.

Thaler, R., and S. Rosen. 1976. "The Value of Saving A Life: Evidence from the Labor Market," in N. Terleckyj, ed., *Household Production and Consumption* (New York, National Bureau of Economic Research), p. 265.

Toyama, T. 1964. "Air Pollution and Health Effects in Japan," *Archives of Environmental Health* vol. 8, p. 153.

Tromp, S. W. 1968. "Influence of Weather and Climate on Asthma and Bronchitis," *Review of Allergy* vol. 22, p. 1027.

U.S. Bureau of the Census. 1973. *Census of Population: 1970. Subject Reports. Mobility by States and the Nation,* PC (2)-2B (Washington, GPO).

U.S. Department of Agriculture. 1941. *Climate and Man, 1941 Yearbook of Agriculture* (Washington, GPO).

U.S. Department of Health, Education and Welfare. 1970. *Air Quality Criteria for Sulfur Oxides,* National Air Pollution Control Administration no. AP-50.

U.S. Environmental Protection Agency. 1972. *The Economics of Clean Air.* Annual Report of the EPA.

U.S. National Center for Health Statistics. 1962. *International Classification of Diseases, Adapted for Indexing Hospital Records by Diseases and Operations.* U.S. Public Health Service no. 719.

Ury, H. K., N. M. Perkins, and J. R. Goldsmith. 1972. "Motor Vehicle Accidents and Vehicular Pollution in Los Angeles," *Archives of Environmental Health* vol. 25, p. 314.

Usher, D. 1973. "An Imputation to the Measure of Economic Growth for Changes in Life Expectancy," in M. Moss, ed., *The Measurement of Economic and Social Performance* (New York, National Bureau of Economic Research), p. 193.

Verma, M. P., F. J. Schilling, and W. H. Becker. 1969. "Epidemiological Study of Illness Absences in Relation to Air Pollution," *Archives of Environmental Health* vol. 18, p. 536.

Waddell, T. E. 1974. *The Economic Damages of Air Pollution,* EPA Publication, Socioeconomic Environmental Studies, series report EPA-600/5-74-012 (Washington, GPO).

Wallace, T. D., and A. Hussain. 1969. "The Use of Error Components Models in Combining Cross-section with Time-series Data," *Econometrica* vol. 37, p. 55.

Waller, R. E. 1971. "Air Pollution and Community Health," *Journal of the Royal College of Physicians (London)* vol. 5, p. 362.

————, and P. J. Lawther. 1955. "Some Observations on London Fog," *British Medical Journal* vol. 2, p. 1356.

————, and ————. 1957. "Further Observations on London Fog," *British Medical Journal* vol. 4, p. 1473.

Wayne, W. S., and P. F. Wehrle. 1969. "Oxidant Air Pollution and School Absenteeism," *Archives of Environmental Health* vol. 19, p. 315.

————, ————, and R. E. Carroll. 1967. "Oxidant Air Pollution and Athletic Performance," *Journal of the American Medical Association* vol. 199, p. 901.

Weidensaul, T. C., and N. L. Lacasse. 1970. *Statewide Survey of Air Pollution Damage to Vegetation—1969.* (University Park, Pennsylvania State University, Center for Air Environment Studies).

Weill, H., M. M. Ziskind, V. Derbes, R. Lewis, R. J. M. Horton, and R. O. McCaldin. 1964. "Further Observations on New Orleans Asthma," *Archives of Environmental Health* vol. 8, p. 184.

Wicken, A. J., and S. F. Buck. 1964. *Report on a Study of Environmental Factors Associated with Lung Cancer and Bronchitis Mortality in Areas of North East England* (London, Tobacco Research Council) research paper no. 8.

Wieand, K. F. 1973. "Air Pollution and Property Values: A Study of the Saint Louis Area," *Journal of Regional Science* vol. 13, p. 91.

Wilkens, E. T. 1954. "Air Pollution and the London Fog of December, 1952," *Journal of the Royal Sanitary Institute* vol. 74, p. 1.

Winkelstein, W., Jr., and M. L. Gay. 1971. "Suspended Particulate Air Pollution," *Archives of Environmental Health* vol. 22, p. 174.

Winkelstein, W., Jr., and S. Kantor. 1969a. "Prostatic Cancer: Relationship to Suspended Particulate Air Pollution," *American Journal of Public Health* vol. 59, p. 1134.

————, and ————. 1969b. "Respiratory Symptoms and Air Pollution in an Urban Population of Northeastern United States," *Archives of Environmental Health* vol. 18, p. 760.

————, and ————. 1969c. "Stomach Cancer: Positive Association with Suspended Particulate Air Pollution," *Archives of Environmental Health* vol. 18, p. 544.

————, ————, E. W. Davis, C. S. Maneri and W. E. Mosher. 1967. "The Relationship of Air Pollution and Economic Status to Total Mortality and Selected Respiratory System Mortality in Men, pt. I: Suspended Particulates," *Archives of Environmental Health* vol. 14, p. 162.

————, ————, ————, ————, and ————. 1968. "The Relationship of Air Pollution and Economic Status to Total Mortality and Selected Respiratory System Mortality in Men, pt. II," *Archives of Environmental Health* vol. 16, p. 401.

World Health Organization. 1972. "Air Quality Criteria and Guides for Urban Air Pollutants," Report of a WHO Expert Committee, Geneva, WHO Technical Report Series, no. 506: 21.

Yocum, J. E., and R. O. McCaldin. 1968. "Effects of Air Pollution on Materials and the Economy, in A. C. Stern, ed., *Air Pollution*, vol. 1 (2nd ed., New York, Academic Press), p. 617.

Yoshida, K., H. Oshima, and M. Imai. 1966. "Air Pollution and Asthma in Yokkaichi," *Archives of Environmental Health* vol. 13, p. 763.

————, Y. Takatsuka, and M. Kitabatake. 1969. "Air Pollution and its Health Effects in Yokkaichi Area: Review on Yokkaichi Asthma," *Mie Medical Journal* vol. 18, p. 195.

Yoshii, M., J. Nonoyama, H. Oshma, H. Yamagiwa, and S. Takeda. 1969. "Chronic Pharyngitis in Air-polluted Districts of Yokkaichi in Japan," *Mie Medical Journal* vol. 19, p. 17.

Young, W. A., D. B. Shaw, and D. V. Bates. 1963. "Pulmonary Function in Welders Exposed to Ozone," *Archives of Environmental Health* vol. 7, p. 337.

Zeckhauser, R., A. Harberger, R. Haveman, L. E. Lynn, Jr., W. A. Niskanen, and A. Williams, eds. 1975. *Benefit–Cost and Policy Analysis, 1974* (Chicago, Aldine).

Zeidberg, L. D., R. J. M. Horton, and E. Landau. 1967a. "The Nashville Air Pollution Study, pt. V: Mortality from Diseases of the Respiratory System in Relation to Air Pollution," *Archives of Environmental Health* vol. 15, p. 214.

————, ————, and ————. 1967b. "The Nashville Air Pollution Study, pt. VI: Cardiovascular Disease Mortality in Relation to Air Pollution," *Archives of Environmental Health* vol. 15, p. 225.

————, and R. A. Prindle. 1963. "The Nashville Air Pollution Study, pt. II: Pulmonary Anthracosis as an Index of Air Pollution," *American Journal of Public Health* vol. 53, p. 185.

————, ————, and E. Landau. 1961. "The Nashville Air Pollution Study, pt. I: Sulfur Dioxide and Bronchial Asthma," *American Review of Respiratory Diseases* vol. 84, p. 489.

————, ————, and ————. 1964. "The Nashville Air Pollution Study, pt. III: Morbidity in Relation to Air Pollution," *American Journal of Public Health* vol. 54, p. 85.

SECTION V

Appendixes

A review of the literature relating air pollution to health

The first portion of this review deals with cross-sectional studies and is organized by disease. The diseases include bronchitis and emphysema; pneumonia, tuberculosis, and asthma; total respiratory disease; lung cancer; total and non-respiratory-tract cancers; cardiovascular disease; and total and miscellaneous morbidity and mortality. The next section provides a review of time-series studies that have used daily, weekly, and monthly observations. The final part of the review examines studies that have related mobile-source pollution to health effects. In addition, appendix G classifies all the studies discussed in the appendixes, as well as those discussed in the text, by specific air pollutants. It includes the page number on which the major discussion of each study is located. For specific publication information, the interested reader is referred to the References (pages 251–270).

CROSS-SECTIONAL STUDIES BY DISEASE

Bronchitis and emphysema

Many studies have investigated the association between air pollution and bronchitis. One difficulty in comparing such studies is that a disease like chronic bronchitis is not always consistently defined (see Goldsmith, 1968). In addition, many different measures of pollution have been considered, ranging from actual measurements of sulfur dioxide and suspended particulates to "presumptive pollution," as measured by fog density.[1]

United States. Winkelstein and his coauthors (1967) collected data from twenty-one areas in and around Buffalo, New York, and compared those areas in terms of the level of air pollution (suspended particulates), income level,

[1] Goldsmith (1965) also presented a general discussion of factors influencing the disease. A comparison between the prevalence of bronchitis in Britain and the United States can be found in Reid and his coauthors (1964). Fletcher (1958) discussed the relationships between exposure to dust and morbidity and mortality from chronic bronchitis.

and the mortality rate for chronic respiratory disease (asthma, bronchitis, chronic interstitial pneumonia, bronchiectasis, and emphysema), making use of cross tabulations. Many physical characteristics were controlled; the death rates were age–race–sex-specific. Some attempt was made to control for socioeconomic characteristics; the median family income of an area was classified into one of five levels and used as a control in the analysis. While this method is less powerful in controlling income than if income data had been treated quantitatively, it does provide some control. Other socioeconomic factors (median number of years of school completed, percentage of laborers in the labor force, and percentage of sound housing) were also mentioned. The only environmental factor controlled was air pollution, as measured by suspended particulates. No data on personal factors were available.

The results indicated a close association between air pollution (suspended particulates) and chronic respiratory disease mortality, since a trend existed between pollution and mortality for each economic level. When areas ranging from pollution level 1 to level 4 were compared, the mortality rate increased by more than 100 percent in white males aged fifty to sixty-nine years.[2] The other socioeconomic factors were compared across areas, and, despite some differences, it appeared unlikely that they could account for the observed patterns in the mortality rate. Unfortunately, since no multivariable statistical analysis was performed, one cannot estimate the increase in mortality associated with air pollution, while controlling for these other factors. However, the study does provide evidence of a causal relationship between air pollution and chronic respiratory disease mortality, even though it is difficult to estimate the magnitude of the association.[3]

Using similar methods, Zeidberg, Horton, and Landau (1967a) found no association between air pollution levels and mortality from bronchitis and emphysema in Nashville, Tennessee. Air pollution was measured by sulfation (sulfur trioxide), soiling (concentration of haze and smoke), dustfall, and twenty-four-hour sulfur dioxide concentrations. The factors possibly responsible for the lack of significant results were discussed by the authors. We discuss some of these in chapter 2 (pages 17–18).

In another study, Zeidberg and Prindle (1963) investigated a total of 641 consecutive autopsies (excluding subjects under five years of age) for evidence of pulmonary anthracosis. Among Nashville residents, deposition of anthracotic pigment increased with length of residence and, in females. was more severe

[2] The five economic levels, based on median family income in a census tract, were as follows: $3,005–$5,007; $5,175–$6,004; $6,013–$6,614; $6,618–$7,347; and $7,431–$11,792. The four air pollution levels (in micrograms) of suspended particulates (per cubic meter per twenty-four hours) were as follows: less than 80; 80–100; 100–135; and more than 135. For economic level 1, the death rates (per 100,000) for pollution levels 2 through 4 were 126, 271, and 392, respectively. For economic level 2, the death rates for air pollution levels 1 through 4 were 136, 145, 172, and 199, respectively. For economic level 3, the death rates for air pollution levels 2 through 4 were 74, 110, and 128, respectively. For economic level 4, the death rates for pollution levels 1 through 3 were 70, 80, and 177, respectively. For economic level 5, the death rates for air pollution levels 1 through 3 were 79, 109, and zero, respectively.

[3] Winkelstein and coauthors (1968) performed a similar study using sulfur oxide concentrations as an index of air pollution. A positive association was found between sulfation and chronic respiratory disease mortality in the two lowest economic groups (the only two groups with sufficient data).

in those who had lived in the most polluted areas of the city (as measured by concentration of haze and smoke). Examination of socioeconomic class (based on hospital pay status) and history of other related diseases failed to indicate patterns that would account for the findings.

Ishikawa and coauthors (1969) estimated the incidence of emphysema in Winnipeg, Canada, and Saint Louis. They examined the lungs of 300 victims of accidental death in each city, matching the samples in terms of age, sex, race, and smoking habits. Thus, they controlled for physical characteristics, compared air pollution exposure by contrasting residents of the two cities, and controlled for smoking habits. Other personal factors and socioeconomic characteristics were not controlled. The incidence and severity of emphysema was higher in Saint Louis, the city with the more polluted air, for each comparison group (over twenty-five years of age). For example, in the forty-five-year-old age group, 5 percent of those in Winnipeg and 46 percent of those in Saint Louis showed evidence of emphysema.

Hammond (1967) did a retrospective study of emphysema mortality and morbidity among males aged forty-five to seventy-four. In addition to age, he collected information on occupational exposure to pollution, probable urban exposure, and smoking habits. Although his analysis controlled for physical characteristics of the population and exposure to pollution and smoking habits, it did not control for many socioeconomic characteristics or other personal factors. Cross tabulations revealed a significant effect of occupational exposure to pollution as well as a strong interaction between occupational exposure and smoking. There was some indication that, among nonsmokers (with and without occupational exposure), rural rates were higher than metropolitan rates; however, these differences were very small.

Great Britain. Bronchitis mortality rates in England and Wales have been correlated with pollution.[4] Stocks (1959), after eliminating the effects of population density, found significant correlations between bronchitis (sex-specific rates) and both a deposit index and smoke. In another study, which controlled for both population density and an index of social class, Stocks (1960) found significant correlations of bronchitis death rates with smoke density. Ashley (1967) also found a positive correlation between mortality from bronchitis (combining sexes) and air pollution (smoke and sulfur dioxide), while controlling for population density. In a later study, which controlled for population density, social class, and type of town, Ashley (1969a) found a significant positive association between air pollution (particularly smoke) and the bronchitis death rate in males. The only physical characteristic sometimes controlled for in these studies was sex. The various social indexes used accounted for several important socioeconomic factors. Air pollution was the only environmental factor controlled. No personal factors were considered.

In an attempt to isolate the independent effects of the factors represented in these studies, we performed a multivariable regressions analysis on data reported by Stocks (1959, 1960) and Ashley (1967), as shown in table A.1. We fit Equation A.1 to the data:

$$MR_i = a_0 + a_1 P_i + a_2 SE_i + e_i \hspace{3cm} \text{A.1}$$

where MR_i is the mortality rate for a particular disease in county borough i,

---

[4] For a review of some of the early British studies, see Martin (1961).

TABLE A.1. Bronchitis Mortality (Data from England and Wales)

	A.1-1[a] M	A.1-2[a] F	A.1-3[b] M	A.1-4[b] F	A.1-5[a] M	A.1-6[c] F	A.1-7[c] M	A.1-8[c] F	A.1-9[d] M	A.1-10[d] M
R^2	.386	.332	.433	.412	.766	.559	.783	.601	.377	.300
Constant	58.158	62.523	58.630	44.307	18.645	34.543	−1.533	13.303	63.518	67.808
Air pollution variables										
Deposit index	.182 (4.80)	.182 (4.55)								
Smoke			1.891 (3.79)	1.756 (3.23)	.310 (3.77)	.303 (2.84)	.301 (5.86)	.213 (3.30)	.199 (4.07)	
Sulfur dioxide										.161 (3.05)
Socioeconomic variables										
Persons per acre	.016 (.22)	−.031 (−.42)	.180 (1.86)	.252 (2.40)	.062 (.53)	−.038 (−.25)			.160 (3.02)	.151 (2.64)
Social class							.176 (1.44)	.248 (1.59)		

Note: The numbers in parentheses below the regression coefficients are t statistics.
Abbreviations: M, males; F, females.
[a] Based on data for fifty-three county boroughs.
[b] Based on data for twenty-eight county boroughs.
[c] Based on data for twenty-six areas.
[d] Based on data for fifty-three urban areas.

P_i is a measure of air pollution in that borough; SE_i is a measure of socio-economic status in borough i; and e_i is an error term with a mean of zero.[5]

The first regression in table A.1 relates the bronchitis mortality rate for men to a deposit index and to the population density in each of the fifty-three county boroughs. Almost 39 percent of the variation in the mortality rate (across boroughs) was "explained" by the regressions. A unit increase in the deposit index (1 gm per 100 m² per month) was associated with an increase of 0.18 percent in the bronchitis mortality rate (with population per acre held constant). An increase in the population density of 0.10 persons per acre was associated with an increase of 0.02 percent in the mortality rate (with air pollution held constant). As indicated in table A.1 by the t statistics, the air pollution variable was extremely significant, whereas the socioeconomic variable contributed little to the explanatory power of the regression.

The ten regressions in table A.1 attempt to explain the bronchitis death rate. Four different data sets were used, along with three measures of pollution and two socioeconomic variables. The coefficients of determination, R^2 (the proportion of the variation in the mortality rate explained by the regression), ranged from 0.300 to 0.783. Air pollution was a significant explanatory variable in all cases. In only three cases was the socioeconomic variable significant.

The implication of the first regression is that a 10 percent decrease in the deposit rate (37.5 gm per 100 m² per month) was associated in this sample with a 7 percent decrease in the bronchitis death rate. Or, for the same sample, improving the quality of air to that enjoyed by the borough having the best air of the total sample (a standard deposit rate for all boroughs of 96 gm per 100 m² per month), would be associated with a fall in the average mortality rate from 129 to 77. Thus, cleaning the air to the level enjoyed by the area with the best air could mean a 40 percent drop in the bronchitis death rate among males. In regression A.1-5 the pollution variable was a smoke index, and a different set of areas was considered. This is more successful in terms of the percentage of variation explained ($R^2 = 0.766$). As before, the air pollution coefficient was extremely significant, and the suggestion is that cleaning the air to the level exhibited by the area with the best air (15 mg per 100 m³) would be associated with a fall in the average bronchitis mortality rate from 106 to 30, a drop of 70 percent. Results of the other regressions based on the mortality data had similar implications. Note that the effect was almost identical for males and females. This indicates reliability and suggests that the effect is independent of occupational exposure, although other explanations are not ruled out.

Other studies in Great Britain have also revealed a positive association between bronchitis mortality and air pollution. Gardner, Crawford, and Morris (1969) utilized linear multivariable regression analysis to examine death rates across sixty-one county boroughs in England and Wales in terms of five independent variables: social score (the first principal component of nine social indexes), air pollution (coal bought for domestic consumption), latitude, water calcium, and rainfall. They had data on four age–sex rates (males and females,

---

[5] Each of the relations in table A.1 was estimated in alternative ways, including transformation into logarithms, a general quadratic, and a "piecewise" linear form. The implications as to the roles of air pollution and of the socioeconomic variables were unchanged by use of the different functional forms.

aged forty-five to sixty-four and sixty-five to seventy-four) for two time periods. For bronchitis mortality they found statistically significant effects of air pollution for each of the four age–sex categories in six of the eight data sets.

Buck and Brown (1964) found that sex-specific bronchitis mortality had a significant, positive association with smoke and sulfur dioxide concentrations in areas of England and Wales. Persons per acre, and a social index (proportion of unskilled workers among adult males) were used as socioeconomic controls. Inclusion of a variable representing current smoking habits did not alter the results. No other personal or environmental factors were controlled.

Wicken and Buck (1964) studied bronchitis mortality in six areas of northeast England. The fact that rates were relatively higher in the two urban districts compared with those of four rural districts could not be fully accounted for by age composition, smoking habits, or social-class distribution (based on occupation) of the respective populations. The urban district with the highest bronchitis death rate also had the highest levels of air pollution (smoke). Furthermore, within that district, the locality with the higher measured level of air pollution (smoke and sulfur dioxide) had higher bronchitis mortality among males. Similar results were reported for the other urban district; however, they were based on presumptive rather than measured pollution. The authors also noted that bronchitis mortality appeared to be more strongly associated with the level of air pollution than with smoking habits.

In a later paper, Buck and Wicken (1967) employed a multiplicative model to explain bronchitis mortality rates for males in Northern Ireland. Using variables representing urban–rural residence and the combined effects of smoking and family history of bronchitis, they found that the model fit the data quite closely and that increased mortality was significantly associated with increased urbanization. Two similar models were used to explain male bronchitis death rates for northeast England. One used variables representing urban–rural residence and smoking habits; the other substituted social class (based on occupation) for smoking habits. The models were estimated separately because of data limitations. Again, urbanization was positively related to bronchitis mortality when the other factors were controlled.

Daly (1959) found significant correlations between bronchitis mortality for males aged forty-five to sixty-four years and indexes of domestic and industrial pollution.[6] When the effects of two social indexes were eliminated by using the combined partial correlation coefficient, a correlation coefficient of 0.47 was obtained between mortality and pollution. Unfortunately, the exact social indexes were not specified, although they were taken from the following four socioeconomic factors: social class, overcrowding, population density, and education. As in the previous studies, "air pollution" was the only environmental factor controlled. No personal factors were accounted for.

Fairbairn and Reid (1958), in a study of thirty-seven areas of the United Kingdom, found a highly significant association between a fog index and bronchitis mortality in both sexes at ages forty-five to sixty-four, using second-order, product-moment correlations. These correlations allowed for variation in only two social factors, population density and domestic overcrowding. It should be noted that the use of a fog index is only an indirect control for air

[6] These indexes were only proxies for actual air pollution levels.

pollution levels and climatological characteristics. Other environmental factors and personal factors were left uncontrolled.

Pemberton and Goldberg (1954) found a significant correlation between sulfur dioxide pollution and bronchitis mortality rates for men aged forty-five and older in the county boroughs of England and Wales. Less consistent results were found for women and for associations with suspended particulate pollution. Correlations between sulfur dioxide pollution and two social indexes (the number of persons per room and an income classification) were not significant. However, the failure to use a multivariable statistical technique means that the independent or supplementary effects of pollution cannot be assessed. Other environmental factors or personal characteristics were not controlled.

Hewitt (1956) found a significant correlation ($r = 0.79$) between bronchitis mortality (standardized) and an air pollution index (based on sulfur dioxide concentration and duration of exposure) in nine public health divisions of London. Correlations were also presented between aggregate respiratory disease mortality and several social indexes in London boroughs; however, no multivariable analysis was performed to account for the combined effects of these factors.

Gorham (1958) computed a logarithmic correlation of 0.32 (significant at the 5 percent level) between the five-year bronchitis mortality rates in fifty-three county and metropolitan boroughs of Great Britain and winter sulfate deposits. No specific controls were imposed. (The correlation with acidity of urban precipitation was -0.49.)

Burgess and Shaddick (1959) did not find a significant relationship between sex-specific bronchitis mortality rates and pollution (smoke and sulfur dioxide) for eight areas in and around London. Although they had data on social class and the percentage of subjects born in London, they did not control for these effects in their analysis. Only simple correlations were considered. No other factors affecting health care were accounted for in the analysis.

Dean (1966) interviewed the families of bronchitis and lung cancer decedents in Northern Ireland to control for such factors as smoking, area of residence, social class (occupation), and previous history of illness (in subjects and relatives). He found that bronchitis mortality was associated mainly with urbanization and smoking habits; for example, among male nonsmokers bronchitis mortality rates were three to four times as high in Belfast as in "truly rural" districts, even when social class was controlled.

Another group of studies in Great Britain used measures of morbidity to explore the association between bronchitis and air pollution. Several of these have been made on homogeneous occupation groups, such as postal employees (Holland and Reid, 1965; Reid, 1956, 1958; Reid and Fairbairn, 1958; Fairbairn and Reid, 1958). The results are relatively pure in that the members of the sample had comparable incomes, working conditions, and social status. Researchers analyzing absences, questionnaires, and lung-function tests concluded that postmen become disabled by bronchitis in areas where fog and specific types of air pollution are prevalent.[7] Cornwall and Raffle (1961) tabulated absences due to bronchitis among London Transport employees during a

[7] In the studies controlling for smoking habits, socioeconomic characteristics, occupational factors, residence, or age, the effect was still significant.

four-year period and found a close association between sickness absence and fog (a surrogate for air pollution). Workers were classified by type of job, age, and work site (London was divided into four areas); the researchers believed that workers resided near their place of work.

Lammers, Schilling, and Walford (1964) compared English and Dutch cotton workers (males fifteen to sixty-four years of age) on the basis of questionnaires and medical examinations. The prevalence of chronic bronchitis and other respiratory symptoms was higher (but not significantly so after controlling for age) in the English than in the Dutch workers. These differences were discussed in relation to smoking habits, occupational exposure (cotton dust), and air pollution (smoke and sulfur dioxide). Differences in pollution were judged the most likely explanation of the observed differences in the incidence of respiratory disease. Other socioeconomic and environmental factors were not controlled; however, it was noted that the social security system in the Netherlands might encourage relatively more illness absence among the Dutch workers.

To determine the prevalence of chronic bronchitis, Higgins (1966) compared readings of lung function for more than 1,300 men in five towns of the United Kingdom. Peak expiratory flow rate was lower in urban than in rural areas and lower still among urban miners and ex-miners. As noted previously, however, attributing such a finding to differences in air pollution levels is problematic, since many important factors not controlled for may be systematically related to urban residence.

Lambert and Reid (1970) obtained information from more than 18,000 men and women (a random sample of a "healthy" population aged thirty-five to sixty-nine) by means of postal questionnaires. Unlike the study above (Higgins, 1966), smoking was controlled. They found that the urban–rural gradient in bronchitis symptoms could not be explained by smoking differences alone, although local pollution seemed to have little effect on nonsmokers. Because of the many uncontrolled factors, one cannot have great confidence in the association between bronchitis symptoms (in smokers) and air pollution. (The air pollutants mentioned included smoke, sulfur dioxide, and an index of coal consumption.)

Other countries. Similar studies have taken place in other countries. Petrilli, Agnese, and Kanitz (1966), studying mortality and morbidity data for Genoa, Italy, found that the frequency of bronchitis was highly correlated with pollution levels (especially sulfur dioxide). The subjects considered were nonsmoking women over sixty-five years of age who had lived for a long period in the same area and who had never worked in industry. Emphasis was also given to domestic heating facilities, overcrowding, and the height of dwelling. Although other personal factors were not considered, the study should be lauded for the number of controls exerted.

In Japan, Toyama (1964) looked at bronchitis mortality for twenty-one districts in Tokyo and discovered a significant correlation ($r = 0.41$) with monthly dustfall. Yoshida, Oshima, and Imai (1966) found two to six times the number of chronic bronchitis cases in districts polluted primarily from dustfall and sulfur dioxide as relatively unpolluted districts of Yokkaichi, Japan (see also Yoshida, Takatsuka, and Kitabatake, 1969). Unfortunately, these studies failed to account for factors other than pollution that may have varied across the areas being compared.

Cederlöf (1966) performed a clever investigation of Swedish twins of the same sex. Information was collected on the twins' zygosity, smoking habits, residential history, and certain disease symptoms. The prevalence of bronchitis symptoms was higher among smoking men in urban areas than for those in rural areas,[8] which suggested that a specific urban factor, such as air pollution, was interacting with smoking. Generally commendable because of the number of factors controlled, this study is particularly noteworthy as one of the few instances in which genetic factors were controlled.

Biersteker (1969) failed to find a significant association between bronchitis mortality or morbidity symptoms and pollution (measured by years of residence) in male municipal employees in Rotterdam, the Netherlands, when smoking habits were accounted for. Again, pollution was measured indirectly. Other personal characteristics were not considered.

Finally, in a study across twenty countries, Stocks (1967) found, only for the United Kingdom, a significant correlation between bronchitis mortality and solid fuel consumption. Fuel consumption was used as a surrogate for pollution, and all the other factors that might vary across countries were left uncontrolled.

Pneumonia, tuberculosis, and asthma

United States. Mills (1943), in a classic study of wards in Pittsburgh and Cincinnati, during 1929–30, reported significant correlations between pneumonia death rates and pollution as measured by sootfall. For white males, the correlation was 0.47 in Pittsburgh and 0.79 in Cincinnati. The actual variation in the corresponding death rates was zero to 7,852 per 100,000 population for Pittsburgh and 41 to 165 for Cincinnati. Mills also found that death rates fell significantly as the altitude of an individual's residence increased; there was a drop of approximately 10 percent in death rate for every 100 ft (30 m) of elevation. He argued that since the male rates were generally higher than those for females, omitted socioeconomic variables could not account for the observed correlations; however, he made no attempt to control such variables in the study. Similarly, no other environmental differences between the cities or personal factors of the populations were considered. In another study, Mills (1952) investigated age–sex–race-specific death rates for pneumonia in Chicago and found that rates were always higher in the more polluted (sootfall and sulfur dioxide) areas of the city. Differences were greatest for the youngest age group studied (thirty to thirty-nine year olds). No socioeconomic or other controls were used.

Sultz and coauthors (1970) analyzed children under sixteen years of age in Erie County, New York, who were hospitalized for asthma and eczema.

[8] This observation was made on the first-born twin in each set (treating them as a random sample), as well as on the pairs with similar smoking habits but different residential histories.

TABLE A.2. Pneumonia Mortality (Data from England and Wales)

	A.2-1 M	A.2-2 F	A.2-3 M	A.2-4 F
R^2	.477	.253	.475	.242
Constant	90.569	95.268	71.714	77.374
Air pollution variables Smoke	.118 (1.34)	.068 (.58)	.159 (2.81)	.124 (1.64)
Socioeconomic variables Persons per acre	.121 (.97)	.137 (.83)		
Social class			.126 (.93)	.106 (.58)

Note: All regressions based on data for twenty-six areas. The numbers in parentheses below the regression coefficients are *t* statistics.
Abbreviations: M, males; *F,* females.

They found "a striking association between air pollution [suspended particulates] level and the incidence of asthma and eczema among boys under five years of age (page 4)."[9] Cross tabulations were presented in which social class (based on median income, education, and the unemployment rate in 1960) was used to account for some important socioeconomic characteristics. No other factors were considered.

Great Britain. A number of British investigators who examined the relationship between bronchitis mortality and air pollution also looked at the association between pneumonia death rates and air pollution.

Stocks (1960) reported data on pneumonia mortality, by sex, for twenty-six areas of northern England and Wales. As shown by our reworking of his data (table A.2), there appeared to be a positive relationship between a smoke index and pneumonia mortality. The relationship was much stronger for men than for women.

Daly (1959) published simple correlations of 0.60 for pneumonia mortality and consumption of domestic fuels and 0.52 for pneumonia mortality and consumption of industrial fuels. For tuberculosis mortality, the correlations were 0.59 and 0.22, respectively. Although simple correlations of both types of mortality with four socioeconomic indexes (social class, overcrowding, population density, and education) were presented, no multivariable method was used.

Fairbairn and Reid (1958) found that mortality from pneumonia (in males aged forty-five to sixty-four) was significantly correlated with a fog index. The correlation for mortality in females was not statistically significant. As previously discussed, they controlled for population density and domestic overcrowding, but not for other socioeconomic factors or personal habits, such as smoking.

[9] The air pollution levels were the same as those used in the study by Winkelstein and coauthors (1967).

Gorham (1959) found that winter sulfate deposits showed a significant correlation with the five-year pneumonia mortality rates in fifty-three areas of Great Britain ($r = 0.35$). As in his previous 1958 study, no specific controls were considered.

Hewitt (1956) found significant correlations between air pollution (as measured by sulfur dioxide and duration of exposure) and both pneumonia and tuberculosis mortality across nine public health divisions in London. For pneumonia, the correlation was 0.65; for tuberculosis, 0.82.

Other countries. In Japan, a type of asthma has been documented that some investigators say differs clinically from the usual symptoms of the disease.[10] It is usually termed Tokyo–Yokohama asthma and has been related to air pollution of the industrialized Kanto Plain. Phelps, Sobel, and Fisher (1961) reported its effects on U.S. Army personnel and their families stationed in the area. More than 100 patients were studied; three cases were discussed in detail. In a later report, Phelps (1961) noted that all patients had a marked airflow obstruction. Another distinguishing characteristic of the disease was the prompt relief experienced by patients removed from the area. However, in a subsequent paper, Phelps and Koike (1962) observed that a number of patients continued to show symptoms of the disease after returning to the United States. A final follow-up study by Phelps (1965), on some of the patients after they left Japan, concluded that Tokyo–Yokohama respiratory disease was a bronchitic illness induced by the combined effects of cigarette smoking and the severe air pollution present in the Tokyo–Yokohama area.[11]

Yoshida, Takatsuka, and Kitabatake (1969) looked at bronchial asthma among Japanese inhabitants in the Yokkaichi area of Japan and found similarities to the situation in the Tokyo–Yokohama region. Asthmatic attacks among thirteen patients were correlated with weekly sulfur dioxide concentrations recorded in the immediate vicinity of the patients' residences ($r = 0.88$). Unfortunately, no controls were mentioned.

Total respiratory disease

United States. Winkelstein and Kantor (1969b) used questionnaires to analyze the relationship between cough and air pollution among 842 white females in the Buffalo, New York, area.[12] A positive association was found between suspended particulates and cough (with phlegm) in nonsmokers (aged forty-five and older) and among smokers who had not moved within the previous five years; among smokers who had moved, the association was inverse. No associations were found between cough and sulfur oxides. In addition

[10] Spotnitz (1965) compared forty-two patients who first developed asthma in the region with thirty-two patients who had asthma prior to coming to Japan and concluded that "it is doubtful that recognition of Yokohama asthma as a distinct clinical entity is justified (p. 374)."

[11] Other studies that discuss the incidence of Tokyo–Yokohama asthma include Ladd and Phelps (1963), Motley and Phelps (1964), Smith and coauthors (1964), and Toyama (1964). Toyama (1964) also examined pneumonia mortality, but did not find a significant correlation with monthly dustfall.

[12] Also, for an excellent discussion of the literature relating air pollution to respiratory disease, see Holland (1972).

to age, sex, race, smoking, and residential mobility, years of schooling and history of bronchitis were considered.

Zeidberg, Horton, and Landau (1967a) studied mortality in Nashville and found that total respiratory disease mortality (age–sex–race-adjusted) was directly related to the degree of sulfation (sulfur trioxide) and soiling (concentration of haze and smoke), although death rates for some specific diseases followed no definite pattern. Neither twenty-four-hour sulfur dioxide levels nor measures of dustfall were significantly related to total respiratory disease mortality. Mortality rate differences were higher for men than women and for nonwhites than whites. Socioeconomic differences (based on occupational level, schooling, domestic overcrowding, and median family income) could not explain the observed associations.

Lepper and coauthors (1969) undertook a similar study in Chicago. Using cross tabulations, they reported that total respiratory deaths varied with the concentration of sulfur dioxide across areas of the city when socioeconomic class (based on median income, education, and unemployment) was controlled. No other factors influencing health were considered. Restricting the comparison to adults or to whites weakened the evidence of association.

Shy and coauthors (1970a, 1970b, 1973) studied the relationship between acute respiratory illness and nitrogen dioxide exposure across areas of Chattanooga, Tennessee, using a biweekly survey between November 1968 and April 1969. A total of 871 families with 4,043 individuals participated. They were selected from three schools in a high exposure area and from two other neighborhoods experiencing lower exposures. At the time of the survey, nitrogen dioxide concentrations were determined by a method which was subsequently shown to be unreliable; however, alternative data were obtained for a corresponding period one year earlier (December 1967 to November 1968). Acute respiratory illness rates were higher among families residing in the area of relatively high nitrogen dioxide exposure, although the rates were not consistently correlated with the nitrogen dioxide exposure gradient among the three schools in the high exposure area. The relative excess could not be explained by differences in family composition, economic levels (as measured by market value of home), education (of family head), or prevalence of chronic conditions. Parental smoking habits did not appear to influence respiratory illness rates among children, but the effects on the parents themselves were not mentioned. No meteorological factors were controlled in the analysis.[13]

A subsequent study in Chattanooga was undertaken by Pearlman and coauthors (1971). They investigated the relationship between illness of the lower respiratory tract and nitrogen dioxide exposure in 3,217 school children and infants. Using the areas designated in the above analysis and controlling for years of exposure, the study found that one or more episodes of bronchitis were reported significantly more often by school children residing for two and three years in areas subjected to high and intermediate nitrogen dioxide levels. This pattern was not consistent for infants, and in no case did the high and intermediate exposure cohorts differ significantly. Similar results were found

---

[13] Levels of suspended nitrates, sulfates, and total particulates were also given. Except for sulfates, they followed the same gradient as did the concentrations of nitrogen dioxide.

for children reporting three or more episodes of bronchitis. Neither morbidity from croup and pneumonia nor hospitalization records differed significantly among the three exposure areas. No specific controls except for exposure were mentioned in the study. In yet another Chattanooga study, Chapman and co-authors (1973) investigated the prevalence of chronic respiratory disease among parents of high-school students residing in the exposure areas. The prevalance of chronic bronchitis among these adults was not associated with the nitrogen dioxide pollution gradient (current or past) across the three areas.

Several studies have compared the prevalence of respiratory disease between two small towns. Ferris and Anderson (1962) examined chronic respiratory disease in Berlin, New Hampshire, analyzing questionnaires as well as measuring respiratory function. Although they found cigarette smoking habits were strongly related to the occurrence of respiratory disease, the relation between chronic respiratory symptoms and air pollution (based on area of residence) was not conclusive. Incidence of disease was considered by sex for various age categories. No other factors affecting health were analyzed. Later Ferris and Anderson (1964) compared their findings in Berlin with the incidence of respiratory disease in Chilliwack, British Columbia (a town with less air pollution, as measured by sulfur dioxide, dustfall, and soiling). After smoking habits were accounted for, the town with higher pollution seemed to have a greater incidence of chronic respiratory disease. No other differences between the two towns were considered, although the authors cautioned that ethnic distributions might play a role.[14] Prindle and coauthors (1963) compared two Pennsylvania towns, Seward and New Florence, in the same fashion. Statistically significant differences in airway resistance and airway resistance volume were found between the samples (persons thirty years of age and older) in the two communities; age, sex, and height were controlled. The authors noted that these differences might reflect the differences in air pollution (dustfall, sulfation, suspended particulate) levels. Other pulmonary function measurements and X-ray examinations did not reveal important differences. Smoking habits, occupational exposures, and length of residence in the two towns were mentioned but not analyzed in detail.

Schoettlin (1962) studied both long-term and acute effects of air pollution on elderly male patients admitted to a VA Hospital in Los Angeles for treatment of chronic respiratory disease. The size of the city in which the patient previously resided was not associated with increased disease symptoms. Several categories of occupational exposure were important, as was the patient's smoking history. In studying acute effects, multivariable regression analysis failed to reveal any significant associations between a physiological measure (vital capacity) and environmental measures (temperature, humidity, oxidants, sulfur dioxide, oxides of nitrogen, and pollen).

[14] See the summary discussion of these studies in Ferris and Whittenberger (1966) and also Anderson and Ferris (1965). In a later study, Ferris (1970) looked at absences from seven elementary schools in Berlin. School absences did not differ significantly among schools despite considerable differences in levels of air pollution (sulfur dioxide and suspended particulates). However, pulmonary function tests did show significant differences. Occupational class of parents could not explain these observations.

Motley, Smart, and Leftwich (1959) studied sixty-six volunteers (forty-six of whom had pulmonary emphysema) in Los Angeles. The severity of emphysema (as measured by lung-volume measurements) was aggravated by smoggy air, whereas improvement was noted when the subjects breathed filtered air. Little effect was seen in lung-volume measurements of "normal" subjects from breathing filtered air compared with smoggy air. The personal characteristics of the volunteers were not considered.

Speizer and Ferris (1963) analyzed sixty road-tunnel employees in Boston, Massachusetts. Chronic respiratory disease was more prevalent in men who had worked in the tunnel and thus had been exposed to automobile exhaust for over ten years than in those with a shorter length of employment. The sample size did not permit adequate evaluation of age and smoking effects; however, these effects were in the expected direction.

Young, Shaw, and Bates (1963) examined seven welders and could not detect effects on pulmonary function measurements from low levels of exposure to ozone. Physiological characteristics, smoking habits, and past history of respiratory disease were accounted for.

Great Britain. Douglas and Waller (1966) found significant relationships between air pollution (estimated from domestic coal consumption) and lower-respiratory-tract infections (coughs, bronchitis, bronchopneumonia, lobar pneumonia) in 3,866 British school children. Boys and girls were similarly affected, and no difference was found between children from middle-class and working-class families. Upper-respiratory-tract infections did not show a significant association with the indexes of air pollution.

Lunn, Knowelden, and Handyside (1967) studied 819 entering school children (five years old) in four areas of Sheffield, England, who were exposed to various levels of pollution (smoke and sulfur dioxide). They collected information on disease history, housing characteristics (for example, size, number of persons sharing subject's room), social class (based on father's occupation), and number of other children in family, and conducted examinations that included pulmonary function measurements. Upper- and lower-respiratory-tract illness showed associations generally reflecting the pollution levels; for example, history of persistent and frequent cough was more than twice as high in the "dirtiest" area as in the cleanest (50.0 versus 22.9 percent). For colds, the percentages were 53.7 and 34.7 percent, respectively. Socioeconomic factors had much less influence. In a follow-up study, Lunn, Knowelden, and Roe (1970) reexamined 558 of the children and also presented evaluations of 1,049 eleven-year-olds examined during the original study. While the eleven-year-olds had a lower prevalence of respiratory illness than the five-year-olds, there was still an excess of respiratory illness in those children living in the more polluted areas. However, the children reexamined four years later (now nine years old) showed less respiratory illness than the eleven-year-olds had shown at the time of the original study. This was attributed, in part, to substantial decreases in pollution levels in the four areas.

Rosenbaum (1961) compared rates of respiratory disease in British servicemen with their home localities before call-up and discovered that the men from industrial regions were more susceptible to respiratory diseases. Despite the lack of controls for past histories of the individuals, the current circumstances of the servicemen were likely to be similar, and diagnoses and treatments were also reasonably constant.

Holland and coauthors (1965) examined the British excess over American levels in the prevalence of respiratory disease among men of the same age in similar occupations. They compared English Post Office van drivers (for the telephone branch of the General Post Office in three country towns) with London Central Post Office van drivers and Bell Telephone drivers in Washington, D.C., Baltimore, Maryland, and Westchester County, New York. The higher prevalence of respiratory symptoms, the lowered ventilatory function, and the increased sputum production in the Englishmen could not be explained by differences in smoking habits. The primary distinction in environment between the areas in England and those in the United States was the higher air pollution levels (as measured by sulfur dioxide and suspended particulates) in London and the three English towns. (See also Holland and Stone, 1965.)

Holland and coauthors (1969b) studied respiratory disease in 2,205 families with newborn children living in two suburbs of London. One-third of the families underwent ventilatory function tests. With smoking habits, domestic overcrowding, and social class (based on father's occupation) controlled, the prevalence of respiratory symptoms in both mothers and children was higher in the area which had a past history of higher pollution (smoke and sulfur dioxide). Present levels in the two areas were similar. (See also Colley and Holland, 1967.)

In another study, Holland and coauthors (1969a) examined 10,971 school children residing in four areas of Kent, England, and found that area of residence, social class, family size, and past respiratory disease history were independently associated with peak expiratory flow (adjusted for age, sex, height, and weight). In general, the flow rates were lowest in the area with the highest levels of smoke and sulfur dioxide pollution.

Colley and Reid (1970) surveyed over 10,000 children (aged six to ten) living in England and Wales. Among the two lowest social classes (based on father's occupation), there was a distinct gradient from the lowest rates of past bronchitis in the rural areas to the highest rates in the more polluted cities. The same trend held for frequency of chronic cough. Results for upper-respiratory-tract infections were less consistent. After adjustment for the different numbers of children in each area, there was no geographic variation in persons per room, persons per dwelling, or rooms per dwelling that could explain the observed gradients. No other socioeconomic or personal factors were evaluated.

Collins, Kasap, and Holland (1971) investigated child mortality in England and Wales. In considering the relation between death rates and population concentration for the years 1950–53 and 1959–63, they found that children under the age of one year living in conurbations were relatively at risk from bronchitis and tuberculosis of the respiratory system. Childhood mortality from all causes, and from respiratory and nonrespiratory causes, was also analyzed for the years 1958–64 in relation to indexes of domestic pollution, industrial pollution, sulfur pollution (from power stations), population density, overcrowding, social class, and education. For children under one year, all indexes (except sulfur pollution from power stations) were significantly correlated with total mortality and mortality from both bronchopneumonia and all respiratory diseases. Associations were weaker for older children. This study illustrates the confounding of factors and the difficulty of drawing confident conclusions.[15]

Other countries. In the USSR, Manzhenko (1966) looked at upper-respiratory-tract infections in 3,009 children (seven to twelve years old) from two school districts with different pollution levels (from dust, sulfur dioxide, and tarry substances). Family income and living conditions were similar in the two areas (the more polluted district actually had better sanitary facilities). The prevalence of chronic rhinitis was 4.7 times as great in the polluted district as in the relatively unpolluted district. Frequencies for upper-respiratory-tract conditions and chronic sinusitis were 1.9 and 9.0 times as high, respectively. X-ray findings also indicated that the incidence of pulmonary conditions was higher in the polluted area.

In Japan, Toyama (1964) surveyed pulmonary ventilatory function in children from two schools in Kawasaki, one in a heavily polluted area, the other in a relatively unpolluted one. The airflow rate of children in the polluted area varied with the level of monthly air pollution (sulfur dioxide, dustfall); the airflow rate of the other children showed a normal increase due to growth. Vital capacity did not show similar differences. In addition, the children in the polluted area complained of occasional nonproductive cough (40 percent), mucous membrane irritation (30 percent), and frequent mucus secretion (35 percent). The figures for the other children were 10 percent, 2 percent, and 3 percent, respectively. The only other factor mentioned was the occupation of the parents. Toyama also reported on school children from six schools in the Tokyo area. The mean peak airflow rate of children in polluted areas (dustfall, sulfur dioxide, suspended particulates) fluctuated from month to month in an irregular pattern; less variation was observed in airflow rates of children in the cleaner areas (again, vital capacity did not show similar associations). Other important factors influencing health were not considered.

Oshima and coauthors (1964) compared workers from a casting company in the Tokyo–Yokohama area with workers from an oil company in the Nigata area (a less industrialized region). Interviews (including pulmonary function tests) were performed for 2,765 persons. Residents of the Tokyo–Yokohama area had greater incidence of sputum production, chronic cough, and throat irritation. Cigarette smokers and persons with a history of allergies experienced the most difficulty. In addition to smoking and disease history, age and length of residence were evaluated. It was concluded that prolonged exposure to the heavily polluted air of the Tokyo–Yokohama regions was associated with an increase in respiratory symptoms.

Yoshii and coauthors (1969) studied 5,331 outpatients of a clinic in Yokkaichi and correlated the incidence of chronic pharyngitis (sore throat) with levels of air pollution (sulfur dioxide). The incidence of common and specific pharyngitis was 4.14 and 2.50 percent, respectively, in outpatients of the heavily or moderately polluted districts; in those from the relatively unpolluted

---

[15] For a general discussion of some of the literature examining the relationship between air pollution and childhood respiratory disease, see Colley (1971).

districts, the incidence was 3.19 and zero percent, respectively. Further evidence based on the incidence of the disease in school children and biopsy specimens of outpatients was presented. No socioeconomic or personal factors were evaluated.

In Norway, Skalpe (1964) compared two groups of pulp mill workers and found that those under fifty years of age who were exposed to sulfur dioxide had a significantly higher frequency of cough, expectoration, and dyspnea, and a significantly lower maximal expiratory flow rate than those who were not exposed. Above this age there were no significant differences. Vital capacity did not differ between groups. Age composition and smoking habits were said to be comparable between the two groups.

Lung cancer

Most of the early studies relating air pollution to lung cancer compared urban rates of lung cancer with rural rates, with the underlying hypothesis that the "urban factor" could, in part, be ascribed to air pollution.[16] One cannot have confidence in these conclusions.

United States. Hammond and Horn (1958) studied 187,783 white males (fifty to sixty-nine years of age) and reported that the age-standardized rate of deaths due to lung cancer was thirty-four (per 100,000) in rural areas, compared with fifty-six in cities of population over 50,000. When standardized with respect to both smoking habits and age, the rate was thirty-nine in rural areas and fifty-two in cities of over 50,000. None of the other factors affecting mortality was considered.[17]

Haenszel, Loveland, and Sirken (1962) analyzed 2,191 lung cancer deaths among white males in forty-six states, and data for a control group of males who died from other causes. They found the crude rate of death from lung cancer in urban areas to have been 1.56 times as high as in rural areas in 1958 and 1.82 times as high in 1948–49 (in subjects thirty-five years of age and older, with adjustments made for age). When adjustments were made for both age and smoking history, the ratio was 1.43. The ratio also increased with duration of residence in the urban or rural area, from 1.08 for residence of less than one year to 2.00 for lifetime residence. Birthplace and census region of residence were also considered. No other socioeconomic characteristics or environmental factors were discussed. Haenszel and Taeuber (1964) reported similar results for white females.[18]

Levin and coauthors (1960) found significant differences between urban and rural age-adjusted mortality rates (for periods around 1950) in New York

[16] For a recent survey of much of the literature relating air pollution to lung cancer, see Carnow and Meier (1973).

[17] See also Hammond (1958), who compared lung cancer death rates in the United States with those in England and Wales.

[18] Haenszel and Taeuber (1964) analyzed data for 683 white American females who died of lung cancer and for a control group as well. They found the crude rate of death from lung cancer to be 1.32 times as high in urban areas as in rural areas for 1958–59 and 1.29 times as high for 1948–49 (in subjects thirty-five years of age and older, with adjustments made for age). When adjustments were made for both age and smoking history, the ratio was 1.27. This ratio increased with the duration of residence in the urban or rural area, from 0.80 for residence of less than one year to 1.76 for lifetime residence.

State (exclusive of New York City), Connecticut, and Iowa. For males, the death rates were 41 percent higher in urban areas of New York, 57 percent higher in Connecticut, and 184 percent higher in Iowa. For females, the differences were 7 percent, 24 percent, and 47 percent, respectively. Factors other than age and sex (for example, smoking habits and occupation) were not controlled.

Buell, Dunn, and Breslow (1967) utilized 69,868 questionnaires covering 336,571 man-years in their study of lung cancer in California veterans. Controlling for length of residence, they found rates of death from lung cancer (adjusted for differences in age and smoking habits) to be 25 percent higher in the major metropolitan areas than in the less urbanized areas. Among nonsmokers, the rates of death from lung cancer in major metropolitan areas were 2.8 to 4.4 times as high as for more rural areas. Other differences among the areas and among the veterans were not considered.[19]

Winkelstein and coauthors (1967) found that although an association existed between areas of high pollution and high lung cancer mortality, the relation was not consistent when economic status was controlled. Similarly, neither Hagstrom, Sprague, and Landau (1967) nor Zeidberg, Horton, and Landau (1967a) were able to isolate an air pollution effect on lung cancer mortality from data for Nashville for the years 1949–60.

Greenburg and coauthors (1967a) investigated 1,190 cancer deaths that occurred in areas of Staten Island, New York, between 1959–61 and found a relationship between age-adjusted, lung cancer death rates and probable air pollution levels. The areas were described in terms of various socioeconomic indexes (income, housing, and education); however, no attempt was made to evaluate the individual effects of the factors influencing health.

Mills (1960) investigated rates of death from lung cancer in Cincinnati, Ohio. Stratifying according to the amount of driving done, area of residence, and smoking history of the deceased, he found that all three factors were associated with higher mortality rates. Mills (1943) found that the lung cancer mortality was almost four times as high in the polluted districts of Cincinnati as in the less polluted ones. Mills (1952) also examined age–sex–race-specific, respiratory-tract cancer mortality in Chicago and observed that high rates for elderly males occurred a decade earlier in the most polluted (sootfall and sulfur dioxide) sections of the city than in the cleaner sections.

Great Britain. Stocks (1947) analyzed lung cancer mortality from towns in England and Wales and found nonsignificant correlations with domestic overcrowding, a social index (based on occupation), and other disease rates. One factor significantly correlated with the mortality rates was mean annual sunshine hours (even with the social index held constant). Stocks concluded that either sunshine was an important factor in preventing lung cancer or that smokiness of the atmosphere was an important factor in producing it.

Stocks and Campbell (1955) utilized environmental histories of persons dying from lung cancer and compared percentage distributions according to smoking habits and residence. They found a tenfold difference between the

---

[19] A number of additional U.S. studies have found that urban lung cancer rates are significantly higher than rates in rural or nonmetropolitan areas (Manos and Fisher, 1959; Mancuso and Coulter, 1958; Griswold and coauthors, 1955; Hoffman and Gilliam, 1954; and Hueper, 1956).

TABLE A.3.   Lung Cancer Mortality (Data from England and Wales)

	$A.3\text{-}1^a$ B	$A.3\text{-}2^b$ B	$A.3\text{-}3^c$ M	$A.3\text{-}4^c$ M	$A.3\text{-}5^d$ M	$A.3\text{-}6^d$ M
R^2	.445	.576	.781	.805	.344	.379
Constant	67.259	68.168	48.215	25.424	87.589	88.903
Air pollution variables						
Deposit index	.041 (2.09)					
Smoke		.864 (4.02)	.137 (2.84)	.162 (5.59)	−.086 (−2.42)	
Sulfur dioxide						−.105 (−3.00)
Socioeconomic variables						
Persons per acre	.154 (4.23)	.161 (3.89)	.115 (1.70)		.184 (4.83)	.198 (5.23)
Social class				.172 (2.47)		

Note: The numbers in parentheses below the regression coefficients are t statistics.
Abbreviations: B, both sexes; *M*, males.
[a] Based on data for fifty-three county boroughs.
[b] Based on data for twenty-eight county boroughs.
[c] Based on data for twenty-six areas.
[d] Based on data for fifty-three urban areas.

death rates for rural and for urban areas and suggested a relationship with air pollution by showing that concentrations of smoke, 3:4 benzopyrene, other polycyclic hydrocarbons, and sulfur dioxide increased with urbanization.

Hewitt (1956) found a significant correlation between an air pollution index (duration of exposure to sulfur dioxide) and lung cancer mortality ($r = 0.70$) across nine public health divisions in London.

Daly (1959) compared mortality rates in urban and rural areas of England and Wales and found a partial correlation coefficient of 0.31 between death rates and air pollution after eliminating the effects of various social factors.

Regressions A.3-1 through A.3-6 (table A.3) show our reworking of the Stocks (1959, 1960) and Ashley (1967) data for lung cancer mortality for England and Wales (there was no smoking information). Regressions A.3-1 through A.3-4 imply that, if the quality of air of all boroughs were improved to that of the borough with the best air, one would expect the rate of death from lung cancer to fall by between 11 and 44 percent. Regressions A.3-5 and A.3-6 show a relationship between air pollution and lung cancer that is either nonsignificant or inverse. The only contrary results come from Ashley's data.[20] In the absence of more complete evidence, we must remain curious

[20] In a subsequent study, Ashley (1969b) employed multivariable regression analysis and found a significant negative association between sulfur dioxide and the mortality of men from lung cancer. Gardner and Waller (1970) attributed Ashley's negative coefficient to his inappropriate modification of the standardized mortality ratio to account for town size. They also questioned his use of mean monthly values of pollution.

about these results. Use of such small samples and inadequate controls is certain to lead to some contrary results, but they are disconcerting when they appear.

Additional evidence from Great Britain relating lung cancer mortality to urbanization is found in Curwen and Kennaway (1954), in which standardized mortality ratios for lung cancer in both sexes were positively related to an index of increasing urbanization in England and Wales. For males, lung cancer mortality was also shown to be correlated with a measure of population density. Dean (1966) also found that among male nonsmokers in Northern Ireland, lung cancer mortality was lower in rural than in urban areas.

Gardner, Crawford, and Morris (1969), using regression analysis, found that air pollution (measured by domestic coal consumption) was significantly associated with four age–sex rates of lung cancer mortality in seven out of eight data sets.

Wicken and Buck (1964) examined lung cancer mortality in six areas of northeast England. Controlling for age, smoking habits, and social class, they found lung cancer death rates to be associated with urbanization and air pollution (smoke) across areas and with air pollution exposure (smoke and sulfur dioxide) within the two urban districts. They noted that the relationship of lung cancer with smoking was stronger than the relationship with air pollution. In a later paper, Buck and Wicken (1967) fit a multiplicative model including an urban–rural residence variable and a variable representing the combined effects of smoking and morning cough to data on male lung cancer mortality in Northern Ireland. Increasing urbanization was closely associated with increasing mortality. Two similar models were fit to mortality data from northeast England, one with variables representing urban–rural residence and smoking habits, the other with social class (based on occupation) substituted for smoking (data constraints necessitated the separate estimation). Again, urbanization was associated with increasing mortality when the other relevant variables were controlled.

A contrary result was reported by Buck and Brown (1964), who found no association between smoke and lung cancer; the relationship between sulfur dioxide and lung cancer was not consistent. Negative results were also reported by Fairbairn and Reid (1958), who uncovered no relationship between lung cancer mortality among civil servants and a fog index across thirty-seven areas of the United Kingdom (see also Reid, 1958).

Other countries. Studies from other parts of Europe include Stocks (1966), who used three sets of data to isolate the effect of air pollution on lung cancer. Contrasting data for eight northern European cities, he found a correlation between lung cancer and air pollution of 0.60, and correlations between lung cancer and smoking that ranged between 0.27 and 0.36. Contrasting data for nineteen countries, he found that an index of solid fuel consumption was a much stronger variable than cigarette consumption per capita (see also Stocks, 1967). Finally, with data from northern England, he found confirmation of an association between lung cancer and air pollution. Numerous other factors that vary across areas were not controlled for in these studies.[21]

[21] See also Firket's (1958) discussion of the prevalence of lung cancer in the Liège area of Belgium.

In Norway, Kreyberg (1956) attributed the higher rates of lung cancer among males in urban areas than in more rural areas to differences in occupation and life habits, such as smoking, rather than to differences in general, unspecified air pollution.

In Japan, Hitosugi (1968) interviewed families of 259 lung cancer victims as well as a random sample of 4,500 adults (thirty-five through seventy-four years of age). Factors collected included age, sex, smoking habits, occupation, residence, and previous medical history. Several measures of air pollution (dustfall, sulfur dioxide, suspended matters, benzopyrene) were related to areas of residence. The results for males, stratified by smoking habits, indicated that increases in the lung cancer mortality among smokers and ex-smokers were generally associated with higher levels of pollution. Results for females were less consistent, possibly due to small samples. Toyama (1964) found a positive but statistically nonsignificant correlation between lung cancer mortality and dustfall across districts of Tokyo. In addition, he discovered a higher incidence of fibrotic lung disease in polluted areas of Tokyo than in unpolluted areas.

Another group of studies examined lung cancer death rates in migrants from one country to another. Eastcott (1956) studied male and female migrants from the United Kingdom to New Zealand, who presumably experienced decreased air pollution exposure. Comparing them with native New Zealanders, he found rates to be 30 percent higher among migrants who moved before they were thirty years old and 75 percent higher among migrants who moved after they were thirty years old. General smoking patterns were compared in the two countries, and New Zealand residents were found to have a slightly higher per capita tobacco consumption. No other differences between countries or among migrants were evaluated. Dean (1959, 1961, 1962, 1964) scrutinized British migrants (white males) to South Africa and Australia and discovered that their lung cancer mortality rate was lower than that of their counterparts remaining in England, but higher than that of the native South Africans and Australians. Cigarette consumption was known to be higher in Australia and South Africa, and specific smoking practices (for example, average butt length) would have suggested that if smoking were the primary factor contributing to lung cancer mortality, rates would have been higher rather than lower in South Africa and Australia. In addition, there were figures suggesting that migrants came from a higher social class (based on occupation) on average than did the general male population of England and Wales. Similar results were reported by Reid and coauthors (1966) for British migrants to Norway.[22]

Buell and Dunn's (1967) review of the evidence on lung cancer and air pollution is summarized in table A.4. For smokers, death rates (adjusted for age and smoking) ranged from 25 to 123 percent higher in urban areas than in rural areas. For nonsmokers, all differences exceeded 120 percent. "The etiological roles for lung cancer of urban living and cigarette smoking seem to be complete," they said, "in that the urban factor is evident when viewing nonsmokers exclusively, and the smoking factor is evident when viewing rural

[22] Mancuso and Coulter (1958) also report lung cancer mortality rates among immigrants from various countries to Ohio. See also Haenszel (1961).

TABLE A.4. Summary of Lung Cancer Mortality Studies

| | | Number of lung cancer deaths per 100,000 population | | | | | |
| | | Standardized for age and smoking | | | Nonsmokers | | |
Study	Population sample	Urban	Rural	Urban/rural	Urban	Rural	Urban/rural
Buell, Dunn, and Breslow (1967)	California men	101	80	1.26	36	11	3.27
Hammond and Horn (1958)	American men	52	39	1.33	15	0	∞
Stocks (1957)	England and Wales	189[a]	85[a]	2.23[a]	50	22	2.27
Dean (1966)	Northern Ireland	—	—	—	38	10	3.80
Golledge and Wicken (1964)	England	149	69	2.15	23	29	0.79
Haenszel, Loveland, and Sirken (1962)	American men	100	50	2.00	16	5	3.20

Source: Buell and Dunn (1967).
[a] No adjustment for smoking.

TABLE A.5. Non-respiratory-tract Cancer Mortality (Data from England and Wales)

| | Stomach cancers | | | | Intestinal cancers | | Other cancers | | | |
	$A.5\text{-}1^a$ M	$A.5\text{-}2^a$ F	$A.5\text{-}3^b$ M	$A.5\text{-}4^b$ F	$A.5\text{-}5^a$ B	$A.5\text{-}6^b$ B	$A.5\text{-}7^c$ M	$A.5\text{-}8^c$ F	$A.5\text{-}9^c$ M	$A.5\text{-}10^c$ F
R^2	.167	.175	.257	.454	.041	.129	.454	.044	.396	.002
Constant	89.133	89.406	88.793	75.946	101.629	97.270	88.030	101.541	82.216	106.299
Air pollution variables										
Deposit index	.066 (2.72)	.070 (3.08)			.018 (1.45)	.174 (1.26)				
Smoke			.714 (2.57)	.883 (4.13)			.019 (.59)	.039 (.92)	.060 (2.75)	.005 (.17)
Socioeconomic variables										
Persons per acre	.005 (.12)	−.023 (−.56)	.065 (1.21)	.066 (1.60)	−.012 (−.52)	.036 (1.35)	.073 (1.60)	−.062 (−1.03)		
Social class									.017 (.33)	−.013 (−.19)

Note: The numbers in parentheses below the regression coefficients are t statistics.
Abbreviations: M, males; F, females; B, both sexes.
[a] Based on data for fifty-three county boroughs.
[b] Based on data for twenty-eight county boroughs.
[c] Based on data for twenty-six areas.

dwellers exclusively" (Buell and Dunn, 1967, page 296). They argued that differences in the quality of diagnosis could not account for the observed differences between urban and rural areas.

Total and non-respiratory-tract cancers

United States. Winkelstein and Kantor (1969c) found the mortality from stomach cancer in Buffalo, New York, was more than twice as great in areas of high pollution as in areas of low pollution.[23] For prostatic cancer, Winkelstein and Kantor (1969a) found that the mortality rate was 2.7 times as high in the most polluted zone as it was in the least polluted.

Hagstrom, Sprague, and Landau (1967) tabulated rates of death from cancer among middle-class residents of Nashville. Using four measures of air pollution, they found the cancer mortality rate to be 25 percent higher in polluted areas than in areas of relatively clean air.[24] They also found significant mortality-rate increases associated with individual categories of cancer, such as cancer of the stomach, esophagus, and bladder. The individual mortality rates were more closely related to air pollution after the data were broken down by sex and race. (See also Sprague and Hagstrom, 1969.)

Levin and coauthors (1960) reported the following relationships for all types of cancer: the age-adjusted cancer-incidence rate was 24 percent higher for urban males than for rural males in New York State (exclusive of New York City), 36 percent higher in Connecticut, and 40 percent higher in Iowa; the incidence rate was 14 percent higher for urban females than for rural females in New York State, 28 percent higher in Connecticut, and 34 percent higher in Iowa. For both males and females, the incidence rate for each of sixteen categories of cancer was higher in urban than in rural areas.[25]

[23] For economic level 1, the mortality rate per 100,000 for gastric cancer in white males, aged fifty to sixty-nine years, changed from zero to 63, and 136 as the air pollution level rose from level 2 to level 4 (see fn. 2, p. 274). For economic level 2, the rates were 45, 41, 48, and 84, respectively, for the four pollution levels. For economic level 3, the rates were 39, 51, and 51 for air pollution levels 2 through 4. For economic level 4, the rates were 15, 38, and 63, respectively, for air pollution levels 1 through 3. For economic level 5, the rates were 26, 16, and zero for air pollution levels 1 through 3. For white women, aged fifty to sixty-nine years, the death rates for economic level 1 were zero, 33, and 24 per 100,000 for air pollution levels 2 through 4. For economic level 2, the rates were 8, 18, 25, and 40, for air pollution levels 1 through 4. For economic level 3, the rates were 30, 16, and 49 for air pollution levels 2 through 4. For economic level 4, the rates were 5, 21, and zero, for air pollution levels 1 through 3. For economic level 5, the rates were 14, zero, and zero, for air pollution levels 1 through 3.

[24] The four measures of pollution were suspended particulates (soiling), dustfall, sulfur trioxide, and sulfur dioxide. For all cancer deaths, the number per 100,000 for middle-class residents (defined to include about 75 percent of all residents) fell from 153 for high-pollution areas, to 130 for moderate-pollution areas, to 124 for low-pollution areas; a soiling index (concentration of haze and smoke per 1,000 linear feet) was used to classify air pollution. When sulfur trioxide (milligrams per 100 cm^2 per day) was used as a basis for classification, the corresponding death rates were 150, 129, and 145, respectively. With dustfall as a measure, the figures were 145, 130, and 131; with twenty-four-hour sulfur dioxide, in parts per million, they were 141, 129, and 138.

[25] In an older study done in Massachusetts, Lombard and Doering (1927) discovered that the apparent association between cancer death rates and population density largely disappeared after adjusting for age and sex and limiting comparisons to native born (of native parents).

In Ohio, Mancuso, MacFarlane, and Porterfield (1955) investigated cancer mortality (standardized for age, sex, and race) among white males aged twenty-five to sixty-four. For cancer of the esophagus, buccal cavity and pharynx, larynx, central nervous system, and bladder, mortality rates were higher in metropolitan counties of Ohio than in nonmetropolitan counties. They did not detect a difference for cancer of the stomach, pancreas, lymphatic and hematopoietic tissues, or prostate, or for leukemias. No other controls were imposed in the study.

Mills (1943) found that mortality from cancers of the upper air passages were 56 percent higher in polluted (sootfall) areas of Cincinnati than in relatively "clean" areas. Cancers of the stomach and rectum also showed increased rates, although breast cancer did not (see also Manos and Fisher, 1959).

Great Britain. Gardner, Crawford, and Morris (1969) presented regressions explaining the incidence of stomach cancer across county boroughs in England and Wales. For males aged forty-five to sixty-four, air pollution (based on domestic coal consumption) was significantly related to the death rates from stomach cancer in both time periods analyzed. For older males (sixty-five to seventy-four), the air pollution measure was significant for one period. The air pollution index was not significantly associated with the female mortality rates.

Curwen and Kennaway (1954) found that the standard mortality ratio for cancer of the larynx in males increased with increasing urbanization in areas of England and Wales. For females, an inverse relationship was observed; however, the number of deaths was quite small and the authors mention the possibility of sampling error. No other socioeconomic or environmental controls were considered.

Our reworking of data from England on rates of death from non-respiratory-tract cancers is presented in table A.5. In the regressions, stomach cancer was significantly related to a deposit index and a smoke index. The effects were nearly identical for males and females. Intestinal cancer appears to have been only marginally related to indexes of either deposit or smoke. For twenty-six areas in northern England and Wales, there appears to have been little relationship between non-respiratory-tract cancers and a smoke index. The single exception in the four regressions occurred for males when the socioeconomic variable was social class: in that case, the smoke index explained a significant amount of variation in the cancer mortality rate. (Apparently, population density and the smoke index were so highly related in these twenty-six areas that neither had significant power to explain much variation in the presence of the other.[26])

Cardiovascular disease

United States. Zeidberg, Prindle, and Landau (1964) found morbidity rates for cardiovascular disease to be associated with air pollution levels across Nashville, Tennessee. In white, middle-class males, fifty-five years and older, a consistent pattern of increasing morbidity with increasing values for soiling (coefficient of haze) and twenty-four-hour sulfur dioxide concentrations was

[26] In his later study of the fifty-three towns, Ashley (1969a), employing multivariable regression analysis, found a positive association between gastric cancer and air pollution (smoke and sulfur dioxide).

observed. Cardiovascular morbidity in white, middle-class females, fifty-five years and older, showed a direct relationship with soiling and sulfur dioxide as well as with mean annual sulfation (sulfur trioxide), dustfall, and twenty-four-hour suspended particulate levels. Results were less consistent for nonwhites. In a later study, Zeidberg and coauthors (1967b) looked at cardiovascular mortality in Nashville and found a consistent pattern between middle-class (age-adjusted) death rates and particulate pollution (as measured by a soiling index). When comparisons were made by pollution exposure for each sex, a regular pattern of association was noted for females, but not for males. Rates were also higher for each pollution level among nonwhites than among whites of the same socioeconomic class.

Other studies have merely related the prevalence of cardiovascular disease to urbanization. Enterline and coauthors (1960) found a higher mortality from heart disease among whites aged forty-five to sixty-four in U.S. center-city counties than in suburban counties; it was also higher in suburban counties than in nonmetropolitan counties. In metropolitan counties with central cities, death rates from coronary heart disease were 37 percent higher for males and 46 percent higher for females than those in nonmetropolitan counties. No specific factors were controlled in the comparisons.

Sauer and coauthors (1966) performed a similar analysis for the states of Georgia and North Carolina and found that metropolitan areas had higher death rates (white males aged forty-five to sixty-four and thirty-five to seventy-four, age-adjusted) than nonmetropolitan areas. Again, no other factors were accounted for.[27]

Friedman (1967) correlated the rate of mortality from coronary heart disease in white males aged forty-five to sixty-four with the proportion of this group living in urban areas. The simple correlation for thirty-three states was 0.79. When cigarette consumption was held constant, the partial correlation was 0.67.

Great Britain. Gardner, Crawford, and Morris (1969) could not find a consistent relationship in their regression analysis of mortality from cardiovascular disease in England and Wales. Although a positive and significant association existed between death rates of males aged forty-five to sixty-four and air pollution (based on domestic coal consumption) for two time periods, rates for males, aged sixty-five to seventy-four, exhibited a negative relationship (statistically nonsignificant), and the results for females were also mixed and statistically nonsignificant.

Other countries. Cederlöf's (1966) study of twins of the same sex in Sweden found that the prevalence of angina pectoris was higher among smoking men in urban than in rural areas. The effect of urbanization was greater for firstborn twins (regarding them as sampled from a "normal" population) than for sets of twins with similar smoking habits but different residential histories.

Total and miscellaneous morbidity and mortality

United States. McDonald and Schwing (1973) employed ridge regression analysis to investigate the association between the age-adjusted total mortality

[27] Buechley, Oechsli, and Stallones (1966) also found excess coronary heart disease deaths in the relatively urban states. See also Manos and Fisher (1959).

rate (in 1959–61) and air pollution (as measured by 1963 pollution potentials) across sixty SMSAs. A number of climate and socioeconomic variables were also included in the multivariable analysis. Ridge regression analysis was used because of collinearity among the explanatory variables. It was argued that the technique produces better estimates than do ordinary least squares of the "true" effects of the explanatory variables in cases of extreme multicollinearity. Unfortunately, evaluation of this claim is somewhat arbitrary, although McDonald and Schwing did present estimates for the "special case" of ordinary least squares. Pollution potentials were used because of deficiencies in the data for the three pollutants of interest: hydrocarbons, oxides of nitrogen, and sulfur dioxide. These "potentials" were based on emissions and weather factors in each area. Using the ridge regression technique and two different criteria for the elimination of explanatory variables, the authors found that in both cases the variable representing sulfur dioxide potential was quite significant in explaining variations in the total mortality rate across areas. The other variables positively and significantly related to the death rate (in both cases) were mean annual precipitation and the percentage of the urbanized nonwhite population. For those over twenty-five, the mean January temperature and median school years completed were negatively and significantly related to the death rate (in both cases).

Zeidberg, Prindle, and Landau (1964) found significant correlations between levels of air pollution (soiling index and sulfur dioxide) and total morbidity among middle-class persons fifty-five years of age and older. Looking at sex- and race-specific rates, they noted that housekeeping white females (aged fifteen to sixty-four) exhibited significant correlations, whereas employed white females showed none. Nonwhite females exhibited significant correlations in both categories.

Across areas of Buffalo, New York, Winkelstein and Gay (1971) looked at mortality from cirrhosis of the liver. They found a graded positive association with air pollution (suspended particulates) when economic status (median income) was controlled. Other socioeconomic, personal, or environmental factors were not controlled.

Manos and Fisher (1959) calculated simple linear correlations between fifty disease-specific mortality rates (for seven age–sex–race-adjusted categories) and thirty indexes of pollution (based on sources of air pollution, as well as city and socioeconomic characteristics). Among these, four causes of death produced a large number of high positive correlations: cancers of the esophagus or stomach; cancers of the trachea, bronchus, or lung; arteriosclerotic heart disease (including coronary disease); and chronic endocarditis (not specified as rheumatic) and other myocardial degeneration.

Great Britain. Gardner, Crawford, and Morris (1969) used multivariable regression analysis to estimate the association of total mortality with air pollution (domestic coal consumption) and found that, in those regressions pertaining to males aged forty-five to sixty-four, "air pollution" was the most important explanatory variable. The explanatory powers of the regressions for the two time periods were $R^2 = 0.80$ and $R^2 = 0.84$. In addition, the pollution variable was significant for the death rate for males aged sixty-five to seventy-four. The variable was not statistically significant in explaining the female death rate.

TIME-SERIES STUDIES
Acute air pollution episodes

Greenburg and coauthors (1962a) investigated a November 1953 episode in New York City during which sulfur dioxide and smokeshade reached unusually high levels. Using analysis of variance to compare the period with six control years, and assuming a three-day lag in the effect of air pollution on mortality,[28] they found a statistically significant increase in the number of deaths, generally distributed over all age groups. In a subsequent study, Greenburg and coauthors (1962b) studied pediatric and adult clinic visits in this period. Using the same control periods and, again, assuming a three-day lag, they found an increase in upper-respiratory-tract illnesses and cardiac visits at the four hospitals under observation. A 1962 air pollution episode in New York City was studied by the same group but with less consistent results. No significant increase was found in emergency clinic visits for cardiac conditions at five major hospitals, although visits for upper-respiratory-tract infections significantly increased at four old-age homes (see Greenburg and coauthors, 1963). Analysis by Greenburg and coauthors (1965) of the frequency of visits to emergency clinics in New York City for treatment of asthma failed to reveal an increase related to air pollution. Greenburg and coauthors (1967b) also compared the number of deaths during a January 29–February 12, 1963, air pollution episode in New York City with that for the same time period in other years. (The control years were characterized by the prevalence of influenza and cold weather, but had no substantial sulfur dioxide or smokeshade pollution.) For the period in question, they found an excess of between 200 and 400 deaths, which they attributed to air pollution. These deaths occurred in people over forty-five from influenza-pneumonia, vascular lesions, cardiac, and "all other" causes. No significant increases were noted for accidents, homicides, suicides, or in deaths among infants under twenty-eight days of age.

Heimann (1970) examined the situation in Boston during November 1966. He analyzed various types of data and found no significant effects of air pollution on total mortality, on mortality or hospitalization of 9,697 elderly nursing-home residents, on the frequency of fetal deaths, or on the number of emergency room visits in one hospital for treatment of heart or respiratory disease. He did find that patients with chronic nonspecific respiratory disease made more visits to their chest clinics. The specific pollutants analyzed were suspended particulates, sulfur dioxide, and a soiling index.

Gore and Shaddick (1958) examined sex-specific mortality (total and five categories) in London during four episodes of fog and high pollution (sulfur dioxide and smoke), as well as the two-year period encompassing these episodes. They concluded that during the episodes with fog and high pollution, a critical level of four times the winter average of pollution caused marked excess mortality. For the two-year period, no significant relationship between mortality and exposure to smoke and sulfur dioxide was demonstrated (three

---

[28] This method was based on investigations of the Donora episode discussed in chapter 9.

of a possible twelve simple correlations were statistically significant). When length of residence (percentage born in London) was combined with each index of pollution, significant correlations were found between both smoke and sulfur dioxide and male and female bronchitis mortality. Simple correlations were also presented between the various mortality rates and an index of social class.

Daily illness and absences

Cassell and coauthors (1969)—over a period of three years (61,000 person-weeks of information)—collected data on daily illness symptoms among 1,747 persons living in New York City (using weekly interviews with families). These data were correlated with four pollutants (sulfur dioxide, carbon monoxide, suspended particulates, and hydrocarbons) and seven meteorologic factors (precipitation, solar radiation, temperature, humidity, sky cover, barometric pressure, and wind speed). Cough was positively correlated with particulates, carbon monoxide, and sulfur dioxide, and negatively correlated with hydrocarbons. In addition, the level of carbon monoxide was positively correlated with headache, eye symptoms, colds, and sore throat. There was some indication that the respiratory symptoms were less strongly related to sulfur dioxide than to particulates. Unfortunately, the analysis did not take account of lag effects or any day-of-the-week patterns. A principal component analysis was also performed, but its interpretation was not clear.

Hospital admissions

Sterling and coauthors (1966) correlated hospital admissions in Los Angeles with a number of pollutants (oxidants, carbon monoxide, sulfur dioxide, nitrogen dioxide, nitric oxide, total oxides of nitrogen, ozone, oxidant precursor, and suspended particulates), humidity, and temperature over a period of 223 days in 1961. After controlling for day of the week, they found significant correlations between admissions for "highly relevant" diseases and all pollutants.[29] For admissions for "relevant" diseases, there were fewer significant correlations.[30] For diseases which were not expected to exhibit an association with pollution, the correlations were generally nonsignificant or negative. In a subsequent paper, Sterling, Pollack, and Phair (1967) looked at length of hospitalization for the patients admitted. Again, controlling for day of the week, they discovered that, for "highly relevant, relevant, heart, and central nervous system disease categories," there were significant correlations between length of stay in the hospital and levels of sulfur dioxide, nitrogen dioxide, total oxides of nitrogen, and suspended particulates.[31] In a later study, Sterling, Pol-

[29] The disease groupings were defined as follows: Highly relevant, allergic disorders, inflammatory diseases of the eye, acute upper-respiratory-tract infections, influenza, and bronchitis; Relevant, diseases of the heart, rheumatic fever and vascular diseases, and other diseases of the respiratory system; Total relevant, combined both of the above categories; and Irrelevant, all other illnesses not mentioned above.

[30] Correlations with carbon monoxide, nitric oxide, total oxides of nitrogen, oxidant precursors, and suspended particulates dropped out.

[31] They also found significant negative correlations between ozone and the length of stay for "relevant" and heart-disease categories.

lack, and Weinkam (1969) again analyzed the admission and hospitalization data, this time using stepwise multivariable regression. The results indicated that a number of pollutants, as well as interactions between pollutants and between pollutants and meteorological factors, exhibited significant associations (sometimes nonlinear and lagged) with both the frequency and duration of hospitalization for various disease categories.

Using multivariable statistical techniques, Silverman (1973b) studied daily emergency admissions at twenty-two Pittsburgh (Allegheny County) hospitals. Controlling for temperature, precipitation, and day of the week, he found that admissions for treatment of respiratory diseases (particularly bronchitis and pneumonia) were significantly associated with a soiling index (a measure of suspended particulates). A doubling of the index was estimated to be associated with an additional 3.3 respiratory emergency admissions (there were an average of 14.7 respiratory emergency admissions each day across hospitals). The air pollution variable was also associated with emergency admissions for heart disease, but not with emergency admissions for deliveries, appendectomies, and other diseases not expected to be causally related. Results of breakdowns by age, sex, and type of insurance coverage were also presented.

Holland, Spicer, and Wilson (1961) found significant correlations between hospital admissions for treatment of respiratory diseases and air pollution (smoke concentration) in London when various meteorological variables were controlled; they could not find significant correlations between hospital admissions for treatment of heart disease and either the air pollution or the meteorological variables.

Time-series studies of respiratory diseases

A number of additional studies have looked at the effects of air pollution on asthmatics over time. Lewis, Gilkeson, and McCaldin (1962) investigated asthma in New Orleans by reviewing daily admissions to an emergency clinic. Various pollutants and other environmental factors were compared with the prevalence of asthma outbreaks, but only one, a combustion particle with associated silica, showed a statistically significant relationship (see also Weill and coauthors, 1964). In a later study, Kenline (1966) analyzed hospital admissions for asthma in New Orleans. Giving special attention to particle size and sampling instrumentation, he found that the presence of certain small particles ($5-10\mu$ in diameter) in the air had a significant positive correlation with admissions. A number of pollutants did not exhibit significant associations. Schoettlin and Landau (1961) investigated 137 asthma patients in Los Angeles during the fall months. They found that 14 percent of the variance in daily attacks ($n = 3,435$) could be explained by the maximum atmospheric concentrations of oxidants for that day. Lower correlations were also noted for temperature, relative humidity, and water vapor pressure. No significant correlations were found between the number of persons affected and levels of carbon monoxide or suspended particulates. Zeidberg, Prindle, and Landau (1961) studied forty-nine adult and thirty-five child asthma patients for a year and found that the attack rate (attacks per person per day) for adults rose from 0.070 on days when atmospheric concentrations of sulfates were low to 0.216 when concentrations were high. The effect was not significant for children.

Brown and Ipsen (1968) observed 314 patients with allergic rhinitis and asthma in New York City from August 1 to November 1, 1963. They related the mean severity of symptoms to ten measurements of air pollution, climatic factors, and mold and pollen counts. Chemical air pollution showed an inconsistent relationship. Girsh and coauthors (1967) studied asthmatic children in a Philadelphia hospital and found a threefold-greater incidence of bronchial asthma during days of high pollution than on days with low pollution levels. Asthmatic students at the University of Minnesota were studied by Smith and Paulus (1971). Of the various pollution indexes, only that for smoke spot (soiling from grain handling operations, as well as incomplete combustion) was significantly correlated with asthma incidence. Various climate variables were also controlled (see also Paulus and Smith, 1967).

Finally, Derrick (1970) found no significant correlation between asthma-induced hospital visits in Brisbane, Australia, and the mean weekly smoke density (using either the seasonal or the short-term variation in the prevalence of asthma from 1960 to 1962). Account was taken of weather variables. Loudon and Kilpatrick (1969) correlated antitussive prescriptions dispensed in two Dallas hospitals with meteorological factors and total suspended particulates, but they failed to demonstrate a relationship between "cough" and air pollution.

Other researchers have evaluated diaries of patients suffering from chronic bronchitis and emphysema (Lawther, Waller, and Henderson, 1970; Waller, 1971; Waller and Lawther, 1955, 1957; Lawther, 1958; Pemberton, 1961). In most cases, a close association was found between the patient's condition and the atmospheric pollution levels (usually measures of smoke and sulfur dioxide). When other weather factors were taken into account, pollution seemed to display the dominant effect. A study on patients with chronic bronchitis and emphysema, carried out by Burrows, Kellogg, and Buskey (1968), showed that severity of daily symptoms correlated with sulfur dioxide and total oxides of nitrogen. When both seasonal and daily temperatures were held constant, hydrocarbons showed an independent correlation with symptoms. Carnow and coauthors (1969) investigated 561 patients with chronic bronchopulmonary disease in Chicago. A daily air pollution index, based on sulfur dioxide levels in the square mile surrounding both employment and residence, was analyzed in conjunction with patient diaries. The researchers found that symptoms in patients aged fifty-five and older with "advanced bronchitis" were exacerbated by increased levels of sulfur dioxide on the day of exposure and on the day following.

Dohan and Taylor (1960) and Dohan (1961) studied absences (of more than seven days) of female employees in eight Radio Corporation of America plants and found a correlation of 0.96 between atmospheric concentrations of air pollution (sulfates) and absences due to respiratory disease in the five cities for which complete data were available. Dohan, Everts, and Smith (1962) analyzed the frequency of respiratory disease in employees of the Curtis Publishing Company in Philadelphia and the Radio Corporation of America in Camden, New Jersey. Frequencies in the two plants in these adjacent cities exhibited a high correlation, suggesting the role of an environmental factor. No conclusive results implicating pollution were stated, although a relationship was noted with the mean weekly sulfate concentrations.[32] Gregory (1970) investigated absences of male employees of a steelworks and found that smoke (but not sulfur dioxide) was correlated with the incidence of bronchitis exacerbations. Temperature and humidity were controlled, but Holland (1971) criticized the study for not controlling for personal factors or large-scale seasonal fluctuations.

Respiratory function studies

Another group of studies compared measurements of respiratory function with levels of air pollution. In Dublin, Ireland, Chapman (1965) analyzed pulmonary function among fifteen male bronchitis patients and found a significant correlation with smoke pollution. Angel and coauthors (1965) observed eighty-five Englishmen working in two factories and an office (most of whom had evidence of chronic bronchitis) during the winter months of 1962–63. Each man was seen every three weeks by a clinician, who questioned him as to the prevalence of respiratory illness and took various measurements including, for example, forced expiratory volume (FEV). The number of new respiratory illnesses occurring each week among the men was found to be correlated with both smoke and sulfur dioxide concentrations. The total number of men affected by respiratory illness each week was more closely related to smoke than to sulfur dioxide levels. (Partial correlations were presented in which temperature was also controlled.)

In Los Angeles, Rokaw and Massey (1962) took monthly measurements of respiratory function for thirty-one patients with severe, chronic obstructive lung diseases, as well as for hospital personnel with no known respiratory impairment. They correlated these measurements with weather conditions and levels of air pollution (including nitric oxide, nitrogen dioxide, carbon monoxide, ozone, and total oxidants), but their results were inconclusive.

Spicer and coauthors (1962) found that a Baltimore group of 150 heterogeneous patients with chronic obstructive airway disease became better or worse together, although no particular pollutant was found responsible for their illnesses. Spicer and Kerr (1966) noted day-to-day variation in respiratory function in seventeen patients with chronic obstructive lung disease and in eleven normal subjects. Spicer, Reinke, and Kerr (1966) also measured the daily pulmonary function of fourteen patients with chronic obstructive lung disease. Of the various pollutants monitored, only sulfur dioxide exhibited a lag effect on asthmatic patients. Spodnik and coauthors (1966), studying 106 seminary students, found that variations in respiratory function occurred together and were correlated significantly with temperature, but no specific association was found with air pollution (suspended particulates). Spicer and Kerr (1970) analyzed a random sample of the seminary students in a search for significant correlations. No meaningful relationships were found between variations in respiratory function and measured air pollution (see also Spicer 1967).

---

[32] Ipsen, Deane, and Ingenito (1969) also analyzed absences in these two plants. They found that none of the three air pollutants studied (sulfates, suspended particulates, and smokeshade) had an effect greater than that of any one of the three climate variables studied (temperature, wind velocity, and humidity), although their sum was positively correlated with the prevalence of upper-respiratory-tract infection.

McMillan and coauthors (1969) examined the peak expiratory flow rate (PEFR) in children in two Los Angeles schools over a period of eleven months. Since the schools experienced different levels of oxidant pollution, the researchers were able to compare its effects at the two schools, as well as to examine the relationship between daily levels of air pollution and daily PEFR. They also tabulated symptoms of upper-respiratory-tract infection. The study was carefully done with controls exerted for important factors affecting respiratory function, and, since school children made up the study group, smoking and occupation were not relevant factors. Despite these controls, they reported that "no significant changes in PEFR were found which correlated with acute changes in air pollution. Higher PEFR means and greater variance were found in the school exposed to higher ambient oxidant concentrations (page 949)."

Daily mortality

Several other studies investigated the relationship between daily mortality and air pollution in Great Britain. Pemberton (1961) found a positive association between bronchitis mortality and air pollution (smoke and sulfur dioxide) and a significant association between lung cancer mortality and smoke pollution. Martin and Bradley (1960) did not find a significant association between daily pneumonia deaths and atmospheric pollution (suspended particulates and fog) in the greater London area. The results of Martin (1964) in relating bronchitis mortality to air pollution (smoke and sulfur dioxide) were inconclusive.

Glasser and Greenburg (1971) examined daily deaths in New York City between 1960 and 1964 (excluding April to September). They attempted to explain deviations in daily deaths from a five-year "normal" by air pollution measures (sulfur dioxide and smokeshade), and climatological variables (temperature deviation from normal, wind speed, sky cover, and rainfall). Using descriptive statistics, cross tabulations, and regression analyses, they found a relationship between daily mortality and air pollution (primarily as measured by sulfur dioxide). One must be curious about their omitting six months from each year. Seasonal factors and air pollution might be confounded during the summer months, but regression analyses including both the relevant climate and pollution variables should sort out the individual effects. If the two semiannual periods differ in some respects, two models can be developed and tested in order to determine whether the underlying structures are similar. Analysis of this time of year is of particular interest in view of the number of inversions and high pollution episodes occurring during the summertime. Glasser and Greenburg also measured mortality in terms of deviations from a fifteen-day moving average. The measure suggests cycles in the data and lags in the effects of pollution, but no explanations are presented. Lagged variables (particularly pollution) were not utilized; hence, the investigation never questioned the timing of the effects.

Schimmel and Greenburg (1972) performed a more elaborate time-series study of New York City, examining a data base that included daily observations on total mortality and nine disease-specific mortality rates over the period 1963–68. In addition to two pollution measures (twenty-four-hour sulfur dioxide and smokeshade readings), data on several weather variables (minimum, mean, and maximum temperature, minimum and maximum humidity, wind speed, and precipitation) were available. Using a linear model, they regressed daily mortality on same-day pollution levels and levels of pollution on previous days.[33] The mode of analysis was novel and deserves comment. Instead of including measures of climate and other factors as independent variables in the regressions, Schimmel and Greenburg chose to adjust the air pollution variables to remove these effects. For example, the temperature adjustment was done by regressing each air pollution variable on mean temperature, using a fourth-degree polynomial. The residuals from these regressions were then used as variables in the analysis and termed "temperature-corrected pollution variables." Similar adjustments were made for seasonal trends and day-of-the-week effects.

The adjustment procedure was employed to eliminate spurious correlations between daily mortality and daily air pollution that might arise because of climatological factors or day-of-the-week patterns. The technique eliminates most of the variation in the air pollution variables associated with these factors. However, we question the appropriateness of this method for adjusting the air pollution measures. Not all of the variation should be eliminated if the goal of the analysis is to obtain unbiased estimates of the effects of air pollution on mortality.[34]

Schimmel and Greenburg estimated that if air pollution in New York City were reduced to zero, there would be (on average) from 18.12 to 36.74 fewer deaths each day.[35] This represents about 12 percent of the over half-million deaths occurring during the six-year period. Examining the individual effects of the two pollutants, they concluded that 80 percent of the excess deaths could be attributed to smokeshade, and only 20 percent to sulfur dioxide. In view of their estimation procedure, we are hesitant to accept this allocation.

MOBILE-SOURCE AIR POLLUTION AND HEALTH EFFECTS

Probably the largest group of studies relating to automobile emissions concerns the health effects of carbon monoxide. Breathing carbon monoxide increases the level of the carboxyhemoglobin (COHb) in the blood, thus reducing the amount of free hemoglobin available for carrying oxygen to body tissues for normal activity. The saturation of the blood with COHb is known to put a strain on the heart, as well as affecting performance on standardized tests (impaired coordination, inability to judge time, slowing down reaction time, and affecting mental abilities). However, these effects have been demonstrated for relatively high levels of carbon monoxide in the air (or COHb in the blood). The critical question is whether the levels resulting from the emissions of mobile sources are sufficient to generate important health effects.

[33] Three types of pollution variables were used: crude, temperature-corrected (using daily mean temperature), and fully adjusted (using temperature, time-trend, and day-of-the-week effects).

[34] This method of adjustment, similar to our interactions test of the 1960 cross-sectional work, is known to produce biased estimates which understate the effect of air pollution.

[35] The range results from the different pollution variables that were tried. The estimates include the sum of air pollution effects over a seven-day period.

The health effects of total oxidants are hypothesized to be similar to those of carbon monoxide, although the detailed physiological mechanism, thought to be different, is not fully understood. Little work has been done on the health effects of the oxides of nitrogen or of hydrocarbons. What follows is a brief review of some of the studies concerning effects from air pollution related to mobile-source emissions.

Beard and Wertheim (1967) performed experiments with human subjects and rats to determine the effect of carbon monoxide on time perceptions. The ability of subjects to ascertain whether a second tone lasted longer, shorter, or for the same time compared with a previous tone (for small differences in duration of the tone) fell uniformly with the level of carbon monoxide breathed. Although the error rate was closely related to concentration (which ranged from zero to 250 ppm), the subjects suffered no noticeable physiological reactions to the carbon monoxide. Hence, even though the experiment appeared to isolate a subtle effect of exposure to carbon monoxide at low concentrations, it is not evident what the implications are for its effect on human behavior in the activities of daily life.

Stewart and coauthors (1970) exposed subjects to carbon monoxide under experimental conditions and recorded physical data as well as performance on a driving simulator, and hand-steadiness and manual dexterity tests. "The most important finding was that an eight-hour exposure to 100 parts per million of carbon monoxide, resulting in a COHb saturation of 11 percent to 13 percent, produced no impairment of performance in the tests studied in this select, healthy group of volunteers. The tests chosen for investigation were those felt to be of practical significance in the performance of vocational endeavors and automobile driving, where significant impairment of visual or auditory acuity, coordination, reaction time, manual dexterity, or time estimation would be intolerable (page 163)".

Curphey, Hood, and Perkins (1965) found an association between COHb level in the blood of 1,075 cadavers and the atmospheric levels of carbon monoxide in the areas where the subjects had lived. Controls were exercised for both the sex and smoking habits of the deceased; however, the evidence did not indicate a strong relationship.

Chovin (1967) examined the level of COHb in Paris traffic policemen and found that levels rose for nonsmokers over the period when they were directing traffic, but it fell for smokers. Thus, smoking caused such a high level of saturation that ambient carbon monoxide concentrations (from traffic) were below those required to raise the level of saturation.[36]

Schulte (1963) examined performance on four standard tasks in forty-nine subjects who were exposed to controlled levels of carbon monoxide. The subjects were tested four times in an experimental design that exposed them to controlled and concentrated levels of carbon monoxide according to a random ordering. The number of errors and the completion times for the tasks were recorded and correlated with the COHb level in the subject's blood. In general, a significant relationship was found and it appeared that COHb levels below

---

[36] Göthe and coauthors (1969) found similar results in three Swedish towns.

5 percent still had an identifiable effect on error rates. Unfortunately, there appeared to be errors in the measurement of COHb levels.[37]

Aronow and Rokaw (1972) examined the effect on ten persons with angina pectoris of breathing freeway air (with high concentrations of carbon monoxide, nitrogen dioxide, hydrocarbons, and oxidants). Each patient was driven twice on a Los Angeles freeway for 90 minutes during heavy traffic. The patients breathed ambient air during the first run and compressed air during the subsequent trip. Aronow and Rokaw found an increase in both the level of carbon monoxide in expired air and the level of COHb after the first drive, but no such elevations were noted after the second drive. In the laboratory the patients exercised to the onset of symptoms; breathing ambient air (as opposed to compressed air) reduced the capacity to exercise. Two points should be made concerning this study. First, the sample was small and carefully selected. One cannot conclude that a larger population of patients with angina pectoris would react in this way, nor can one judge what the effects would be on the population at large. Second, the COHb level rose (on average) from 1.12 to 5.08 percent when patients switched from compressed air to ambient air. These levels are quite low compared with previous experiments in terms of finding significant effects on performance. It must be recognized that this was an experiment involving a study group hypothesized to be extremely sensitive to air pollution.

Cohen, Deane, and Goldsmith (1969) examined daily fatality rates for 3,080 patients admitted with myocardial infarction to thirty-five Los Angeles hospitals during 1958. Two types of rates were calculated. The first was the number of patients admitted on day i who subsequently died divided by the total number of patients admitted on day i. The second was the number of patients dying on a given day divided by the number of patients at risk in the hospital. Hospitals were divided into those located in high-pollution areas and low-pollution areas based on carbon monoxide levels.[38] Weekly fatality rates were then calculated separately for the high- and low-pollution areas.

A significant difference between area rates occurred only during the quartile of weeks having the highest carbon monoxide concentrations. Age, man–woman ratio, and insurance coverage of the patients were examined, but did not explain the observed differences. In addition, a separate correlation analysis was undertaken to examine possible day-of-the-week effects.[39] For the first fatality rate, five out of a possible ten correlations with carbon monoxide levels were statistically significant in the high-pollution area; none was significant in the low-pollution area. For the second fatality rate, two out of ten correlations were statistically significant in the high area; again, none was significant in the low area (all significant correlations were positive). Given

[37] "These studies [Schulte and others] although widely quoted, were marred by technical defects in experimental method" (World Health Organization, 1972, p. 21).

[38] The majority of hospitals were located in the high-pollution area; 2,484 admissions for myocardial infarction occurred there and 596 occurred in the low-pollution area.

[39] All days, weekends, weekdays, and each individual day were considered separately.

these mixed results and the fact that personal characteristics (such as smoking, income, and occupation) and other environmental factors (such as temperature, humidity, and precipitation) were not controlled, the study only suggests a possible association between patients admitted with myocardial infarction and levels of carbon monoxide.

Another study, by Kuller and coauthors (1975), made it possible to partially replicate the previous Los Angeles study. For a two-year period (1970–72), Kuller and his associates analyzed the relationship between 522 sudden deaths from arteriosclerotic heart disease (ASHD), 539 transural myocardial infarctions, and 226 non-sudden ASHD deaths and ambient carbon monoxide levels in Baltimore. Their results indicated that there was no evidence of any clustering of deaths or infarctions on specific days. Consequently, it was concluded that ambient carbon monoxide levels in an urban area such as Baltimore are not a major factor in the onset of sudden deaths or myocardial infarctions. It was noted, however, that the "negative" results from Baltimore as compared with Los Angeles may have been due, in part, to the relatively lower levels of carbon monoxide in Baltimore.

Seskin (1976) analyzed health-care utilization, air pollution, and weather data for 1973 and 1974 in examining the association between air pollution levels in metropolitan Washington, D.C., and health effects. Using multivariate discriminant and regression analyses, the only association found to be consistent and statistically significant for both 1973 and 1974 was between daily unscheduled ophthalmologic visits and levels of photochemical oxidant pollution. In addition, a relationship between urgent clinic visits and photochemical oxidant levels during 1974 was noted. Isolated positive and significant associations were also found between photochemical oxidant levels and unscheduled pediatric visits, carbon monoxide levels and both unscheduled ophthalmologic and unscheduled pediatric visits, and sulfur dioxide levels and both unscheduled internal medicine and unscheduled ophthalmologic visits. The magnitude of the associations suggested that air pollution levels in Washington, D.C., had a very limited effect on the health-care utilization of the sample population.

Durham (1974) investigated the health effects of air pollution on student populations at seven California universities during the 1970–71 academic year. The data consisted of morbidity rates at student health centers,[40] daily peak and mean concentrations of twenty-four-hour averages for eight pollutants (oxidants, nitric oxide, nitrogen dioxide, total oxides of nitrogen, carbon monoxide, hydrocarbons, sulfur dioxide, and suspended particulates), and information on nine meteorological factors. Analysis of the data indicated that, within each region, variations in air pollution from one campus to another overshadowed any variation in climatic factors. In addition, any differences in sociological attributes (sex ratios, smoking habits, athletic activity, commuting distance, and health center usage) were accounted for by analyzing separate subpopulations.

---

[40] Confounding factors such as prescheduled appointments, long-term and genetic conditions, and the effects of weekends, holidays, and examination periods were controlled in analyzing the health data. Tests also indicated the representativeness of the health center samples.

Attempts were first made to use stepwise multivariable regression to analyze the data. However, these failed to reveal significant patterns among the variables. Correlation techniques were then adopted. Consistent illness-specific differences were found in the relative magnitude, duration, and optimal time lag of the air pollution–health correlations. A partial correlation analysis indicated that most respiratory illnesses yielded 20 to 25 percent significant correlations with pollutants when weather factors were controlled; whereas, fewer than 5 percent of the partial correlations involving nonrespiratory illnesses were significant. The most highly pollution-related illnesses were found to be (in order): pharyngitis, bronchitis, tonsillitis, colds, and sore throat. Oxidants, sulfur dioxide, and nitrogen dioxide were the pollutants most highly associated with respiratory illnesses.

Factor analysis was also applied to the data. Results for the schools in the Los Angeles area indicated that the highest correlations for sore throat, pharyngitis, and tonsillitis occurred at the University of Southern California, while the lowest correlations were observed at the University of California at Irvine.[41] Common cold symptoms and eye irritation were similar in the two schools. This was attributed to the relatively high levels of photochemical oxidant concentrations in the two areas. Strong associations between respiratory illness and pollution variables were not found for schools in the San Francisco Bay area. This was attributed to the relatively low levels of pollution in the bay area.

Hammer and coauthors (1974) carried out a study of daily symptoms in student nurses at two Los Angeles nursing schools during a three-year period (October 1961–June 1964).[42] An average of sixty-one students per day completed symptom diaries on the incidence of headache, eye discomfort, cough, and chest discomfort.[43] The daily percentage of students reporting each symptom was calculated as follows:[44]

$$\frac{\text{number of students reporting a symptom on a given day}}{\text{number of students completing diaries on that day}} \times 100$$

These daily percentages were then compared to daily maximum hourly measurements of photochemical oxidants, carbon monoxide, nitrogen dioxide as well as daily maximum temperature. Threshold functions were calculated for both the "simple" and "adjusted" symptom rates in relation to photochemical oxidants. The daily symptom data could not be explained by functions of carbon monoxide, nitrogen dioxide, or maximum temperature. Despite the fact that

[41] The data suggested that a 16.7 percent respiratory illness excess among students at the University of Southern California over students at Irvine may be due to higher levels of atmospheric pollutants.

[42] The sample consisted of students with a median age of 18.6 years (at school entry), mostly women, and 94 percent white. The students came from families with an average of 3.2 children and a median family income of $5,000 to $7,500 per year. Students were not informed that the relation of symptoms to air pollution was of major interest.

[43] Space was provided in the diaries to grade each symptom as mild, moderate, or severe; virtually all symptoms were reported as mild.

[44] Separate calculations were also made in which symptoms accompanied by fever or chills were excluded. These were referred to as "adjusted."

the results indicated associations between the various symptoms and oxidant pollution, the findings would have been more convincing if other factors such as day-of-the-week effects were controlled explicitly and if symptom relationships with other meteorological variables such as humidity, precipitation, and temperature were examined.

In an earlier report of the student nurse study, Hammer and coauthors (1965) analyzed daily symptoms in three groups of 120 nurses living in Santa Barbara and Los Angeles.[45] Daily symptoms during a twenty-eight-day period were compared with concurrent levels of photochemical oxidants. A time-associated relationship between daily maximum oxidant levels and the daily frequency of eye discomfort was observed for Los Angeles during the study period. The daily frequencies of other symptoms were similar between the two cities and appeared to vary randomly with oxidant levels in Los Angeles.[46] Given the lack of other controls (for example, other meteorological factors) and the lack of complete pollution data, this study has very little independent informational content. It does offer limited support to the later study discussed above.

Cohen and coauthors (1972) examined 441 nonsmoking whites aged forty-five to sixty-four who lived in the San Gabriel Valley and in San Diego. The study populations were selected because of their active participation in the Seventh-Day Adventist church and because they had not smoked for at least twenty years and had never smoked heavily. Exposure differences to average oxidant concentrations were relatively small, although substantial differences existed in exposure to peak oxidant levels. Average nitrogen dioxide exposures differed by a factor of two.

Respiratory symptoms were evaluated and ventilatory tests were taken. The two study groups showed no statistically significant differences in the prevalence of chronic respiratory disease or in the lung function tests which were performed. In addition to smoking habits, sex, social class (based on education and occupation), and height were controlled. While controls for other personal habits were not used, the common church membership of the individuals presumably controlled for other important factors.

Wayne and Wehrle (1969) examined the association between daily oxidant levels and school absenteeism at two elementary schools in Los Angeles during the period September 1962 to June 1963.[47] They hypothesized that oxidant air pollution caused respiratory symptoms, which would be reflected in increased absence rates. However, they were unable to detect a statistically significant relationship between absences due to respiratory illness and concurrent or one-day lag measures of oxidant levels.[48] Wayne, Wehrle, and Carroll (1967) assessed the effects of air pollution (oxidants and carbon monoxide) on the performance of high-school males at track meets. They related the times for various events (accounting for the individual's previous performance) with the pollutant levels at the time of the meets. Oxidant levels were

[45] The groups were said to be similar in terms of age, race, sex, family size, family income, and past medical history.
[46] These symptoms included hoarseness, cough, sputum, and chest discomfort.
[47] The school areas differed in socioeconomic characteristics and ethnic origins.
[48] This was true for analyses of the data by day, week, and season.

significantly correlated with decreased performance; carbon monoxide, temperature, and humidity were not. Unfortunately, the sample size was so small that it is difficult to extrapolate the results.

Ury, Perkins, and Goldsmith (1972) examined the association between automobile accidents and both carbon monoxide and oxidant levels in Los Angeles. The basic analysis involved a comparison of the pollution level and the number of motor vehicle accidents during the same one-hour period one week apart. Thus, hour-of-the-day and day-of-the-week effects were controlled explicitly. If the day with the higher pollution level also had more accidents, a score of +1 was assigned (a score of −1 was assigned for the opposite case). The researchers detected no association between carbon monoxide levels and the frequency of accidents; however, when readings for oxidants were used in place of carbon monoxide, a significant association appeared. This association disappeared when a lag of one hour or more was used between pollution readings and accident occurrences.

Although the experiment was ingeniously contrived, it left one important factor uncontrolled. Since the pollutants in question are found primarily in automobile emissions, increased concentrations would result from increased traffic. The increased traffic would also be expected to result in increased accidents. Ury and his associates argued that this possibility could not account for their findings, but they could not rule it out.

Clayton, Cook, and Frederick (1960) also looked at the relationship between traffic accidents and carbon monoxide levels. Since only 3 of 237 people involved in traffic accidents had COHb levels of 10 percent or more, they concluded that carbon monoxide did not significantly impair driving ability in Detroit.

Taken together, these studies offer no convincing proof that traffic accidents are caused in part by carbon monoxide. On the other hand, they provide no adequate tests of the proposition. Instead of attempting to relate accident rates to air pollution readings or blood concentrations, such studies must find a way to control for the number of cars at risk. This might be done in an experiment similar to Schulte's (1963), in which subjects were put through a driving simulator and the number of accidents recorded as a function of COHb levels in the subject's blood. A cruder way of relating COHb levels and accident rates would be to compare the accident records of smokers with those of nonsmokers. Since cigarette smokers have higher COHb levels than nonsmokers, one would expect smokers to have a higher accident rate if a significant effect did exist.

APPENDIX B

The implications of our findings on the national ambient air quality standards

The Clean Air Amendments of 1970 (PL 91-604) required that the Environmental Protection Agency establish primary and secondary national ambient air quality standards (NAAQS) for each air pollutant for which criteria had been issued under the 1967 Clean Air Act (sulfur dioxide, suspended particulates, carbon monoxide, photochemical oxidants, hydrocarbons, and nitrogen dioxide.)[1] The proposed rules establishing these standards were published June 30, 1971, and final rules were promulgated on April 30, 1971 (see table B.1).

PRIMARY STANDARD

The *primary standard* was to be that level of ambient air quality which, in the judgment of the administrator of the EPA, was "requisite to protect the public health." The Senate Committee on Public Works (where the concept first arose) described the standard as follows:

In requiring that national ambient air quality standards be established at a level necessary to protect the health of persons, the Committee recognizes that such standards will not necessarily provide for the quality of air required to protect those individuals who are otherwise dependent on a controlled internal environment such as patients in intensive care units or newborn infants in nurseries. However, the Committee emphasizes that included among those persons whose health should be protected by the ambient standard are particularly sensitive citizens such as bronchial asthmatics and emphysematics who in the normal course of daily activity are exposed to the ambient environment. In establishing an ambient standard necessary to protect the health of these persons, reference should be made to a representative sample of persons comprising the sensitive group rather than to a single person in such a group. Ambient air quality is sufficient to protect the health of such persons whenever there is an absence of adverse effect on the health of a statistically related sample of persons in sensitive groups from exposure to the ambient air. An ambient air quality standard, therefore, should be the maximum permissible ambient air level of an air pollution agent or class of such agents (related to a period of time) which will protect the health of any group of the population.

[1] Background information for this discussion was obtained from Jorling (1974).

312

For purposes of this description, a statistically related sample is the number of persons necessary to test in order to detect a deviation in the health of any person within such sensitive group which is attributable to the condition of the ambient air.

Furthermore, in establishing the primary standard, the administrator was to apply an "adequate margin of safety." Thus, if conflicting or ambiguous evidence was presented, he was to resolve the issue on the side of protecting the public health.

SECONDARY STANDARD

In establishing the secondary ambient air quality standard, the administrator was directed to establish numerical indexes for those parameters of air quality which are necessary to protect "public welfare," defined in the act as "any effects on soils, waters, crops, vegetation, man-made materials, animal wildlife, weather, visibility and climate, damage to or deterioration of property and hazards to transportation, as well as effects on economic values and on personal comfort and well being." Thus, its purpose was to establish (for areas having poor air quality) the level of ambient air quality that in no way would affect man or the environment.

SUSPENDED PARTICULATES

As shown in table B.1, the primary standard for suspended particulates is 75 μg per cubic meter of air; based on an annual geometric mean, and 260 μg per cubic meter, based on a maximum twenty-four-hour reading. By looking at table D.1 (page 321), one can determine to some extent the levels of particulate pollution prevailing in the areas we examined. For example, the average of the mean (arithmetic) biweekly suspended particulate readings across the 117 SMSAs in 1960 was approximately 118 μg per cubic meter. Furthermore, the average of the maximum biweekly suspended particulate readings across the same areas during 1960 was over 268 μg per cubic meter.[2] In 1969 the average of the mean biweekly suspended particulate readings across the 112 SMSAs was 96 μg per cubic meter. The average of the maximum biweekly suspended particulate readings for this time period was 244 μg per cubic meter. Clearly, many of the areas included in our samples experienced readings in excess of the primary standards.[3] Since one of our basic conclusions was that suspended particulate levels were significantly related to the mortality rates and since a linear specification seemed to "fit" the data as well as alternative forms, it seems likely that if one is willing to accept the notion of a national standard as meaningful (see below), then the present primary standard for suspended particulates may not be stringent enough.

SULFATES AND SULFUR DIOXIDE

Measures of sulfates were the primary form of air pollution involving sulfur for which we had extensive empirical results. However, at this time

[2] This figure is an underestimate of the true maximum twenty-four-hour readings experienced in these areas since it is based on an arbitrary biweekly measurement.

[3] Specifically, 104 SMSAs in 1960 and 88 SMSAs in 1969 experienced average annual means of suspended particulate pollution in excess of 75 μg per cubic meter (based on an arithmetic mean). Since the arithmetic mean is always larger than a geometric mean, these SMSAs failed to meet the primary standard.

TABLE B.1.   National Primary and Secondary Ambient Air Quality Standards

Air pollutant	Federal standard	
	Primary	Secondary
Sulfur dioxide	80 μg per cubic meter (0.03 ppm) annual arithmetic mean 365 μg per cubic meter (0.14 ppm) maximum in twenty-four hours	60 μg per cubic meter (0.02 ppm) annual arithmetic mean[a] 260 μg per cubic meter (0.1 ppm) maximum in twenty-four hours[a] 1,300 μg per cubic meter (0.5 ppm) maximum in three hours
Suspended particulates.	75 μg per cubic meter annual geometric mean 260 μg per cubic meter maximum in twenty-four hours	60 μg per cubic meter annual geometric mean 150 μg per cubic meter maximum in twenty-four hours
Carbon monoxide	10 mg per cubic meter (9 ppm) maximum in eight hours 40 mg per cubic meter (35 ppm) maximum in one hour	10 mg per cubic meter (9 ppm) maximum in eight hours 40 mg per cubic meter (35 ppm) maximum in one hour
Photochemical oxidants	160 μg per cubic meter (0.08 ppm) maximum in one hour	160 μg per cubic meter (0.08 ppm) maximum in one hour
Hydrocarbons (corrected for methane)	160 μg per cubic meter (0.08 ppm) maximum in three hours, 6 A.M. to 9 A.M.	160 μg per cubic meter (0.08 ppm) maximum in three hours, 6 A.M. to 9 A.M.
Nitrogen dioxide	100 μg per cubic meter (0.05 ppm) annual arithmetic mean	100 μg per cubic meter (0.05 ppm) annual arithmetic mean

Note: Maximum concentrations are not to be exceeded more than once per year.
[a] In 1973 EPA relaxed the secondary standard for sulfur dioxide by withdrawing the requirement of annual mean measurement and confining the secondary standard to a three-hour measurement.

there is no national standard for sulfates despite the fact that this type of air pollution is of considerable concern to the EPA. This concern arises from increasing evidence as to the deleterious effects of sulfates.

Nevertheless, given the tenuous relationship between sulfur dioxide and sulfates, we do not feel justified in discussing the national standard for sulfur dioxide in terms of our findings for sulfates. Rather, our limited findings on sulfur dioxide itself, may shed some light on this subject.

In the 1969 cross-sectional analysis (see chapter 7), sulfur dioxide data were available for sixty-nine areas. The average of the mean biweekly sulfur dioxide readings for these areas was 33 μg per cubic meter (see table D.1). This is considerably below the primary standard of 80 μg per cubic meter. Further, the average of the maximum biweekly sulfur dioxide readings was approximately 116 μg per cubic meter; whereas, the primary standard based on the maximum twenty-four-hour reading is 365 μg per cubic meter. Thus, in general, the sulfur dioxide levels experienced in the areas under scrutiny were below the standard.[4] Our cross-sectional findings, however, indicated that these levels of sulfur dioxide were still significantly related to mortality rates across the SMSAs (see tables 7.8, 7.9, and 7.10).[5] Putting aside for the moment the question of whether setting standards to protect health is a useful exercise, these limited results provide some evidence that the current annual sulfur dioxide standard may not be sufficiently stringent.[6]

NITROGEN DIOXIDE

The 1969 cross-sectional analysis on additional air pollutants also included data on nitrogen dioxide. For the sample of sixty-nine SMSAs, the average of the mean biweekly nitrogen dioxide readings was slightly over 136 μg per cubic meter. The primary standard is set at 100 μg per cubic meter.[7] The results depicted in tables 7.8, 7.9, and 7.10 indicated that nitrogen dioxide was significantly related to the unadjusted and adjusted total mortality rates, but not to the race-adjusted infant mortality rates. However, the cross-sectional, time-series analysis in chapter 8 did not indicate that annual changes in nitrogen dioxide levels were significantly related to annual changes in the mortality rates (tables 8.4, 8.5, and 8.6). Further, the daily time-series analysis in chapter 9 did not detect consistent, significant associations between the daily levels of nitrogen dioxide and daily deaths in any of the cities examined.[8] Given these mixed and somewhat limited results, it is difficult to draw any policy conclusions regarding the national standard for nitrogen dioxide. At the same time, the evidence would seem to indicate that some control of nitrogen dioxide levels is warranted.

CARBON MONOXIDE AND HYDROCARBONS

The two remaining criteria air pollutants, for which our findings are relevant, are carbon monoxide and hydrocarbons. The only empirical results relating to these pollutants are found in chapter 9. As reported there, neither air pollutant was found to be statistically significant in explaining daily deaths for the cities examined. However, the measurements of both of these air pollutants that were reported and used in the analysis do not correspond to the measure-

[4] In fact only two SMSAs, Chicago and Providence, exceeded the primary standard based on an annual average of 80 μg per cubic meter, and both of them, as well as New Haven, exceeded the primary standard based on the maximum twenty-four-hour reading of 365 μg per cubic meter. (However, see fn 2.)

[5] The reader is also reminded that our findings generally indicated that the association between levels of sulfur dioxide and the mortality rates was weaker than the association between levels of sulfates and the mortality rates.

[6] In general, this conclusion is supported by the cross-sectional time-series findings of chapter 8 (see tables 8.4, 8.5, and 8.6). In addition, the daily time-series analysis for Chicago (chapter 9) found sulfur dioxide to be significantly related to daily deaths, although the levels of sulfur dioxide were considerably in excess of the national standards (see table D.13).

[7] Fifty-two of the sixty-nine SMSAs failed to meet the primary standard in 1969.

[8] The average level of nitrogen dioxide in the four-pollutant data set examined for Chicago was 0.04 ppm (see table D.13). The national standard for nitrogen dioxide is 0.05 ppm.

ments on which the national standards are based.[9] Hence, it is difficult to infer the implications of our findings with regard to these air pollutants and the levels at which the standards are set. Our results cannot be used to support or refute the standards.

ON THE USE OF STANDARDS

As discussed previously, our results do not lend support to the threshold concept. When we examined alternative specifications, we found that generally a simple linear specification "fit" the data as well as other functional forms.[10] We found (for the air pollutants under consideration) little indication that specific levels could be considered "safe" levels, below which no health effects could be detected. Given our findings, we feel that the notion of an air pollution standard (or threshold) for a pollutant that will "protect the public health or welfare" is not meaningful. It translates into setting standards on the basis of damages (or benefits) alone. Instead, we would argue that standards should be based on benefit–cost tradeoffs. That is, we believe that society must weigh the costs and benefits of achieving various levels of air quality, and once a desired level is selected, the standards corresponding to it should be determined.

[9] Both air pollutants were measured, and analyzed, on the basis of daily averages. In addition, total hydrocarbons, rather than nonmethane hydrocarbons, were monitored and analyzed.

[10] See chapters 3 and 7 on alternative specifications.

SMSAs used in the analyses

TABLE C.1. SMSAs Used in the Analyses

SMSA	Basic 1960 and 1961 data sets (n=117)	Identical 1960 and 1969 data sets (n=81)	Basic 1969 data set (n=112)	1969 data set with additional air pollutants (n=69)	Basic 1960–69 data set (n=241)[a]	1962–68 data set with additional air pollutants (n=105)[b]
Albany, N.Y.			✕	✕		
Albuquerque, N.Mex.	✕	✕	✕	✕		
Allentown, Pa.	✕	✕	✕	✕		
Atlanta, Ga.	✕	✕	✕	✕		
Atlantic City, N.J.	✕					
Augusta, Ga.	✕					
Austin, Tex.	✕					
Baltimore, Md.	✕	✕	✕	✕	✕	
Baton Rouge, La.	✕	✕	✕			
Beaumont, Tex.	✕					
Birmingham, Ala.	✕					
Boston, Mass.[c]	✕	✕	✕			
Bridgeport, Conn.[c,d]	✕		✕			
Brockton, Mass.[c]	✕					
Buffalo, N.Y.			✕	✕		
Canton, Ohio	✕	✕	✕	✕		
Charleston, S.C.	✕					
Charleston, W.Va.	✕	✕	✕	✕		
Charlotte, N.C.	✕	✕	✕			
Chattanooga, Tenn.	✕	✕	✕	✕	✕	
Chicago, Ill.	✕	✕	✕	✕	✕	
Cincinnati, Ohio	✕	✕	✕	✕	✕	
Cleveland, Ohio*	✕	✕	✕	✕	✕	✕
Columbia, S.C.	✕	✕	✕			
Columbus, Ga.	✕	✕	✕			
Columbus, Ohio	✕	✕	✕	✕	✕	

(Continued)

TABLE C.1. (Continued)

SMSA	Basic 1960 and 1961 data sets (n=117)	Identical 1960 and 1969 data sets (n=81)	Basic 1969 data set (n=112)	1969 data set with additional air pollutants (n=69)	Basic 1960–69 data set (n=241)[a]	1962–68 data set with additional air pollutants (n=105)[b]
Dallas, Tex.	X	X	X	X		
Davenport, Iowa			X			
Dayton, Ohio	X	X	X	X		
Denver, Colo.*†	X	X	X	X	X	X
Des Moines, Iowa*	X	X	X	X	X	X
Detroit, Mich.*	X	X	X	X	X	X
Duluth, Minn.	X	X	X			
Durham, N.C.			X			
El Paso, Tex.	X					
Erie, Pa.			X			
Evansville, Ind.			X	X		
Fall River, Mass.[c]	X	X	X			
Fargo, N.Dak.			X			
Flint, Mich.	X	X	X	X		
Fort Wayne, Ind.			X			
Fort Worth, Tex.	X	X	X			
Fresno, Calif.	X	X	X			
Galveston, Tex.	X					
Gary, Ind.	X		X	X		
Grand Rapids, Mich.			X	X		
Greensboro, N.C.	X	X	X	X		
Greenville, S.C.	X	X	X			
Hamilton, Ohio	X					
Harrisburg, Pa.	X	X	X			
Hartford, Conn.*[c]	X	X	X	X	X	X
Honolulu, Hawaii			X			
Houston, Tex.	X		X	X		
Huntington, W.Va.	X	X	X			
Huntsville, Ala.			X			
Indianapolis, Ind.	X	X	X	X	X	X
Jackson, Mich.	X					
Jackson, Miss.	X					
Jacksonville, Fla.	X	X	X	X		
Jersey City, N.J.	X	X	X	X		
Johnstown, Pa.	X	X	X	X		
Kansas City, Mo.	X					
Kenosha, Wis.			X			
Knoxville, Tenn.	X	X	X			
Lansing, Mich.	X					
Las Vegas, Nev.	X	X	X			
Little Rock, Ark.	X	X	X	X		
Lorain, Ohio	X					
Los Angeles, Calif.	X	X	X			
Louisville, Ky.			X	X		
Macon, Ga.	X					
Madison, Wis.	X	X	X			
Manchester, N.H.[c]	X					
Memphis, Tenn.	X	X	X	X		
Miami, Fla.	X	X	X	X		

318

TABLE C.1. *(Continued)*

SMSA	Basic 1960 and 1961 data sets (n=117)	Identical 1960 and 1969 data sets (n=81)	Basic 1969 data set (n=112)	1969 data set with additional air pollutants (n=69)	Basic 1960–69 data set (n=241)ª	1962–68 data set with additional air pollutants (n=105)ᵇ
Milwaukee, Wis.*	X	X	X	X	X	X
Minneapolis, Minn.*	X	X	X	X	X	X
Mobile, Ala.	X	X	X	X		
Montgomery, Ala.	X	X	X	X		
Nashville, Tenn.*	X	X	X	X	X	X
Newark, N.J.	X	X	X	X	X	X
New Haven, Conn.*c	X	X	X	X	X	X
New Orleans, La.	X	X	X	X		
Newport News, Va.			X			
New York City, N.Y.*	X	X	X		X	
Norfolk, Va.	X	X	X	X		
Oklahoma City, Okla.	X					
Omaha, Nebr.	X	X	X	X		
Orlando, Fla.d	X					
Paterson, N.J.			X	X		
Peoria, Ill.			X			
Philadelphia, Pa.	X	X	X	X	X	
Phoenix, Ariz.	X	X	X	X		
Pittsburgh, Pa.*‡	X				X	
Portland, Maine	X					
Portland, Oreg.*	X	X	X		X	
Providence, R.I.*c	X	X	X	X	X	X
Racine, Wis.			X			
Raleigh, N.C.	X					
Reading, Pa.	X					
Richmond, Va.	X	X	X	X		
Roanoke, Va.	X					
Rochester, N.Y.			X	X		
Rockford, Ill.	X	X	X	X		
Sacramento, Calif.	X	X	X			
Saginaw, Mich.	X	X	X	X		
Saint Louis, Mo.	X	X	X	X		
Salt Lake City, Utah*d	X	X	X	X	X	X
San Antonio, Tex.	X	X	X	X		
San Bernardino, Calif.			X	X		
San Diego, Calif.	X	X	X	X		
San Francisco, Calif.	X	X	X	X		
San Jose, Calif.	X	X	X	X		
Savannah, Ga.	X	X	X	X		
Scranton, Pa.	X					
Seattle, Wash.*	X	X	X	X	X	
Shreveport, La.	X	X	X			
Sioux Falls, S.Dak.	X					
South Bend, Ind.	X	X	X			
Springfield, Ill.			X			
Springfield, Mass.c	X	X	X	X		
Springfield, Ohio	X					

(Continued)

TABLE C.1. (*Continued*)

SMSA	Basic 1960 and 1961 data sets (n = 117)	Identical 1960 and 1969 data sets (n = 81)	Basic 1969 data set (n = 112)	1969 data set with additional air pollutants (n = 69)	Basic 1960–69 data set (n = 241)[a]	1962–68 data set with additional air pollutants (n = 105)[b]
Spokane, Wash.			×			
Syracuse, N.Y.			×	×		
Tacoma, Wash.	×	×	×			
Tampa, Fla.	×		×	×		
Terre Haute, Ind.	×					
Toledo, Ohio	×	×	×			
Topeka, Kans.	×	×	×	×		
Trenton, N.J.			×			
Tucson, Ariz.			×			
Tulsa, Okla.			×	×		
Utica, N.Y.			×	×		
Waco, Tex.	×					
Washington, D.C.	×	×	×	×	×	
Wheeling, W.Va.	×					
Wichita, Kans.	×	×	×	×		
Wilkes Barre, Pa.	×	×	×			
Wilmington, Del.*	×	×	×		×	×
Winston-Salem, N.C.	×		×			
Worcester, Mass.[c]	×	×	×	×		
York, Pa.	×					
Youngstown, Ohio*	×	×	×		×	×

Note: The 1960 SMSA definitions were used throughout the analyses.

[a] Twenty-six SMSAs studied for ten years with nineteen observations omitted: asterisk (*) denotes that 1961 data were not available; dagger (†) denotes that 1966 data were not available; double dagger (‡) denotes that 1969 data were not available.

[b] Fifteen SMSAs studied for seven years.

[c] State economic areas.

[d] SMSAs dropped from crime rate analysis (see table 6.3, p. 117).

Variables used in the analyses

TABLE D.1. Basic Variables

		1960 (117 SMSAs)		1961 (117 SMSAs)	
Variable	Description	Mean	Standard deviation	Mean	Standard deviation
Air pollution	Min S: Smallest biweekly sulfate reading (μg per cubic meter × 10)	47.239	31.276	47.598	30.796
	Mean S: Arithmetic mean of biweekly sulfate readings (μg per cubic meter × 10)	99.649	52.885	102.342	57.773
	Max S: Largest biweekly sulfate reading (μg per cubic meter × 10)	228.393	124.411	237.427	131.655
	Min P: Smallest biweekly suspended particulate reading (μg per cubic meter	45.479	18.571	44.658	18.592
	Mean P: Arithmetic mean of biweekly suspended particulate readings (μg per cubic meter)	118.145	40.942	113.786	39.573
	Max P: Largest biweekly suspended particulate reading (μg per cubic meter)	268.359	132.073	265.145	131.386
Socioeconomic	P/M²: SMSA population density (per square mile × 0.1)	69.965	135.443	70.738	135.178
	≥65: Percentage of SMSA population at least sixty-five years old (×10)	83.872	21.072	84.376	20.733
	NW: Percentage of nonwhites in SMSA population (×10)	124.812	104.099	125.726	103.290
	Poor: Percentage of SMSA families with incomes below the poverty level (×10)	181.120	65.236	172.581	62.208
	Log Pop: The logarithm of SMSA population (×100)	565.717	40.663	566.401	40.721
Mortality	Unadjusted total mortality rate (per 100,000)	912.316	153.282	895.043	154.014
	Age–sex–race-adjusted total mortality rate (per 100,000)	1015.974	78.045	988.470	74.870
	Unadjusted infant mortality rate (per 10,000 live births)	254.034	36.462	250.325	33.683
	Race-adjusted infant mortality rate (per 10,000 live births)	251.436	30.953	247.162	25.350
	White infant mortality rate (per 10,000 live births)	224.205	27.637		
	Nonwhite infant mortality rate (per 10,000 live births)	382.564	121.279		

Variable	Description	1960 (81 SMSAs)		1969 (81 SMSAs)	
		Mean	*Standard deviation*	*Mean*	*Standard deviation*
Air pollution	Min S: Smallest biweekly sulfate reading (μg per cubic meter $\times$ 10)	45.494	31.149	34.802	20.323
	Mean S: Arithmetic mean of biweekly sulfate readings (μg per cubic meter $\times$ 10)	103.914	55.340	110.062	50.191
	Max S: Largest biweekly sulfate reading (μg per cubic meter $\times$ 10)	234.111	129.621	272.148	154.416
	Min P: Smallest biweekly suspended particulate reading (μg per cubic meter	48.605	18.813	31.790	13.575
	Mean P: Arithmetic mean of biweekly suspended particulate readings (μg per cubic meter)	122.531	40.898	96.123	28.887
	Max P: Largest biweekly suspended particulate reading (μg per cubic meter)	267.790	125.908	239.988	111.888
Socioeconomic	P/M²: SMSA population density (per square mile $\times$ 0.1)	85.016	160.196	93.328	157.006
	$\geq$65: Percentage of SMSA population at least sixty-five years old ($\times$10)	82.136	17.316	88.272	17.222
	NW: Percentage of nonwhites in SMSA population ($\times$10)	122.617	100.067	133.074	96.247
	Poor: Percentage of SMSA families with incomes below the poverty level ($\times$10)	172.049	63.374	93.000	37.918
	Log Pop: The logarithm of SMSA population ($\times$100)	575.895	40.252	581.704	40.816
Mortality	Unadjusted total mortality rate (per 100,000)	901.148	131.426	905.309	140.941
	Age–sex–race-adjusted total mortality rate (per 100,000)	1018.148	68.581	967.667	68.050
	Unadjusted infant mortality rate (per 10,000 live births)				
	Race-adjusted infant mortality rate (per 10,000 live births)				
	White infant mortality rate (per 10,000 live births)				
	Nonwhite infant mortality rate (per 10,000 live births)				

Variable	Description	1969 (112 SMSAs) Mean	1969 (112 SMSAs) Standard deviation	1969 (69 SMSAs) Mean	1969 (69 SMSAs) Standard deviation
Air Pollution	Min S: Smallest biweekly sulfate reading (μg per cubic meter $\times$ 10)	34.625	19.307	34.768	18.608
	Mean S: Arithmetic mean of biweekly sulfate readings (μg per cubic meter $\times$ 10)	109.366	45.947	115.652	47.258
	Max S: Largest biweekly sulfate reading (μg per cubic meter $\times$ 10)	273.294	146.279	286.435	142.852
	Min P: Smallest biweekly suspended particulate reading (μg per cubic meter)	31.045	13.550	32.290	14.691
	Mean P: Arithmetic mean of biweekly suspended particulate readings (μg per cubic meter)	95.580	28.642	99.507	27.436
	Max P: Largest biweekly suspended particulate reading (μg per cubic meter)	244.491	132.666	268.768	149.779
Socioeconomic	P/M^2: SMSA population density (per square mile $\times$ 0.1)	84.054	137.775	97.813	160.781
	≥ 65: Percentage of SMSA population at least sixty-five years old ($\times$ 10)	89.839	20.437	90.913	20.487
	NW: Percentage of nonwhites in SMSA population ($\times$ 10)	126.946	102.641	129.609	92.209
	Poor: Percentage of SMSA families with incomes below the poverty level ($\times$ 10)	88.902	35.087	87.899	35.103
	Log Pop: The logarithm of SMSA population ($\times$ 100)	575.664	39.876	586.181	35.907
Mortality	Unadjusted total mortality rate (per 100,000)	902.250	147.743	910.058	138.238
	Age–sex–race-adjusted total mortality rate (per 100,000)	958.955	69.683	959.812	71.094
	Unadjusted infant mortality rate (per 10,000 live births)	203.964	25.664		
	Race-adjusted infant mortality rate (per 10,000 live births)	203.027	27.355	208.116	23.496
	White infant mortality rate (per 10,000 live births)	181.571	21.481		
	Nonwhite infant mortality rate (per 10,000 live births)	307.000	99.315		

(Continued)

TABLE D.1. (*Continued*)

Variable	Description	1960–69 (26 SMSAs) Mean	1960–69 (26 SMSAs) Standard deviation	1962–68 (15 SMSAs) Mean	1962–68 (15 SMSAs) Standard deviation
Air Pollution	Min S: Smallest biweekly sulfate reading (μg per cubic meter × 10)	43.461	23.431	38.952	21.407
	Mean S: Arithmetic mean of biweekly sulfate readings (μg per cubic meter × 10)	131.071	53.489	116.924	44.373
	Max S: Largest biweekly sulfate reading (μg per cubic meter × 10)	308.851	140.821	285.886	120.922
	Min P: Smallest biweekly suspended particulate reading (μg per cubic meter)	49.523	20.570	48.133	16.909
	Mean P: Arithmetic mean of biweekly suspended particulate readings (μg per cubic meter)	126.473	32.824	122.076	26.685
	Max P: Largest biweekly suspended particulate reading (μg per cubic meter)	292.963	106.759	282.324	112.119
Socioeconomic	P/M²: SMSA population density (per square mile × 0.1)	129.463	102.034	120.125	75.292
	≥65: Percentage of SMSA population at least sixty-five years old (×10)	89.432	11.553	89.295	10.054
	NW: Percentage of nonwhites in SMSA population (×10)	117.004	67.558	95.276	60.419
	Poor: Percentage of SMSA families with incomes below the poverty level (×10)	101.631	34.362	93.752	26.830
	Log Pop: The logarithm of SMSA population (×100)	607.586	40.296	592.958	30.435
Mortality	Unadjusted total mortality rate (per 100,000)	935.581	98.476	916.000	97.142
	Age–sex–race-adjusted total mortality rate (per 100,000)	996.967	57.097	983.533	55.119
	Unadjusted infant mortality rate (per 10,000 live births)				
	Race-adjusted infant mortality rate (per 10,000 live births)	227.004	25.184	227.219	25.244
	White infant mortality rate (per 10,000 live births)				
	Nonwhite infant mortality rate (per 10,000 live births)				

Sources: See the list of data sources at the end of appendix D.

Note: Some variables are scaled to provide for computational accuracy and to provide for the use of a consistent format in reporting the estimated coefficients in the tables.

TABLE D.2. Additional Variables Used in the Analysis of Alternative Specifications, 1960

Variable	Mean	Standard deviation
Log-log		
Log Min S ($\times$ 100)	157.421	33.907
Log Mean P ($\times$ 100)	204.788	14.551
Log P/M^2 ($\times$ 100)	262.701	39.402
Log $\geq$ 65 ($\times$ 100)	191.003	10.917
Log NW ($\times$ 100)	189.092	49.477
Log Poor ($\times$ 100)	223.085	15.332
Log Pop	565.717	40.663
Log unadjusted total mortality rate ($\times$ 100)	295.426	71.115
Quadratic		
(Min S)^2 ($\times$ 0.1)	320.136	500.181
(Mean P)^2 ($\times$ 0.01)	156.202	114.051
(Min S) $\times$ (Mean P) ($\times$ 0.1)	592.584	556.829
Dummy variable		
DS$_1$: 1 if Min S $\leq$ 25 (μg per cubic meter $\times$ 10), 0 otherwise	.231	.423
DS$_2$: 1 if 25 (μg per cubic meter $\times$ 10) $<$ Min S $\leq$ 47 (μg per cubic meter $\times$ 10), 0 otherwise	.359	.482
DS$_3$: 1 if 47 (μg per cubic meter $\times$ 10) $<$ Min S $\leq$ 70 (μg per cubic meter $\times$ 10), 0 otherwise	.256	.439
DS$_4$: 1 if 70 (μg per cubic meter $\times$ 10) $<$ Min S, 0 otherwise	.154	.362
DP$_1$: 1 if Mean P $\leq$ 75 μg per cubic meter, 0 otherwise	.111	.316
DP$_2$: 1 if 75 μg per cubic meter $<$ Mean P $\leq$ 111 μg per cubic meter, 0 otherwise	.367	.484
DP$_3$: 1 if 111 μg per cubic meter $<$ Mean P $\leq$ 165 μg per cubic meter, 0 otherwise	.385	.489
DP$_4$: 1 if 165 μg per cubic meter $<$ Mean P, 0 otherwise	.137	.345
Linear spline		
Min S$_1$: Min S $-$ 25 (μg per cubic meter $\times$ 10) if Min S $\geq$ 25 (μg per cubic meter $\times$ 10), 0 otherwise	24.231	29.288
Min S$_2$: Min S $-$ 47 (μg per cubic meter $\times$ 10) if Min S $\geq$ 47 (μg per cubic meter $\times$ 10), 0 otherwise	11.154	23.811
Min S$_3$: Min S $-$ 70 (μg per cubic meter $\times$ 10) if Min S $\geq$ 70 (μg per cubic meter $\times$ 10), 0 otherwise	5.094	17.729
Mean P$_1$: Mean P $-$ 75 μg per cubic meter if Mean P $\geq$ 75 μg per cubic meter, 0 otherwise	44.017	39.849
Mean P$_2$: Mean P $-$ 111 μg per cubic meter if Mean P $\geq$ 111 μg per cubic meter, 0 otherwise	19.649	30.215
Mean P$_3$: Mean P $-$ 165 μg per cubic meter if Mean P $\geq$ 165 μg per cubic meter, 0 otherwise	3.914	14.062
Mean P split—high		
Min S	55.448	38.494
Mean P	150.586	32.493
P/M^2	100.286	186.481
$\geq$ 65	82.672	19.528
NW	109.741	87.896
Poor	169.017	56.646
Log Pop	577.677	45.491
Unadjusted total mortality rate	924.776	163.017
Mean P split—low		
Min S	39.169	19.143
Mean P	86.254	15.095
P/M^2	40.158	26.282
$\geq$ 65	85.051	22.593
NW	139.627	116.749
Poor	193.017	71.188
Log Pop	553.959	31.458
Unadjusted total mortality rate	900.068	143.409

(*Continued*)

TABLE D.2. *(Continued)*

Variable	Mean	Standard deviation
Census regions		
New England: 1 if SMSA is in this region, 0 otherwise	.094	.293
Mid-Atlantic: 1 if SMSA is in this region, 0 otherwise	.111	.316
Eastern North Central: 1 if SMSA is in this region, 0 otherwise	.196	.399
Western North Central: 1 if SMSA is in this region, 0 otherwise	.077	.268
South Atlantic: 1 if SMSA is in this region, 0 otherwise	.214	.412
Eastern South Central: 1 if SMSA is in this region, 0 otherwise	.068	.253
Western South Central: 1 if SMSA is in this region, 0 otherwise	.120	.326
Mountain: 1 if SMSA is in this region, 0 otherwise	.043	.203
Pacific: 1 if SMSA is in this region, 0 otherwise	.077	.268
Migration		
Migration: percent change in SMSA population from 1950 to 1960 ($\times$ 10)	307.709	260.325
Migration split—high		
Min S	36.483	22.694
Mean P	113.362	40.064
P/M^2	48.243	34.524
≥ 65	73.465	20.088
NW	149.396	109.961
Poor	185.052	70.492
Log Pop	565.681	32.434
Migration	468.448	278.185
Unadjusted total mortality rate	821.690	113.590
Migration split—low		
Min S	57.814	34.939
Mean P	122.847	41.589
P/M^2	91.319	185.963
≥ 65	94.102	16.637
NW	100.644	92.691
Poor	177.254	59.579
Log Pop	565.753	47.678
Migration	149.695	90.826
Unadjusted total mortality rate	1001.407	134.251

Sources: See the list of data sources at the end of appendix D.

TABLE D.3. Additional Mortality Rates Used in the Analyses

	1960 (117 SMSAs)		1961 (117 SMSAs)	
Mortality rate	Mean	Standard deviation	Mean	Standard deviation
Disease specific[a]				
Cancer mortality rates				
Total cancers: Malignant neoplasms, including neoplasms of lymphatic and hematopoietic tissues (per 100,000)	143.376	32.929	145.368	32.364
Buccal and pharyngeal cancers: Malignant neoplasm of buccal cavity and pharynx (per 10,000,000)	344.453	148.525	349.009	134.031
Digestive cancers: Malignant neoplasm of digestive organs and peritoneum, not specified as secondary (per 1,000,000)	472.128	150.878	471.855	145.191
Respiratory cancers: Malignant neoplasm of respiratory system, not specified as secondary (per 1,000,000)	222.393	61.435	232.342	63.095
Breast cancers: Malignant neoplasm of breast (per 1,000,000)	126.009	36.343	132.991	37.564
Cardiovascular disease mortality rates				
Total cardiovascular disease: Diseases of cardiovascular system (per 100,000)	482.308	114.604	476.932	113.630
Heart disease: Diseases of heart (per 100,000)	349.171	118.283	339.274	92.398
Endocarditis: Nonrheumatic chronic endocarditis and other myocardial degeneration (per 1,000,000)	280.009	175.385	262.043	164.449
Hypertensive disease: Hypertensive heart disease (per 1,000,000)	352.419	133.640	334.556	128.571
Respiratory system mortality rates				
Total respiratory diseases: Asthma, influenza, pneumonia, bronchitis, and tuberculosis of respiratory system (per 1,000,000)	453.684	102.607	371.983	96.666
Tuberculosis: Tuberculosis of respiratory system (per 10,000,000)	546.957	270.082	505.769	291.182
Asthma: Asthma (per 10,000,000)	290.034	130.207	260.752	148.124
Influenza: Influenza (per 10,000,000)	339.991	263.972	87.727	124.052
Pneumonia: Pneumonia, except of newborn (per 1,000,000)	313.094	87.451	265.795	80.850
Bronchitis: Bronchitis (per 10,000,000)	228.333	109.083	206.880	114.372

(Continued)

TABLE D.3. *(Continued)*

Mortality rate	1960 (117 SMSAs)		1969 (112 SMSAs)	
	Mean	*Standard deviation*	*Mean*	*Standard deviation*
Age–sex–race-specific (per 100,000)				
All ages				
Males and females, whites and nonwhites	1015.974	78.045	958.955	69.683
White males	1144.590	81.609	1114.429	84.831
White females	900.017	80.721	822.616	58.899
Nonwhite males	1121.085	288.816	1087.813	228.891
Nonwhite females	874.752	214.549	759.982	156.162
Newborn to fourteen years				
Males and females, whites and nonwhites	215.470	31.607	174.384	22.711
White males	215.761	34.672	175.804	24.765
White females	162.812	23.870	128.875	19.253
Nonwhite males	398.692	250.533	329.232	139.178
Nonwhite females	313.812	148.256	256.893	100.643
Fifteen to forty-four years				
Males and females, whites and nonwhites	166.043	22.799	183.348	24.829
White males	192.376	27.430	209.795	32.961
White females	101.658	15.484	107.732	17.633
Nonwhite males	358.231	146.811	475.500	139.935
Nonwhite females	246.658	100.793	247.848	120.019
Forty-five to sixty-four years				
Males and females, whites and nonwhites	1223.145	132.327	1155.813	131.191
White males	1579.222	172.332	1509.170	184.456
White females	745.624	99.283	711.152	67.755
Nonwhite males	2266.359	775.041	2159.134	695.821
Nonwhite females	1634.889	609.414	1332.991	428.854
Sixty-five years and older				
Males and females, whites and nonwhites	6428.786	565.224	6037.705	461.918
White males	7642.778	606.771	7514.330	579.116
While females	5584.171	573.664	5043.304	416.638
Nonwhite males	7385.068	2520.883	6768.089	2122.348
Nonwhite females	5398.991	1559.260	4766.250	1363.393

Sources: See the list of data sources at the end of appendix D.
▪ ICDA (International Classification of Diseases, numbers): Total cancers 140–205; buccal and pharyngeal cancers 140–148; digestive cancers 150–156A, 157–159; respiratory cancers 160–164; breast cancers 170; total cardiovascular diseases 330–334, 400–468; heart disease 400–402, 410–443; endocarditis 421–422; hypertensive disease 440–443; total respiratory diseases 001–008, 241, 480–483, 490–493, 500–502; tuberculosis 001–008; asthma 241; influenza 480–483; pneumonia 490–493; bronchitis 500–502.

TABLE D.4. Occupation Variables Used in the Analyses, 1960

Percentage of civilian labor force × 10	1960 (117 SMSAs)	
	Mean	Standard deviation
Unemployed	50.137	15.380
Males	656.692	30.138
Agriculture	22.326	20.382
Construction	57.881	15.042
Manufacturing (durables)	143.132	97.976
Manufacturing (nondurables)	116.278	64.372
Transportation: transportation, communication, and other public utilities	69.829	21.849
Trade: wholesale and retail trade	180.027	27.488
Finance: finance, insurance, and real estate	43.556	13.927
Education: educational services	49.158	16.366
Public administration	54.161	38.079
White collar: percentage of employed persons in white-collar occupations	435.222	53.204
Use of transit: percentage of employed persons who use public transportation to work	107.991	71.487

Source: See the list of data sources at the end of appendix D.

TABLE D.5. Home-heating Characteristics Used in the Analyses, 1960

Home-heating characteristic	1960 (117 SMSAs)	
	Mean	Standard deviation
Water-heating fuels (percentage of occupied housing units × 10)		
Gas: utility gas	534.529	280.055
Electricity	220.082	218.334
Coal: coal or coke	28.138	86.339
Bottled gas: bottled, tank, or LP gas	42.697	24.324
Oil: fuel oil, kerosine, etc.	90.136	158.771
Other: other water-heating fuel[a]	4.780	7.645
None: without water-heating fuel	79.642	60.941
Home-heating fuels (percentage of occupied housing units × 10)		
Gas: utility gas	491.987	329.679
Oil: fuel oil, kerosine, etc.	315.074	291.318
Coal: coal or coke	110.683	149.846
Electricity	23.666	73.616
Bottled gas: bottled; tank, or LP gas	31.488	32.623
Other: other home-heating fuel[a]	21.340	27.943
None: without home-heating fuel	5.772	23.541
Heating equipment (percentage of total housing units × 10)		
Steam: steam or hot water	192.807	218.110
Warm-air furnace	355.873	222.767
Floor: floor, wall, or pipeless furnace	125.964	125.317
Electric: built-in electric units	17.449	54.767
Flue: other means with flue	178.160	119.940
Without flue: other means without flue	118.811	181.913
None: without heating equipment	10.938	27.088
Without air conditioning (percentage of total housing units × 10)	843.521	115.488

Source: See the list of data sources at the end of appendix D.
[a] Includes purchased steam, waste materials (such as corncobs), and wood.

TABLE D.6.   Climate Variables Used in the Analyses, 1960

	1960 (117 SMSAs)	
Climate variable	Mean	Standard deviation
Min temp: average daily minimum temperature (°F. × 10)	459.735	75.712
Max temp: average daily maximum temperature (°F. × 10)	654.991	79.786
Degree days: heating degree days (× 0.1)	468.253	196.856
Precipitation: total precipitation (inches × 10)	371.045	130.910
1:00 A.M. humidity: average percentage of relative humidity at 1:00 A.M.	76.812	8.114
1:00 P.M. humidity: average percentage of relative humidity at 1:00 P.M.	56.957	7.388
Wind: average hourly windspeed (miles per hour × 10)	91.709	19.048
.01 in. rain: number of days with ≥ .01 inch of precipitation	109.889	26.735
1 in. snow: number of days with ≥ 1 inch of snow or sleet	8.214	6.623
Fog: number of days with heavy fog	27.068	18.968
Max temp ≥ 90°F.: number of days with maximum temperature 90°F. and above	38.231	39.150
Max temp ≤ 32°F.: number of days with maximum temperature 32°F. and below	27.179	28.964
Min temp ≤ 32°F.: number of days with minimum temperature 32°F. and below	94.299	49.573
Min temp ≤ 0°F.: number of days with minimum temperature 0°F. and below	3.504	7.543

Sources: See the list of data sources at the end of appendix D.

TABLE D.7. Suicide and Venereal Disease Variables Used in the Analyses

Variable	1960 (117 SMSAs)		1961 (117 SMSAs)	
	Mean	*Standard deviation*	*Mean*	*Standard deviation*
Suicide rate (per 1,000,000)	106.479	34.062	102.393	34.825
Venereal disease rates				
Primary and secondary syphilis (per 1,000,000)	144.085	231.441	200.513	268.018
All stages of syphilis (per 100,000)	106.273	88.920	114.845	90.008
Gonorrhea (per 100,000)	264.075	251.106	276.174	238.673
Dummy variables				
DV_1 = 1 if county data for both 1960 and 1961, 0 otherwise	.299	.460	.299	.460
DV_2 = 1 if data are for 1962 and 1963, 0 otherwise	.026	.159	.026	.159
DV_3 = 1 if county data for 1960 and city data for 1961, 0 otherwise	.034	.182	.034	.182
DV_4 = 0 if city data for 1960 and county data for 1961, 1 otherwise	.991	.092	.991	.092
DV_5 = 0 if county data for 1960 and city data for 1961, 1 otherwise	.966	.182	.966	.182
DV_6 = 1 if city data for 1960 and county data for 1961, 0 otherwise	.009	.092	.009	.092

Sources: See the list of data sources at the end of appendix D.

TABLE D.8.　Variables Used in the Analysis of Crime Rates

Variable	1960 (114 SMSAs)	
	Mean	Standard deviation
Air pollution variables		
Min S	47.324	31.344
Mean S	100.342	53.310
Max S	228.079	124.923
Min P	45.781	18.650
Mean P	118.728	41.208
Max P	269.675	133.145
Socioeconomic variables		
P/M²	70.235	137.117
≥65	83.833	21.275
NW	126.053	104.659
Poor	181.939	65.073
Log Pop	565.780	41.141
Crime rate variables (per 1,000,000)		
Total offenses	11733.324	4957.581
Murder and nonnegligent manslaughter	55.833	40.496
Forcible rape	82.693	52.428
Robbery	481.947	409.783
Aggravated assault	773.561	736.503
Burglary	5418.035	2487.867
Larceny ($50 and over)	2885.105	1356.306
Auto theft	2036.140	1061.259

Sources: See the list of data sources at the end of appendix D.

TABLE D.9.　Additional Variables Used in the Analysis of Alternative Specifications, 1969

	Mean	Standard deviation
Log-log		
Log Min S (× 100)	146.780	26.231
Log Mean P (× 100)	196.254	12.356
Log P/M² (× 100)	269.882	43.880
Log ≥65 (× 100)	194.255	9.793
Log NW (× 100)	194.537	41.040
Log Poor (× 100)	191.994	15.429
Log Pop	575.664	39.876
Log unadjusted total mortality rate	294.939	7.311
Log age–sex–race-adjusted total mortality rate	298.068	3.194
Quadratic		
(Min S)² (× 0.1)	156.848	173.657
(Mean P)² (× 0.01)	99.446	66.001
(Min S) × (Mean P) (× 0.1)	344.670	255.650

(*Continued*)

TABLE D.9. (*Continued*)

Variable	Mean	Standard deviation
Dummy variable		
DS_1: 1 if Min S $\leq$ 16 (μg per cubic meter $\times$ 10), 0 otherwise	.152	.360
DS_2: 1 if 16 (μg per cubic meter $\times$ 10) < Min S $\leq$ 35 (μg per cubic meter $\times$ 10), 0 otherwise	.482	.502
DS_3: 1 if 35 (μg per cubic meter $\times$ 10) < Min S $\leq$ 54 (μg per cubic meter $\times$ 10), 0 otherwise	.223	.418
DS_4: 1 if 54 (μg per cubic meter $\times$ 10) < Min S, 0 otherwise	.143	.352
DP_1: 1 if Mean P < 67 μg per cubic meter, 0 otherwise	.107	.311
DP_2: 1 if 67 μg per cubic meter < Mean P $\leq$ 95 μg per cubic meter, 0 otherwise	.491	.502
DP_3: 1 if 95 μg per cubic meter < Mean P $\leq$ 123 μg per cubic meter, 0 otherwise	.241	.430
DP_4: 1 if 123 μg per cubic meter < Mean P, 0 otherwise	.161	.369
Linear spline		
Min S_1: Min S − 16 (μg per cubic meter $\times$ 10) if Min S $\geq$ 16 (μg per cubic meter $\times$ 10), 0 otherwise	19.411	18.361
Min S_2: Min S − 35 (μg per cubic meter $\times$ 10) if Min S $\geq$ 35 (μg per cubic meter $\times$ 10), 0 otherwise	7.509	13.187
Min S_3: Min S − 54 (μg per cubic meter $\times$ 10) if Min S $\geq$ 54 (μg per cubic meter $\times$ 10), 0 otherwise	2.250	7.096
Mean P_1: Mean P − 67 μg per cubic meter if Mean P $\geq$ 67 μg per cubic meter, 0 otherwise	29.500	27.399
Mean P_2: Mean P − 95 μg per cubic meter if Mean P $\geq$ 95 μg per cubic meter, 0 otherwise	11.143	20.603
Mean P_3: Mean P − 123 μg per cubic meter if Mean P $\geq$ 123 μg per cubic meter, 0 otherwise	3.491	12.527
Outliers deleted		
Min S	33.281	18.176
Mean P	92.359	22.671
P/M^2	68.706	60.333
$\geq$65	88.660	17.436
NW	124.291	95.294
Poor	88.456	35.643
Log Pop	574.153	37.487
Unadjusted total mortality rate	893.825	134.939
Age–sex–race-adjusted total mortality rate	956.951	67.216

Source: See the list of data sources at the end of appendix D.

TABLE D.10. Index Variables Used in the Analyses

	Mean	Standard deviation
S index (sulfate index)[a]		
For 1969 unadjusted total mortality rate for 112 SMSAs (= .473 Min S + .173 Mean S + .028 Max S)	42.903	18.404
For 1969 age–sex–race-adjusted total mortality rate for 112 SMSAs (= .678 Min S + .085 Mean S + .076 Max S)	53.668	23.545
For 1969 unadjusted total mortality rate for 81 SMSAs (= .401 Min S + .025 Mean S + .050 Max S)	30.379	14.438
For 1969 age–sex–race-adjusted total mortality rate for 81 SMSAs (= .444 Min S + .166 Mean S + .035 Max S)	43.437	19.995
P index (suspended particulate index)[a]		
For 1969 unadjusted total mortality rate for 112 SMSAs (= .199 Min P + .303 Mean P − .018 Max P)	30.597	9.197
For 1969 age–sex–race-adjusted total mortality rate for 112 SMSAs (= .199 Min P + .332 Mean P − .030 Max P)	30.615	9.630
For 1969 unadjusted total mortality rate for 81 SMSAs (= −.555 Min P + .696 Mean P − .081 Max P)	29.937	12.865
For 1969 age–sex–race-adjusted total mortality rate for 81 SMSAs (= −.640 Min P + .714 Mean P − .100 Mean P)	24.211	12.499
SE index (socioeconomic index)[a]		
For 1969 unadjusted total mortality rate for 112 SMSAs (= .083 P/M^2 + 6.880 ≥ 65 + .396 NW + .038 Poor − .276 Log Pop)	519.955	128.050
For 1969 age–sex–race-adjusted total mortality rate for 112 SMSAs (= .052 P/M^2 + .265 ≥ 65 + .145 NW + .139 Poor − .093 Log Pop)	54.955	18.132
For 1969 unadjusted total mortality rate for 81 SMSAs (= .092 P/M^2 + 7.737 ≥ 65 + .496 NW + .138 Poor − .167 Log Pop)	672.926	123.899
For 1969 age–sex–race-adjusted total mortality rate for 81 SMSAs (= .061 P/M^2 + .917 ≥ 65 + .239 NW + .166 Poor − .159 Log Pop)	41.068	28.181
AP_{60}: air pollution index for 1960 (= .401 Min S + .025 Mean S + .050 Max S − .555 Min P + .696 Mean P − .081 Max P)[b]	69.337	24.161
AP_{69}: air pollution index for 1969 (= .401 Min S + .025 Mean S + .050 Max S − .555 Min P + .696 Mean P − .081 Max P)[a]	60.316	23.169
SE_{60}: socioeconomic index for 1960 (= .092 P/M^2 + 7.737 ≥ 65 + .496 NW + .138 Poor − .167 Log Pop)[b]	631.407	114.421
SE_{69}: socioeconomic index for 1969 (= .092 P/M^2 + 7.737 ≥ 65 + .496 NW + .138 Poor − .167 Log Pop)[a]	672.926	123.899

Sources: See the list of data sources at the end of appendix D.
[a] Based on 1969 air pollution and socioeconomic data.
[b] Based on 1960 air pollution and socioeconomic data.

TABLE D.11. Additional Air Pollution Variables Used in the Analyses

Variable	1969 (69 SMSAs)		1962–68 (15 SMSAs)	
	Mean	Standard deviation	Mean	Standard deviation
Min NO_3: smallest biweekly nitrate reading (μg per cubic meter $\times$ 10)	4.377	3.469	5.124	3.143
Mean NO_3: arithmetic mean of biweekly nitrate readings (μg per cubic meter $\times$ 10)	21.609	11.774	22.524	8.198
Max NO_3: largest biweekly nitrate reading (μg per cubic meter $\times$ 10)	61.667	36.029	62.400	31.758
Min NO_2: smallest biweekly nitrogen dioxide reading (μg per cubic meter)	40.319	24.885	46.278	23.920
Mean NO_2: arithmetic mean of biweekly nitrogen dioxide readings (μg per cubic meter)	136.232	53.882	118.181	45.580
Max NO_3: largest biweekly nitrogen dioxide reading (μg per cubic meter)	281.667	119.704	240.181	108.755
Min SO_2: smallest biweekly sulfur dioxide reading (μg per cubic meter)	4.536	3.592	7.743	9.113
Mean SO_2: arithmetic mean of biweekly sulfur dioxide readings (μg per cubic meter)	33.000	29.355	61.924	44.545
Max SO_2: largest biweekly sulfur dioxide reading (μg per cubic meter)	115.812	97.608	205.648	166.670
Mean S $\times$ Mean P ($\times$ 0.01)	123.330	85.187	145.099	66.508
Mean S $\times$ Mean NO_3 ($\times$ 0.01)	25.971	19.579	27.025	15.668
Mean S $\times$ Mean NO_2 ($\times$ 0.01)	163.232	108.774	145.064	89.885
Mean S $\times$ Mean SO_2 ($\times$ 0.01)	44.590	54.005	85.646	80.407
Mean P $\times$ Mean NO_3 ($\times$ 0.01)	22.328	15.199	28.808	15.538
Mean P $\times$ Mean NO_2 ($\times$ 0.01)	138.978	78.260	142.500	59.280
Mean P $\times$ Mean SO_2 ($\times$ 0.01)	35.359	42.599	74.435	54.298
Mean NO_3 $\times$ Mean NO_2 ($\times$ 0.01)	31.308	25.470	26.829	16.148
Mean NO_3 $\times$ Mean SO_2 ($\times$ 0.01)	6.405	6.379	13.312	10.233
Mean NO_2 $\times$ Mean SO_2 ($\times$ 0.01)	51.470	59.453	79.331	72.683

Sources: See the list of data sources at the end of appendix D.

TABLE D.12. Additional Variables Used in the Cross-sectional Time-series Analyses

Variable	1960–69 (26 SMSAs)		1962–68 (15 SMSAs)	
	Mean	Standard deviation	Mean	Standard deviation
Mortality				
U.S. total mortality rate (per 100,000)	957.881	9.488	959.528	9.624
U.S. infant mortality rate (per 10,000 live births)	239.319	16.769	239.871	13.025
Linear time	5.722	2.815		
Dummy time variables				
1960: 1 if observation is for 1960, 0 otherwise	.108	.311		
1961: 1 if observation is for 1961, 0 otherwise	.037	.190		
1962: 1 if observation is for 1962, 0 otherwise	.108	.311		
1963: 1 if observation is for 1963, 0 otherwise	.108	.311		
1964: 1 if observation is for 1964, 0 otherwise	.108	.311		
1965: 1 if observation is for 1965, 0 otherwise	.108	.311		
1966: 1 if observation is for 1966, 0 otherwise	.104	.306		
1967: 1 if observation is for 1967, 0 otherwise	.108	.311		
1968: 1 if observation is for 1968, 0 otherwise	.108	.311		
1969: 1 if observation is for 1969, 0 otherwise	.104	.306		

Sources: See the list of data sources at the end of appendix D.

TABLE D.13. Variables Used in the Analysis of Daily Deaths in Chicago

Variables	9/62–6/63 n = 298 Mean	9/62–6/63 n = 298 Standard deviation
Air pollution variables[a]		
SO_{2t}: Average daily sulfur dioxide reading on day t (parts per million $\times$ 10)	1.668	1.307
NO_{2t}: Average daily nitrogen dioxide reading on day t (parts per million $\times$ 10)		
NO_t: Average daily nitric oxide reading on day t (parts per million $\times$ 10)		
HC_t: Average daily total hydrocarbons reading on day t (parts per million)		
$\prod_{k=0}^{3} SO_{2t-k}$		
$\prod_{k=0}^{3} NO_{t-k}$		
Climate variables		
Mean temp: Average daily temperature (°F. $\times$ 0.1)	4.439	2.159
Rainfall: Total daily precipitation (inches)	.056	.168
Wind: Average daily wind speed (miles per hour $\times$ 0.1)	1.087	.406
Day-of-the-week variables		
Sunday: 1 if observation is for a Sunday, 0 otherwise	.144	.352
Monday: 1 if observation is for a Monday, 0 otherwise	.141	.349
Tuesday: 1 if observation is for a Tuesday, 0 otherwise	.141	.349
Wednesday: 1 if observation is for a Wednesday, 0 otherwise	.141	.349
Thursday: 1 if observation is for a Thursday, 0 otherwise	.144	.352
Friday: 1 if observation is for a Friday, 0 otherwise	.144	.352
Saturday: 1 if observation is for a Saturday, 0 otherwise	.144	.352
Mortality variable		
Average number of daily deaths	121.054	16.936

9/63–6/64 n = 299		9/63–5/64 n = 269		8/63–8/64 n = 392	
Mean	Standard deviation	Mean	Standard deviation	Mean	Standard deviation
1.848	1.458	1.982	1.471		
		.409	.117	.452	.164
		.992	.398	.897	.381
		2.992	.779		
4.759	2.032	4.474	1.925	5.357	2.095
.060	.162	.060	.163	.068	.195
1.130	.381	1.150	.385	1.064	.375
.144	.351	.145	.353	.143	.350
.144	.351	.141	.349	.143	.350
.144	.351	.141	.349	.143	.350
.140	.348	.141	.349	.143	.350
.140	.348	.141	.349	.143	.350
.144	.351	.145	.353	.143	.350
.144	.351	.145	.353	.143	.350
116.371	13.104	116.390	12.960	114.622	13.985

(*Continued*)

Variables	8/63–5/64 n = 300	
	Mean	Standard deviation
Air pollution variables[d]		
SO_{2t}: Average daily sulfur dioxide reading on day t (parts per million $\times$ 10)		
NO_{2t}: Average daily nitrogen dioxide reading on day t (parts per million $\times$ 10)		
NO_t: Average daily nitric oxide reading on day t (parts per million $\times$ 10)		
HC_t: Average daily total hydrocarbons reading on day t (parts per million)	3.005	.819
$\prod\limits_{k=0}^{3} SO_{2t-k}$		
$\prod\limits_{k=0}^{3} NO_{t-k}$		
Climate variables		
Mean temp: Average daily temperature (°F. $\times$ 0.1)	4.746	1.996
Rainfall: Total daily precipitation (inches)	.060	.172
Wind: Average daily wind speed (miles per hour $\times$ 0.01)	1.118	.387
Day-of-the-week variables		
Sunday: 1 if observation is for a Sunday, 0 otherwise	.143	.351
Monday: 1 if observation is for a Monday, 0 otherwise	.140	.348
Tuesday: 1 if observation is for a Tuesday, 0 otherwise	.143	.351
Wednesday: 1 if observation is for a Wednesday, 0 otherwise	.143	.351
Thursday: 1 if observation is for a Thursday, 0 otherwise	.143	.351
Friday: 1 if observation is for a Friday, 0 otherwise	.143	.351
Saturday: 1 if observation is for a Saturday, 0 otherwise	.143	.351
Mortality variable		
Average number of daily deaths	114.803	13.586

9/63–5/64[b] n = 260		9/63–5/64[c] n = 271		9/63–5/64[d] n = 274	
Mean	Standard deviation	Mean	Standard deviation	Mean	Standard deviation
2.031	1.472	1.969	1.474	1.953	1.474
.999	.402	.991	.397	.987	.398
		68.535	173.426		
		1.426	2.165		
4.410	1.921	4.489	1.926	4.517	1.933
.062	.166	.059	.163	.063	.179
1.161	.385	1.147	.385	1.145	.385
.146	.352	.144	.352	.146	.352
.142	.350	.140	.348	.142	.350
.142	.350	.140	.348	.142	.350
.142	.350	.144	.352	.142	.350
.142	.350	.144	.352	.142	.350
.142	.350	.144	.352	.142	.350
.142	.350	.144	.352	.142	.350
.189	11.097	116.284	13.000	116.179	13.007

Sources: See the list of data sources at the end of appendix D.

[a] The means and standard deviations of the lagged air pollution variables were approximately equal to their values for the current readings.

[b] Values for moving average specification (see table 9.3).

[c] Values for episodic pollution specification (see table 9.3).

[d] Values for Almon lag specification (see table 9.4).

TABLE D.14. Variables Used in the Analyses of Data from England and Wales

Variables	Fifty-three county boroughs[a] Mean	Fifty-three county boroughs[a] Standard deviation	Twenty-eight county boroughs[a] Mean	Twenty-eight county boroughs[a] Standard deviation	Twenty-six areas[b] Mean	Twenty-six areas[b] Standard deviation	Fifty-three urban areas[c] Mean	Fifty-three urban areas[c] Standard deviation
Air pollution variables								
Deposit index: Average concentration of deposited matter (grams per 100 m³ per month)	375.057	125.678						
Smoke: Average concentration of suspended matter (milligrams per 100 m³)			24.786	12.270				
Smoke: Average annual concentration (milligrams per 1,000 m³)								
Smoke: Average annual concentration (micrograms per cubic meter)					260.038	146.256	119.075	61.272
Sulfur dioxide: Average annual concentration (micrograms per cubic meter)							129.717	61.370
Socioeconomic variables								
Person per acre: The number of persons per acre ($\times 10$)	163.642	67.445	173.679	63.397	102.923	103.351	158.887	56.746
Social class: An index of social class based on the proportion of males aged fourteen and over, employed in certain (unspecified) occupations					163.692	60.532		
Mortality variables (standardized)								
Bronchitis mortality rate for males	128.925	37.653	136.750	40.502	105.538	58.246	112.642	26.570
Bronchitis mortality rate for females	125.849	38.183	131.571	43.329	109.423	54.782		
Pneumonia mortality rate for males					133.654	41.716		
Pneumonia mortality rate for females					127.077	46.503		
Lung cancers mortality rate for males					95.577	34.958	106.679	18.672
Lung cancers mortality rate for both sexes	107.698	20.377	117.607	20.156				
Stomach cancers mortality rate for males	114.679	20.653	117.786	19.687				
Stomach cancers mortality rate for females	111.717	19.400	109.321	17.687				
Intestinal cancers mortality rate for both sexes	106.264	9.602	107.893	9.077				
Other cancers mortality rate for males					100.538	14.983		
Other cancers mortality rate for females					105.423	14.938		

Sources: [a]Stocks (1959); [b]Stocks (1960); [c]Ashley (1967).

342

SOURCES OF DATA

Air pollution

1960 and 1961: U.S. Department of Health, Education and Welfare. 1962. *Air Pollution Measurements of the National Air Sampling Network. Analyses of Suspended Particulates, 1957–61* (Cincinnati, U.S. Public Health Service), no. 978.

1962: ———. *National Air Sampling Network. Air Quality Data, 1962* (Cincinnati, U.S. Public Health Service).

1963: ———. 1965. *Air Pollution Measurements of the National Air Sampling Network. Analysis of Suspended Particulates, 1963* (Cincinnati, U.S. Public Health Service).

1964 and 1965: ———. 1966. *Air Quality Data from the National Air Sampling Networks and Contributing State and Local Networks, 1964–65* (Cincinnati, U.S. Public Health Service).

1966: ———. 1968. *Air Quality Data from the National Air Sampling Networks and Contributing State and Local Networks, 1966 Edition* (Durham, N.C., National Air Pollution Control Administration), Publication no. APTD 68-9.

1967: U.S. Environmental Protection Agency. 1971. *Air Quality Data for 1967 from the National Air Surveillance Networks and Contributing State and Local Networks, Revised 1971* (Research Triangle Park, N.C., Office of Air Programs), Publication no. APTD 0741.

1968 and 1969: unpublished.[1]

Daily 1962: U.S. Department of Health, Education and Welfare. 1969. *CAMP Daily Average Values, 1962. Chicago, Cincinnati, New Orleans, Philadelphia, Washington, D.C.* U.S. Public Health Service. National Air Pollution Control Administration. Division of Air Quality and Emission Data.

Daily 1963: ———. 1969. *CAMP Daily Average Values, 1963. Chicago, Cincinnati, New Orleans, Philadelphia, Washington, D.C.* U.S. Public Health Service. National Air Pollution Control Administration. Division of Air Quality and Emission Data.

Daily 1964: ———. 1969. *CAMP Daily Average Values, 1964. Chicago, Cincinnati, Philadelphia, Saint Louis, Washington, D.C.* U.S. Public Health Service. National Air Pollution Control Administration. Division of Air Quality and Emission Data.

Daily 1965: ———. 1968. *CAMP Daily Average Values, 1965. Chicago, Cincinnati, Denver, Philadelphia, Saint Louis, Washington, D.C.* U.S. Public Health Service. National Air Pollution Control Administration. Division of Air Quality and Emission Data.

Daily 1966: ———. 1969. *CAMP Daily Average Values, 1966. Chicago, Cincinnati, Denver, Philadelphia, Saint Louis, Washington, D.C.* U.S. Public Health Service. National Air Pollution Control Administration. Division of Air Quality and Emission Data.

---

[1] Sulfate and nitrate data for 1969 from U.S. Environmental Protection Agency. 1973. *Air Quality Data for Nonmetallic Inorganic Ions, 1969 and 1970* (Research Triangle Park, N.C., Office of Air Programs), Publication no. APTD 1466.

Socioeconomic
    1960: U.S. Bureau of the Census. 1962. *County and City Data Book, 1962*
    (Washington, GPO).
    1970: ———. 1971. *Census of Population: 1970. General Population Char-*
    acteristics (Washington, GPO). ———. 1971. *Census of Population: 1970.*
    General Social and Economic Characteristics (Washington, GPO).
    ———. 1972. *Census of Population: 1970. General Social and Economic*
    Characteristics (Washington, GPO).

Mortality (and live births)[2]
    1960: U.S. Department of Health, Education and Welfare. 1963. *Vital Sta-*
    tistics of the United States, 1960 (Washington, GPO).
    1961: ———. 1963. *Vital Statistics of the United States, 1961* (Washington,
    GPO).
    1962: ———. 1964. *Vital Statistics of the United States, 1962* (Washington,
    GPO).
    1963: ———. 1965. *Vital Statistics of the United States, 1963* (Washington,
    GPO).
    1964: ———. 1966. *Vital Statistics of the United States, 1964* (Washington,
    GPO).
    1965: ———. 1967. *Vital Statistics of the United States, 1965* (Washington,
    GPO).
    1966: ———. 1968. *Vital Statistics of the United States, 1966* (Washington,
    GPO).
    1967: ———. 1969. *Vital Statistics of the United States, 1967* (Washington,
    GPO).
    1968: ———. 1971. *Vital Statistics of the United States, 1968* (Washington,
    GPO).
    1969: ———. 1973. *Vital Statistics of the United States, 1969* (Washington,
    GPO).

Occupation mix
    1960: U.S. Bureau of the Census. 1962. *County and City Data Book, 1962*
    (Washington, GPO).

Home-heating characteristics
    1960: U.S. Department of Commerce. 1963. *U.S. Census of Housing, 1960.*
    Vol. 1, States and Small Areas (Washington, GPO), pts. 2–8.

Climate
    1960: U.S. Weather Bureau. 1960. *Climatological Data, National Summary*
    (Washington, GPO), vol. 1.
    Daily: U.S. Department of Commerce. *Local Climatological Data* (for rele-
    vant cities and time periods), (Asheville, N.C., National Climatic Center).

[2] Mortality figures published in vol. II, pt. B; and natality figures published in vol.
I. Natality figures for 1963, 1968, and 1969 were published in 1964, 1970, and 1974,
respectively.

Suicides

    1960: U.S. Department of Health, Education and Welfare. 1963. *Vital Statistics of the United States, 1960* (Washington, GPO).

    1961: ————. 1963. *Vital Statistics of the United States, 1961* (Washington, GPO).

Venereal Disease

    1960 and 1961: Data provided by the Center for Disease Control, Department of Health, Education and Welfare, Atlanta.

Crime Rates

    1960: U.S. Department of Justice. 1961. *Crime in the United States (Uniform Crime Reports—1960)* (Washington, Federal Bureau of Investigation).

Adjustment method for mortality rates

Let MR_i be the SMSA mortality rate for age–sex–race group i and let P_i be the proportion of the total U.S. population in age–sex–race group i. Then the direct method for calculating the age–sex–race-adjusted total mortality rate (ASR) is $ASR = \sum_i MR_i P_i$.[1]

Since the adjustment procedure uses a single age distribution for adjusting the mortality rate of each SMSA, it permits direct comparison of the same age-adjusted, sex–race mortality rate across areas but does not permit comparison of different age-adjusted, sex–race mortality rates.

An example may clarify the issue. Assume there are two age groups, young (Y) and old (O). Suppose that 80 percent of the total population are young and 20 percent are old, and that their mortality rates (MR_Y and MR_O, respectively) are 2 and 9 per 100, respectively; for example, $MR_Y = 2$ and $MR_O = 9$. This gives rise to a national unadjusted total mortality rate of $(0.8 \times 2) + (0.2 \times 9) = 3.4$. Now, let Clean City have a higher proportion of old people than the national average (say, 50 percent) but lower than average mortality rates: MR_Y (Clean City) $= 1$ and MR_O (Clean City) $= 7$, and let Dirty City have a much lower proportion of old people (5 percent) but relatively high mortality rates: MR_Y (Dirty City) $= 2.5$ and MR_O (Dirty City) $= 12$. With these assumptions, the unadjusted total mortality rate in Clean City would be equal to $(0.5 \times 1) + (0.5 \times 7) = 4$, and the unadjusted total mor-

---

[1] Note that $\sum_i P_i = 1$, and that for the entire nation the unadjusted total mortality rate (UMR) and the age–sex–race-adjusted total mortality rate (ASR) are equal. The last equality can be seen from the following relationship:

$$ASR = \sum_i \frac{D_i}{P_i} \times \frac{P_i}{U.S.\ Pop} = \frac{1}{U.S.\ Pop} \sum D_i = UMR$$

where D_i is the number of deaths in age–sex–race group i, and $U.S.\ Pop$ is the total population of the United States.

tality rate in Dirty City would be equal to $(0.95 \times 2.5) + (0.05 \times 12) = 2.975$. Clean City's relatively high unadjusted total mortality rate (compared with Dirty City's and the national average) carries with it the implication that there are factors in Clean City that make it a less healthy environment, an incorrect conclusion. Similarly, Dirty City's relatively low unadjusted total mortality rate suggest that there are factors in Dirty City that make it a healthy place to live. However, if the total mortality rate in each city is adjusted for age, using the age distribution of the national population, the two mortality rates become: ASR (Clean) $= (0.8 \times 1) + (0.2 \times 7) = 2.2$, and ASR (Dirty) $= (0.8 \times 2.5) + (0.2 \times 12) = 4.4$. Thus the adjustment provides for a more valid comparison of the mortality rates.

As a second illustration, assume that 80 percent of whites are young while 90 percent of nonwhites are young (and that 81 percent of the national population is young). Now let MR_Y (White) $= 2$, MR_O (White) $= 9$, MR_Y (Nonwhite) $= 2.4$, and MR_O (Nonwhite) $= 10$. Using the single age distribution of the national population, the two adjusted mortality rates would be ASR(White) $= (0.81 \times 2) + (0.19 \times 9) = 3.33$, and ASR(Nonwhite) $= (0.81 \times 2.4) + (0.19 \times 10) = 3.844$. These two rates are directly comparable and indicate that the adjusted nonwhite mortality rate is approximately 15 percent higher than the adjusted white mortality rate. If the individual age distributions for the two races were used to calculate the adjusted mortality rates, the results would be ASR(White) $= (0.8 \times 2) + (0.2 \times 9) = 3.4$, and ASR (Nonwhite) $= (0.9 \times 2.4) + (0.1 \times 10) = 3.16$. These two rates are *not* directly comparable; they would imply that the nonwhite death rate was lower than the white death rate.

The basic
health-benefit calculation

In chapter 10, we presented our "best" estimate of the benefits associated with an 88 percent abatement of sulfur oxides and a 58 percent abatement of particulates in terms of improvements in health. That benefit estimate was $16.1 billion (1973 dollars) for 1979 and represented 7.0 percent of the total 1979 economic costs of morbidity and mortality (assuming a 6 percent discount rate). Here, we present the details of that calculation.

As stated in chapter 10, the total economic costs are based on 1972 data, analyzed by Cooper and Rice (1976). The two basic components of these costs involve *indirect* costs based on forgone earnings due to sickness and death and *direct* costs based on direct medical care expenditures. In 1972, the total *indirect* costs of morbidity and mortality were estimated to be $99.7 billion (1972 dollars) and the total *direct* costs of morbidity and mortality were estimated to be $75.2 billion (1972 dollars).

We adjusted the 1972 indirect cost estimate to 1973 dollars by applying the change in the consumer price index (CPI): $99.7 billion (1972 dollars) = $99.7 × [CPI (1973)/CPI (1972)] = $99.7 × (133.1/125.3) = $105.9 billion (1973 dollars).[1] The 1979 indirect costs were then estimated by adjusting this value under the assumption that the average annual increase in real per capita income would be equal to 1.5 percent through 1979 and that the population would continue to grow at an annual rate of 0.8 percent through 1979. Thus, $105.9 billion (1973 dollars) was adjusted to a 1970 estimate of [($105.9) × $(1.023)^7$] = $124.2 billion (1973 dollars).[2]

Direct costs in fiscal year 1973 were estimated to be $79.7 billion (1973 dollars) and direct costs in fiscal year 1976 were estimated to be $116.5 billion

---

[1] Data for these calculations are taken from the *Social Security Bulletins* for the relevant years, Social Security Administration, U.S. Department of Health, Education and Welfare.

[2] The exponent is seven, since the adjustment to 1973 dollars does not account for increases in real per capita income or population.

(1976 dollars).[3] The 1979 direct costs were estimated first by calculating the average annual rate of increase in direct costs over the four years 1973–76 and adjusting this for the rise in general prices over the same period; and then by assuming that this adjusted rate of increase would continue through 1979. The average annual rate of increase in direct costs between 1973 and 1976 was 13.5 percent.[4] The average annual rate of increase in general prices throughout the economy over this period was 8.6 percent.[5] Hence, in 1973 dollars, the direct costs increased 4.9 percent per year between 1973 and 1976. Using this factor, together with the 1973 estimate of direct costs, we obtain a 1979 estimate of $[(\$79.7) \times (1.049)^6] = \$106.2$ billion (1973 dollars).

We then added the 1979 estimates of the two components of the total costs of morbidity and mortality, $124.2 billion + $106.2 billion = $230.4 billion (1973 dollars). Seven percent of this total was equal to $16.1 billion (1973 dollars).[6] Thus, the 1979 health benefits associated with an 88 percent reduction in sulfur oxides and a 58 percent reduction in particulates were estimated to be valued at $16.1 billion (1973 dollars).

[3] These figures were obtained by taking the total health expenditures (in current dollars) for fiscal years 1973 and 1976, $95.4 billion and $139.3 billion, respectively, and subtracting from each of those expenditures corresponding to cost categories not allocated by Cooper and Rice (1976, p. 22).

[4] The average rate of increase in direct costs over the four years 1973–76 was calculated by taking the ratio of 1976 direct costs to 1973 direct costs (both in current dollars) and converting this to an annual rate of increase. The relevant ratio is $116.5/79.7 = 1.462$. Since $\sqrt[3]{1.462} = 1.135$, the average annual rate of increase was 13.5 percent.

[5] The average annual rate of increase in general prices over the four years 1973–76 was calculated by taking the ratio CPI(1976)/CPI(1973) and converting this to an annual rate of increase. The relevant ratio is $170.5/133.1 = 1.281$. Since $\sqrt[3]{1.281} = 1.086$, the average annual rate of increase was 8.6 percent.

[6] The 7.0 percent was obtained by applying 88 percent to the sulfate elasticity (0.050) and 58 percent to the suspended particulate elasticity (0.044). (See table 3.4.)

Air pollution–health studies classified by air pollutant

Air pollutant and authors	Major discussion page
Suspended particulates (includes dustfall, soiling indexes, sootfall, etc.)	
Anderson and Ferris (1965)	285 fn
Angel and coauthors (1965)	303
Ashley (1967)	275
Ashley (1969a)	275
Ashley (1969b)	291 fn
Becker, Shilling, and Verma (1968)	190
Biersteker (1969)	281
Boyd (1960)	190
Brown and Ipsen (1968)	302
Buck and Brown (1964)	278
Burgess and Shaddick (1959)	279
Cassell and coauthors (1968)	300
Chapman (1965)	303
Cohen and coauthors (1972)	310
Derrick (1970)	302
Dohan (1961)	302
Durham (1974)	308
Ferris (1970)	285 fn
Ferris and Anderson (1964)	285
Fletcher (1958)	273 fn
Gardner and Waller (1970)	291 fn
Gardner, Crawford, and Morris (1969)	277
Girsh and coauthors (1967)	302
Glasser and Greenburg (1971)	193

Air pollutant and authors	Major discussion page
Glasser, Greenburg, and Field (1967)	189
Gore and Shaddick (1958)	299
Greenburg and coauthors (1962a)	299
Greenburg and coauthors (1962b)	299
Greenburg and coauthors (1963)	299
Greenburg and coauthors (1965)	299
Greenburg and coauthors (1967a)	290
Greenburg and coauthors (1967b)	299
Gregory (1970)	303
Hagstrom, Sprague, and Landau (1967)	294
Heimann (1970)	299
Hitosugi (1968)	293
Hodgson (1970)	190
Holland (1971)	303
Holland and coauthors (1965)	287
Holland and coauthors (1969a)	287
Holland and coauthors (1969b)	287
Holland, Spicer, and Wilson (1961)	301
Holland and Stone (1965)	287

Air pollutant and authors	Major discussion page	Air pollutant and authors	Major discussion page
Ipsen, Deane, and Ingenito (1969)	303 fn	Spodnik and coauthors (1966)	303
Ishikawa and coauthors (1969)	275	Sterling and coauthors (1966)	300
Kenline (1966)	301	Sterling, Pollack, and Phair (1967)	300
Lambert and Reid (1970)	280	Sterling, Pollack, and Weinkam (1969)	301
Lammers, Schilling, and Walford (1964)	280	Stocks (1947)	290
Lave (1972)	212	Stocks (1959)	275
Lave and Seskin (1973)	53 fn	Stocks (1960)	275
Lave and Seskin (1977)	246	Stocks (1966)	292
Lawther (1958)	302	Stocks (1967)	275
Lawther, Waller, and Henderson (1970)	302	Stocks and Campbell (1955)	290
Lewis, Gilkeson, and McCaldin (1962)	301	Sultz and coauthors (1970)	281
London Ministry of Health (1954)	188 fn	Toyama (1964)	280
Loudon and Kilpatrick (1969)	302	Verma, Schilling, and Becker (1969)	190 fn
Lunn, Knowelden, and Handyside (1967)	286	Waller (1971)	302
Lunn, Knowelden, and Roe (1970)	286	Waller and Lawther (1955)	302
Manzhenko (1966)	288	Waller and Lawther (1957)	302
Martin (1964)	304	Weill and coauthors (1964)	301
Martin and Bradley (1960)	304	Wicken and Buck (1964)	278
McCarroll (1967)	188 fn	Wilkens (1954)	188 fn
McCarroll and Bradley (1966)	189	Winklestein and coauthors (1967)	273
McMillan and coauthors (1969)	304	Winklestein and Gay (1971)	298
Mills (1943)	281	Winklestein and Kantor (1969a)	294
Mills (1952)	281	Winklestein and Kantor (1969b)	283
Paulus and Smith (1967)	302	Winklestein and Kantor (1969c)	294
Pemberton (1961)	304	Yoshida, Oshima, and Imai (1966)	280
Pemberton and Goldberg (1954)	279	Yoshida, Takatsuka, and Kitabatake (1969)	283
Prindle and coauthors (1963)	285	Zeidberg and Prindle (1963)	274
Schimmel and Greenburg (1972)	304	Zeidberg, Horton, and Landau (1967a)	274
Schoettlin and Landau (1961)	301	Zeidberg, Horton, and Landau (1967b)	297
Scott (1953)	188 fn	Zeidberg, Prindle, and Landau (1961)	301
Shy and coauthors (1970a)	284	Zeidberg, Prindle, and Landau (1964)	295
Shy and coauthors (1970b)	284		
Shy and coauthors (1973)	284		
Silverman (1973a)	193 fn		
Silverman (1973b)	301		
Smith and Paulus (1971)	302		
Spicer (1967)	303	*Sulfur oxides (includes*	
Spicer and coauthors (1962)	303	*sulfur dioxide,*	
Spicer and Kerr (1966)	303	*sulfur trioxide,*	
Spicer and Kerr (1970)	303	*sulfates, etc.)*	
Spicer, Reinke, and Kerr (1966)	303	Amdur (1977)	236
		Anderson and Ferris (1965)	285 fn

Air pollutant and authors	Major discussion page	Air pollutant and authors	Major discussion page
Angel and coauthors (1965)	303	Gregory (1970)	303
Ashe (1959)	188 fn	Hagstrom, Sprague,	
Ashley (1967)	275	and Landau (1967)	294
Ashley (1969a)	295 fn	Heimann (1970)	299
Ashley (1969b)	291 fn	Hewitt (1956)	279
Becker, Schilling,		Hitosugi (1968)	293
and Verma (1968)	190	Hodgson (1970)	190
Biersteker (1969)	281	Holland (1971)	303
Boyd (1960)	190	Holland and coauthors	
Brinton (1949)	188 fn	(1965)	287
Brown and Ipsen (1968)	302	Holland and coauthors	
Buck and Brown (1964)	278	(1969a)	287
Burgess and Shaddick (1959)	279	Holland and coauthors	
Burrows, Kellogg,		(1969b)	287
and Buskey (1968)	302	Holland and Reid (1965)	279
Carnow and coauthors (1969)	302	Holland and Stone (1965)	287
Cassell and coauthors		Ipsen, Deane, and Ingenito	
(1968)	300	1969)	303 fn
Cohen and coauthors (1972)	310	Ishikawa and coauthors	
Colley and Holland (1967)	287	(1969)	275
Collins, Kasap, and Holland		Kenline (1966)	301
(1971)	287	Lambert and Reid (1970)	280
Daly (1959)	278	Lammers, Schilling,	
Dohan (1961)	302	and Walford (1964)	280
Dohan, Everts, and Smith		Lave (1972)	212
(1962)	302	Lave and Seskin (1973)	53 fn
Dohan and Taylor (1960)	302	Lave and Seskin (1977)	246
Durham (1974)	308	Lawther (1958)	302
Ferris (1970)	285 fn	Lawther, Waller,	
Ferris and Anderson (1964)	285	and Henderson (1970)	302
Firket (1931)	188	Lepper and coauthors (1969)	284
Firket (1958)	292 fn	London Ministry of Health	
Gardner, Crawford,		(1954)	188 fn
and Morris (1969)	298	Lunn, Knowelden,	
Gardner and Waller (1970)	291 fn	and Handyside (1967)	286
Girsh and coauthors (1967)	302	Lunn, Knowelden,	
Glasser and Greenburg		and Roe (1970)	286
(1971)	193	Manzhenko (1966)	288
Glasser, Greenburg,		Martin (1964)	304
and Field (1967)	189	McCabe and Clayton	
Gore and Shaddick (1958)	299	(1952)	188
Gorham (1958)	279	McCarroll (1967)	188 fn
Gorham (1959)	283	McCarroll and Bradley	
Greenburg and coauthors		(1966)	189
(1962a)	299	McMillan and coauthors	
Greenburg and coauthors		(1969)	304
(1962b)	299	Mills (1952)	281
Greenburg and coauthors		Pemberton (1961)	304
(1963)	299	Pemberton and Goldberg	
Greenburg and coauthors		(1954)	279
(1965)	299	Petrilli, Agnese, and Kanitz	
Greenburg and coauthors		(1966)	280
(1967a)	290	Prindle and coauthors (1963)	285
Greenburg and coauthors		Schimmel and Greenburg	
(1967b)	299	(1972)	304

Author Index

Subject Index

For Product Safety Concerns and Information please contact our EU
representative GPSR@taylorandfrancis.com
Taylor & Francis Verlag GmbH, Kaufingerstraße 24, 80331 München, Germany